GULF WAR and HEALTH

VOLUME 8

Update of Health Effects of Serving in the Gulf War

Committee on Gulf War and Health: Health Effects of Serving in the Gulf War, Update 2009

Board on the Health of Select Populations

INSTITUTE OF MEDICINE
OF THE NATIONAL ACADEMIES

THE NATIONAL ACADEMIES PRESS
Washington, D.C.
www.nap.edu

THE NATIONAL ACADEMIES PRESS 500 Fifth Street, N.W. Washington, DC 20001

NOTICE: The project that is the subject of this report was approved by the Governing Board of the National Research Council, whose members are drawn from the councils of the National Academy of Sciences, the National Academy of Engineering, and the Institute of Medicine. The members of the committee responsible for the report were chosen for their special competences and with regard for appropriate balance.

This study was supported by Contract No. V101 (93) P-2136, TO 101-E8709(17) between the National Academy of Sciences and Department of Veterans Affairs. Any opinions, findings, conclusions, or recommendations expressed in this publication are those of the author(s) and do not necessarily reflect the view of the organizations or agencies that provided support for this project.

International Standard Book Number-13: 978-0-309-14921-1
International Standard Book Number-10: 0-309-14921-5

Additional copies of this report are available from the National Academies Press, 500 Fifth Street, N.W., Lockbox 285, Washington, DC 20055; (800) 624-6242 or (202) 334-3313 (in the Washington metropolitan area); Internet, http://www.nap.edu.

For more information about the Institute of Medicine, visit the IOM home page at: **www.iom.edu.**

Printed in the United States of America

The serpent has been a symbol of long life, healing, and knowledge among almost all cultures and religions since the beginning of recorded history. The serpent adopted as a logotype by the Institute of Medicine is a relief carving from ancient Greece, now held by the Staatliche Museen in Berlin.

Suggested citation: IOM (Institute of Medicine). 2010. *Gulf War and Health, Volume 8: Update of Health Effects of Serving in the Gulf War.* Washington, DC: The National Academies Press.

"Knowing is not enough; we must apply.
Willing is not enough; we must do."

—Goethe

INSTITUTE OF MEDICINE

OF THE NATIONAL ACADEMIES

Advising the Nation. Improving Health.

THE NATIONAL ACADEMIES

Advisers to the Nation on Science, Engineering, and Medicine

The **National Academy of Sciences** is a private, nonprofit, self-perpetuating society of distinguished scholars engaged in scientific and engineering research, dedicated to the furtherance of science and technology and to their use for the general welfare. Upon the authority of the charter granted to it by the Congress in 1863, the Academy has a mandate that requires it to advise the federal government on scientific and technical matters. Dr. Ralph J. Cicerone is president of the National Academy of Sciences.

The **National Academy of Engineering** was established in 1964, under the charter of the National Academy of Sciences, as a parallel organization of outstanding engineers. It is autonomous in its administration and in the selection of its members, sharing with the National Academy of Sciences the responsibility for advising the federal government. The National Academy of Engineering also sponsors engineering programs aimed at meeting national needs, encourages education and research, and recognizes the superior achievements of engineers. Dr. Charles M. Vest is president of the National Academy of Engineering.

The **Institute of Medicine** was established in 1970 by the National Academy of Sciences to secure the services of eminent members of appropriate professions in the examination of policy matters pertaining to the health of the public. The Institute acts under the responsibility given to the National Academy of Sciences by its congressional charter to be an adviser to the federal government and, upon its own initiative, to identify issues of medical care, research, and education. Dr. Harvey V. Fineberg is president of the Institute of Medicine.

The **National Research Council** was organized by the National Academy of Sciences in 1916 to associate the broad community of science and technology with the Academy's purposes of furthering knowledge and advising the federal government. Functioning in accordance with general policies determined by the Academy, the Council has become the principal operating agency of both the National Academy of Sciences and the National Academy of Engineering in providing services to the government, the public, and the scientific and engineering communities. The Council is administered jointly by both Academies and the Institute of Medicine. Dr. Ralph J. Cicerone and Dr. Charles M. Vest are chair and vice chair, respectively, of the National Research Council.

www.national-academies.org

COMMITTEE ON GULF WAR AND HEALTH: HEALTH EFFECTS OF SERVING IN THE GULF WAR, UPDATE 2009

STEPHEN L. HAUSER (*Chair*), Professor and Chair of Neurology, University of California, San Francisco, School of Medicine

ALVARO ALONSO, Assistant Professor, Division of Epidemiology and Community Health, School of Public Health, University of Minnesota

ROBERT H. BROWN, JR., Chair and Professor of Neurology, University of Massachusetts School of Medicine

DOUGLAS A. DROSSMAN, Co-director, University of North Carolina Center for Functional GI and Motility Disorder, and Professor of Medicine and Psychiatry, University of North Carolina School of Medicine

W. DANA FLANDERS, Professor of Epidemiology, Biostatistics and Bioinformatics, Emory University Rollins School of Public Health

MATTHEW C. KEIFER, Co-director, Pacific Northwest Agricultural Safety and Health Center, and Professor of Occupational Medicine, University of Washington Harborview Medical Center

FRANCINE LADEN, Associate Professor of Environmental Epidemiology, Harvard School of Public Health, and Assistant Professor of Medicine, Channing Laboratory, Brigham & Women's Hospital

JENNIFER D. PECK, Assistant Professor of Epidemiology, University of Oklahoma Health Sciences Center

BEATE R. RITZ, Professor, Department of Epidemiology, Department of Environmental Health Sciences, and Vice Chair, Department of Epidemiology at the University of California, Los Angeles, School of Public Health

REBECCA P. SMITH, Assistant Clinical Professor, Department of Psychiatry, Mount Sinai Hospital and School of Medicine

EZRA S. SUSSER, Professor of Epidemiology, Mailman School of Public Health and Professor of Psychiatry, College of Physicians and Surgeons at Columbia University

CHRISTINA M. WOLFSON, Director, Division of Clinical Epidemiology, McGill University Health Centre, and Professor, Department of Epidemiology and Biostatistics and Occupational Health, Department of Medicine, McGill University

STUDY STAFF

ROBERTA WEDGE, Study Director
RENEE WLODARCZYK, Senior Program Associate
PATRICK BAUR, Research Associate
JOSEPH GOODMAN, Senior Program Assistant
CHRISTIE BELL, Financial Officer
FREDRICK ERDTMANN, Director, Board on the Health of Select Populations

REVIEWERS

This report has been reviewed in draft form by persons chosen for their diverse perspectives and technical expertise, in accordance with procedures approved by the National Research Council's (NRC's) Report Review Committee. The purpose of this independent review is to provide candid and critical comments that will assist the institution in making its published report as sound as possible and to ensure that the report meets institutional standards for objectivity, evidence, and responsiveness to the study charge. The review comments and draft manuscript remain confidential to protect the integrity of the deliberative process. We wish to thank the following individuals for their review of this report:

Alberto Ascherio, Department of Epidemiology, Harvard University School of Public Health
Floyd E. Bloom, Department of Molecular and Integrative Neuroscience, The Scripps Research Institute
Gregory L. Burke, Division of Public Health Sciences, Wake Forest University School of Medicine
Edward V. Loftus, Jr., Division of Gastroenterology and Hepatology, Mayo Clinic
Anne Louise Oaklander, Center for Shingles and Postherpetic Neuralgia, Massachusetts General Hospital
Robert D. Sparks, California Medical Association Foundation
Carol A. Tamminga, Department of Psychiatry, The University of Texas Southwestern Medical Center
Nancy Fugate Woods, University of Washington School of Nursing

Although the reviewers listed above have provided many constructive comments and suggestions, they were not asked to endorse the conclusions or recommendations, nor did they see the final draft of the report before its release. The review of the report was overseen by **Harold C. Sox,** American College of Physicians of Internal Medicine. Appointed by the NRC and the Institute of Medicine, he was responsible for making certain that an independent examination of the report was carried out in accordance with institutional procedures and that all review comments were carefully considered. Responsibility for the final content of the report rests entirely with the author committee and the institution.

PREFACE

In war, there are no unwounded soldiers.
—José Narosky

The committee began its task with a sense of deep obligation to the servicemen and women who fought so bravely on our behalf in the Gulf War theater. Our appreciation of the risks, privations, and sacrifices that these courageous servicemembers undertook only deepened as our knowledge of the combat mission increased during the course of the committee's meetings. There is no greater service that a human being can provide to one's fellow citizens than to risk life and health on their behalf. We are honored to dedicate this report to these troops.

As scientists and clinicians, the committee members are also aware of our responsibilities not only to those who served in the Gulf War coalition but also to the cause of science and evidence-based medicine. Only by being true to the latter do we serve the former.

There is no doubt that many of the veterans deployed to the gulf region during 1990-1991 have continued to experience troubling constellations of symptoms involving multiple body systems; these have been variously termed multisymptom illness or Gulf War illness, and as such are emblazoned in the public's mind as a consequence of military service in this battleground. Many other veterans have not experienced the full array of Gulf War illness symptoms but continue to suffer from seemingly related symptoms, including persistent fatigue, chronic fatigue syndrome, irritable bowel syndrome, memory problems, headache, bodily pains, disturbances of sleep, as well as other physical and emotional problems. Many of these symptoms are difficult to categorize as they have no known cause, no objective findings on clinical examination, no diagnostic biomarkers, no known tissue pathology, and no curative therapy. The inadequate basic understanding of the root cause of these symptoms highlights the limitations of current medical science and clinical practice. The committee recognizes that symptoms that cannot be easily quantified are sometimes dismissed—incorrectly—as insignificant, and that they receive inadequate attention—and funding—by the medical and scientific establishment. For example, chronic pain is experienced by 81 million people in the United States alone, yet funding to understand the biology of pain is woefully inadequate, clinical care pathways for individuals suffering from pain are underdeveloped, and training in pain medicine for clinicians lags behind the training for far less common maladies.

Many of the complaints experienced by Gulf War veterans, veterans who arrived in the Gulf War theater after the hostilities ended, and nondeployed veterans, are also seen in the general population. It is beyond dispute, however, that the prevalence of symptoms such as headaches, joint pain, and difficulty concentrating is higher in veterans deployed to the Gulf War theater than the others.

During the past decade two groups, the Institute of Medicine (IOM) and the congressionally mandated Research Advisory Committee on Gulf War Veterans' Illnesses (RAC) have been charged with evaluating the health of and research on Gulf War veterans. In the 2006 IOM report *Gulf War and Health, Volume 4: Health Effects of Serving in the Gulf War*, the authoring committee concluded that although Gulf War veterans reported higher levels of symptoms that might be associated with exposures in the field, no associations with any specific exposures could be identified. In contrast, a report issued by the RAC in November 2008 concluded that Gulf War illness resulted from exposure to pyridostigmine bromide, pesticides, and possibly other exposures.

Although not formally charged with investigating evidence that exposure to specific environmental hazards may have been associated with multisymptom illness, this committee was asked by General Shinseki, Secretary of the Department of Veterans Affairs, to comment on it and did so in an appendix. To ignore this question would not serve the larger purpose of our inquiry. We conclude that current evidence is inadequate to determine whether an association exists between multisymptom illness and any specific battlefield exposure or exposures. Veterans who continue to suffer from these discouraging symptoms deserve the very best that modern science and medicine can offer to delineate the true underlying cause of these symptoms in order to speed the development of effective treatments, cures, and, it is hoped, preventions. The committee suggests a path forward to accomplish these goals and we believe that, through a concerted national effort and rigorous scientific input, answers can likely be found.

The committee would like to thank the many Gulf War veterans who spoke with us about their experiences in the gulf and upon their return to the United States. They provided valuable insights into the symptoms and medical conditions that have been the legacy of the Gulf War for many of the men and women who served in the military. The committee also appreciated hearing from representatives from the Department of Veterans Affairs about the facilities and programs available to Gulf War veterans and from representatives of the RAC who presented the findings of that committee and answered this committee's questions. And finally, the committee would like to thank the IOM staff—Patrick Baur, Joseph Goodman, Renee Wlodarczyk—who assisted in this effort. In particular, we thank Roberta Wedge, who guided the entire process with flexibility, provided many invaluable insights, and displayed a sure hand at every step along our path.

Stephen L. Hauser (*Chair*)
Committee on Gulf War and Health:
Health Effects of Serving in the Gulf War,
Update 2009

CONTENTS

Tables and Boxes

ACRONYMS

AChE	acetylcholinesterase
ACR	American College of Rheumatology
AFQT	Armed Forces Qualifying Test
ALS	amyotrophic lateral sclerosis
ANCOVA	analysis of covariance
BAI	Beck Anxiety Inventory
BDI	Beck Depression Inventory
BIRLS	Beneficiary Identification Records Locator System
BMI	body mass index
BSI	Brief Symptom Inventory
BuChE	butyrylcholinesterase
CAPS	Clinician Administered PTSD Scale
CCD	Canadian Cancer Database
CCEP	Comprehensive Clinical Evaluation Program
CDC	Centers for Disease Control and Prevention
CES	Combat Exposure Scale
CFS	chronic fatigue syndrome
CI	confidence interval
CIDI	Composite International Diagnostic Interview
CMD	Canadian Mortality Database
CMI	chronic multisymptom illness
CMV	cytomegalovirus
CNS	central nervous system
COD	cause of death
COSHPD	California Office of Statewide Health Planning and Development
CRP	C-reactive protein
CVLT	California Verbal Learning Test
CWP	chronic widespread pain
DASA	Defence Analytical Services Agency (United Kingdom)
DMDC	Defense Manpower Data Center
DNA	deoxyribonucleic acid
DND	Department of National Defence (Canada)
DoD	Department of Defense
DSM	*Diagnostic and Statistical Manual of Mental Disorders*
DSP	distal symmetric polyneuropathy
DU	depleted uranium
EBV	Epstein-Barr virus
EEG	electroencephalography
ESR	erythrocyte sedimentation rate
FARS	Fatality Analysis Reporting System
FEV_1	forced expiratory volume in 1 second

FGID	functional gastrointestinal disorder
FSH	follicle stimulating hormone
FVC	forced vital capacity
GAD	generalized anxiety disorder
GAO	Government Accountability Office
GHQ-12	12-item General Health Questionnaire
GI	gastrointestinal
GW	Gulf War
GWV	Gulf War deployed veterans
HIV	human immunodeficiency virus
HPA	hypothalamic-pituitary-adrenal axis
HR	hazard ratio
HSC	Health Symptoms Checklist
IBS	irritable bowel syndrome
ICD	International Statistical Classification of Diseases and Related Health Problems
IOM	Institute of Medicine
LH	luteinizing hormone
MANOVA	multivariate analysis of variance
MCH	mean corpuscular hemoglobin
MCS	multiple chemical sensitivity
MCV	mean corpuscular volume
MDD	major depressive disorder
MRR	mortality rate ratio
MS	multiple sclerosis
NART	National Adults Reading Test
NAS	National Academy of Sciences
NDI	National Death Index
NDV	nondeployed veterans
NIH	National Institutes of Health
NIS	neuropathy impairment score
NOAA	National Oceanic and Atmospheric Administration
NTE	neuropathy target esterase
ODTP	Oregon Dual Task Procedure
OPIDP	organophosphate-induced delayed polyneuropathy
OR	odds ratio
PASAT	Paced Auditory Serial Addition Test
PB	pyridostigmine bromide
PCL	patient checklist
PCL-C	Patient Checklist-Civilian
PCL-M	Patient Checklist-Military
PFT	pulmonary function test
PHQ	Patient Health Questionnaire
PIR	proportional incidence ratio
PMR	proportional morbidity ratio
PON1	paraoxonase-1
POW	prisoner of war

PR	prevalence ratio
PRIME-MD	Primary Care Evaluation of Mental Disorders
PTSD	posttraumatic stress disorder
QoLI	quality of life index
RAC	VA Research Advisory Committee on Gulf War Veterans' Illnesses
RoM	ratio of means
RR	relative risk (or risk ratio as indicated in text)
SCAN	Schedule for Clinical Assessment and Diagnosis
SCID	Structured Clinical Interview for *DSM-III-R*
Sd	standard deviation
SF-12	12-Item Short Form Health Survey
SF-36	36-Item Short Form Health Survey
SMR	standardized mortality ratio
SNAP	Schedule for Nonadaptive and Adaptive Personality
SSA	Social Security Administration
TBI	traumatic brain injury
TOMM	Test of Memory Malingering
UK	United Kingdom
VA	Department of Veterans Affairs
WAIS	Wechsler Adult Intelligence Scale
WCST	Wisconsin Card Sorting Test
WHO	World Health Organization
WMS	Wechsler Memory Scale

SUMMARY

On August 2, 1990, Iraq invaded Kuwait. In response, the United States led a coalition of international armed forces in Operation Desert Shield, a buildup of military personnel and materiel in the Persian Gulf area. Operation Desert Storm began on January 16, 1991, with an air offensive; the 4-day ground war ended on February 28, and a ceasefire was signed in April 1991. Of the almost 700,000 US troops deployed to the Persian Gulf region during the height of the buildup, only about 50,000 US troops were still in the region by June 1991.

Many veterans of the Gulf War have reported a multitude of symptoms that began during or shortly after the war and, in many cases, have persisted to the present. The symptoms include fatigue, musculoskeletal pain, sleep disturbance, cognitive dysfunction, and moodiness. Numerous exposures experienced by veterans during the war have been implicated as the causes of these problems, including exposure to oil-well fire smoke and to the anti–nerve-gas agent prophylactic pyridostigmine bromide. The aggregation of the health problems, often called Gulf War illness or Gulf War syndrome, continues to plague as many as one-third of the veterans who were deployed to the war, and the symptoms are seen in veterans of several of the countries that formed the coalition forces, including the United States, the United Kingdom (UK), Australia, Canada, and Denmark.

In 1998, in response to the growing concerns about the health of the Gulf War veterans, Congress passed two laws: PL 105-277, the Persian Gulf War Veterans Act, and PL 105-368, the Veterans Programs Enhancement Act. Those laws directed the secretary of veterans affairs to enter into a contract with the National Academy of Sciences (NAS) to review and evaluate the scientific and medical literature regarding associations between illness and exposure to toxic agents, environmental or wartime hazards, or preventive medicines or vaccines associated with Gulf War service and directed the secretary to consider the NAS conclusions when making decisions about compensation. NAS assigned the study to the Institute of Medicine (IOM).

Given the large number of agents to study, IOM divided the task into several reviews, which are now complete: *Gulf War and Health, Volume 1: Depleted Uranium, Pyridostigmine Bromide, Sarin, Vaccines*; *Gulf War and Health, Volume 2: Insecticides and Solvents*; *Gulf War and Health, Volume 3: Fuels, Combustion Products, and Propellants*; *Gulf War and Health: Updated Literature Review of Sarin*; *Amyotrophic Lateral Sclerosis in Veterans: Review of the Scientific Literature*; *Gulf War and Health, Volume 4: Health Effects of Serving in the Gulf War*; *Gulf War and Health, Volume 5: Infectious Disease*; *Gulf War and Health, Volume 6: Physiologic, Psychologic, and Psychosocial Effects of Deployment-Related Stress*; and *Gulf War and Health, Volume 7: Long-Term Consequences of Traumatic Brain Injury.*

CHARGE TO THE COMMITTEE

In 2005, the Department of Veterans Affairs (VA) requested that IOM appoint a committee, the Committee on Gulf War and Health: A Review of the Medical Literature Relative to Gulf War Veterans' Health (the Volume 4 committee), to review that body of literature and to summarize what was known about the current status of veterans' health. In 2006, the committee produced a report, *Gulf War and Health, Volume 4: Health Effects of Serving in the Gulf War,* which summarized the overall health effects in veterans and noted which health outcomes were more evident in Gulf War veterans than in their nondeployed counterparts irrespective of the specific exposures experienced by the deployed veterans. The present report is an update of *Volume 4* and covers the literature published since 2005 on the health effects seen in veterans deployed to the Persian Gulf in 1990-1991.

The specific charge to the Committee on Gulf War and Health: Health Effects of Serving in the Gulf War, Update 2009 (the Update committee), as requested by VA, was to review, evaluate, and summarize the literature on the following health outcomes that were noted in the 2006 report as seeming to have higher incidence or prevalence in Gulf War deployed veterans: cancer (particularly brain and testicular cancer), amyotrophic lateral sclerosis and other neurologic diseases (such as Parkinson's disease and multiple sclerosis), birth defects and other adverse pregnancy outcomes, and postdeployment psychiatric conditions. The committee was also to review studies of cause-specific mortality in Gulf War veterans as recommended in the 2006 report. Finally, the committee was to examine the literature to identify any emerging health outcomes.

Thus, the Update committee limited its review to epidemiologic studies of health outcomes published since the last literature search conducted for *Volume 4.* The committee included in its review only studies that compared the health status of Gulf War veterans with that of nondeployed veterans or veterans deployed elsewhere, such as in Bosnia or Germany.

COMMITTEE'S APPROACH

During its deliberations, the Update committee held two public sessions at which it heard from numerous interested parties, including representatives of veteran-service organizations and individual Gulf War veterans. VA Secretary Shinseki also asked the committee to invite representatives of the VA Research Advisory Committee on Gulf War Veterans' Illnesses (RAC) to make presentations on the findings and conclusions in its report *Gulf War Illness and the Health of Gulf War Veterans: Scientific Findings and Recommendations*, released in November 2008.

Extensive searches of the epidemiologic literature published since 2005 were conducted with the same search strategy as that used for *Volume 4*; over 1000 new citations were identified. After an assessment of the titles and abstracts found in the initial searches, the committee focused on some 400 potentially relevant epidemiologic studies for further review and evaluation.

The committee adopted a policy of using only peer-reviewed publications as the basis of its conclusions except for some government reports. The process of peer review by fellow professionals increases the likelihood of high quality but does not guarantee the validity of a study or the ability to generalize its findings. Accordingly, committee members read each study critically and considered its relevance and quality. The committee did not collect original data, nor did it perform any secondary data analysis.

To be comprehensive in its approach to the epidemiologic literature, the committee also reviewed the studies that had been included in *Volume 4* as primary or secondary studies. The Volume 4 committee did not draw conclusions about the strength of associations between specific exposures experienced during the Gulf War and particular health effects. However, *Volume 4* did indicate what health outcomes were more prevalent in deployed veterans than in nondeployed veterans. The Update committee has been asked to determine the strength of associations between being deployed to the Gulf War and specific health effects. To make such a determination, the committee needed to review the studies cited in *Volume 4* to assess whether they would still be classified as primary or secondary. The committee also tried to be comprehensive in its review of the literature inasmuch as the strength of an association would rest on a weight-of-the-evidence approach; that is, the committee considered it important to evaluate all primary and secondary studies that identified health outcomes so that a complete picture of the body of evidence could be presented.

The Update committee then considered the epidemiologic studies identified in the updated literature search. Those studies were also reviewed and classified as primary or secondary according to the criteria discussed below. Once the committee had assessed the studies cited in *Volume 4* and evaluated the new studies identified in the more recent literature, it considered the entire body of relevant literature and determined the strength of associations between being deployed to the Gulf War and specific health outcomes on the basis of all the primary studies and supported by the secondary studies.

Because the committee was not attempting to link health outcomes to exposures other than deployment to the Persian Gulf theater, for which there is no known animal model, it did not review toxicologic, animal, or experimental studies comprehensively; however, it did evaluate the key epidemiologic and animal cited in the RAC report (see Appendix A). Epidemiologic studies that attempted to associate health effects in Gulf War veterans with specific exposures, such as oil-well fire smoke or nerve-gas agents, were also considered by the committee.

VOLUME 4 CONCLUSIONS

The Volume 4 committee cataloged the health outcomes that appeared to be more prevalent in veterans who had been deployed to the Gulf War than in veterans who served in the military at the same time but were not deployed to the Persian Gulf area, but it did not evaluate the strength of associations between deployment to the Gulf War and specific health outcomes. Studies were categorized as to whether the health outcomes seen in veterans were based on self-reports (including self-reports of physician diagnoses) or on objective measures, such as results of physical examinations by health-care providers or of laboratory tests. Using that approach, the Volume 4 committee found that on the basis of self-reports, deployed veterans had more symptoms indicative of multisymptom illness (although the symptoms did not appear to constitute a unique syndrome, illness, or symptom complex), such psychiatric disorders as posttraumatic stress disorder (PTSD), gastrointestinal disorders, skin disorders, joint pain, and respiratory disorders. However, when objective measures were used to diagnose the health outcomes seen in deployed and nondeployed veterans, different results were seen. Deployed veterans were more likely than nondeployed veterans to experience injury or death from transportation accidents in the years immediately after the war and possibly were at increased risk for amyotrophic lateral sclerosis (ALS), and in one study deployed veterans' offspring were more likely to have birth defects. Objective measures failed to show an increased prevalence of hospitalizations, cancer (results for testicular cancer were inconsistent), peripheral neuropathy, cardiovascular disease, diabetes, or pulmonary function in active-duty Gulf War veterans. The committee noted that few studies attempted to link specific exposures, such as exposure to oil-well fire smoke and possibly nerve agents released at Khamisiyah, to health outcomes. Only self-reports of exposure to oil-well fires were linked to an increase in self-reported respiratory symptoms that were suggestive of asthma and bronchitis.

CONSIDERATIONS IN IDENTIFYING AND EVALUATING THE LITERATURE

The Update committee sought to characterize and weigh the strengths and limitations of the available evidence presented in the studies that it reviewed. For *Volume 4* of the *Gulf War and Health* series, numerous cohort studies and case control studies were objectively reviewed without preconceptions about health outcomes that might be seen in Gulf War veterans. The Volume 4 committee developed criteria to determine which studies to include in its review. The Update committee reviewed and used those criteria to evaluate the studies that have been published since *Volume 4* and also uses categories of association to determine the strength of associations between deployment to the Gulf War and health outcomes. The categories of association have been used by the other reports in the *Gulf War and Health* series.

Primary and Secondary Studies

To be a primary study, which would be used by the committee to support its conclusions, a study needed to demonstrate rigorous methods (for example, to be published in a peer-reviewed journal, to include details of methods, to have a control or reference group, and to include adjustments for confounders if needed), needed to include information regarding a persistent health outcome, needed to have a medical evaluation conducted by a health professional, and needed to use laboratory testing as appropriate. Those types of studies constituted the committee's primary literature. The committee did not evaluate studies of acute trauma, rehabilitation, medical treatment, or transient illness.

Studies reviewed by the committee that did not necessarily meet all the criteria of a primary study were considered secondary studies. Secondary studies are typically not as methodologically rigorous as primary studies and might present subclinical findings; that is, they are studies of altered functioning consistent with later development of a diagnosis but without clear predictive value.

The present report excludes studies of participants in Gulf War registries established by VA or the Department of Defense (DoD), such as DoD's Comprehensive Clinical Evaluation Program. Registry participants cannot be considered representative of all Gulf War veterans in that they are self-selected subjects, many of whom have joined the registries because they believe that they have symptoms of a new medical syndrome; in addition, they were not randomly selected from all Gulf War military personnel, and there is no nondeployed control group.

Categories of Association

The committee attempted to express its judgment of the available data clearly and precisely. It agreed to use the categories of association that have been established and used by previous Committees on Gulf War and Health and other IOM committees that have evaluated vaccine safety, effects of herbicides used in Vietnam, and indoor pollutants related to asthma. Those categories of association have gained wide acceptance over more than a decade by Congress, government agencies (particularly VA), researchers, and veterans groups.

The five categories below describe different levels of association and present a common message: the validity of an observed association is likely to vary with the extent to which common sources of spurious associations could be ruled out as the reason for the association. Accordingly, the criteria for each category express a degree of confidence based on the extent to which sources of error were reduced. The committee members read each of each the studies carefully, noted the studies' findings and limitations, and discussed the classification of each study (primary or secondary) in plenary session. The committee then discussed the weight of the evidence and reached consensus on the categorization of association to be assigned for each health outcome considered in this report.

Sufficient Evidence of a Causal Relationship

Evidence is sufficient to conclude that a causal relationship exists between being deployed to the Gulf War and a health outcome. The evidence fulfills the criteria for sufficient evidence of a causal association in which chance, bias, and confounding can be ruled out with reasonable confidence. The association is supported by several of the other considerations used to assess causality: strength of association, dose-response relationship, consistency of association, temporal relationship, specificity of association, and biologic plausibility.

Sufficient Evidence of an Association

Evidence suggests an association, in that a positive association has been observed between deployment to the Gulf War and a health outcome in humans; however, there is some doubt as to the influence of chance, bias, and confounding.

Limited/Suggestive Evidence of an Association

Some evidence of an association between deployment to the Gulf War and a health outcome in humans exists, but this is limited by the presence of substantial doubt regarding chance, bias, and confounding.

Inadequate/Insufficient Evidence to Determine Whether an Association Exists

The available studies are of insufficient quality, validity, consistency, or statistical power to permit a conclusion regarding the presence or absence of an association between deployment to the Gulf War and a health outcome in humans.

Limited/Suggestive Evidence of No Association

There are several adequate studies, covering the full range of levels of exposure that humans are known to encounter, that are consistent in not showing an association between exposure to a specific agent and a health outcome at any level of exposure. A conclusion of no association is inevitably limited to the conditions, levels of exposure, and length of observation covered by the available studies. In addition, the possibility of a very small increase in risk at the levels of exposure studied can never be excluded.

MAJOR COHORT STUDIES

Another step that the committee took in organizing its literature was to determine how all the study cohorts were related to one another. Numerous Gulf War cohorts have been assembled from several countries, and it is on the basis of those original cohorts that many derivative studies have been conducted and published. The committee organized the literature into the major cohorts and derivative studies because it did not want to interpret the findings of the same cohorts as though they were results of studies of unique groups.

The largest studies of Gulf War veterans have been conducted in countries that were members of the Gulf War coalition, including the United States, the United Kingdom, Canada, Denmark, and Australia. Most major cohorts, once established, led to numerous studies that examined more detailed questions about Gulf War veterans' health; the committee refers to these as derivative studies. The cohort studies of Gulf War veterans and the derivative studies have contributed greatly to our understanding of veterans' health, but they are beset by limitations that are commonly encountered in epidemiologic studies, including lack of representativeness, selection bias, lack of control for potential confounding factors, self-reporting of health outcomes, outcome misclassification, and self-reporting of exposure.

The committee considered studies that used both population-based cohorts and military-unit–based cohorts. Population-based studies of particular importance included the large nationally representative study of Gulf War deployed and nondeployed veterans conducted by VA to address congressional mandates, a study of Iowa veterans initiated by the Iowa Persian Gulf Study Group, a study of all Canadian Gulf War veterans, studies of Oregon and Washington veterans conducted by the Portland Environmental Hazards Research Center, and a study of Kansas veterans. Two teams of researchers in the United Kingdom studied separate, nonoverlapping samples of the over 53,000 UK military personnel sent to the Gulf War. The first team was from the University of London (Guy's, King's, and St. Thomas Medical Schools), and the second was from the University of Manchester. A third team of researchers from the London School of Hygiene and Tropical Medicine surveyed the entire cohort of 53,000 veterans for birth defects and other reproductive outcomes. Peacekeepers from Denmark were also studied for a variety of health outcomes, as was the entire Australian military contingent deployed to the Gulf War. Military-unit–based studies have been conducted on Air Force National Guard members from Pennsylvania; Fort Devens, MA; and New Orleans, LA; and Seabees, members of a naval reserve unit of a mobile construction battalion. In addition, several studies have looked at hospitalizations and mortality of Gulf War veterans since the war.

HEALTH OUTCOMES

The Update committee reviewed numerous new studies from the epidemiologic literature on Gulf War veterans and identified about 400 studies for in-depth evaluation. The latter studies and those described in *Volume 4* formed the basis of the committee's conclusions regarding associations between deployment to the Gulf War and long-term health outcomes. Most of the studies compared the prevalence of a given medical condition or symptom in the deployed veterans with the prevalence in nondeployed veterans. If the prevalence of a symptom or condition was linked by the study authors to any specific exposures experienced during deployment—such as vaccines, oil-well fire smoke, anti-nerve-gas agents, or combat—the committee reviewed those associations as well. Although for the most part the Update committee considered the same health outcomes as did the Volume 4 committee, there were several differences: the Update committee added two new health outcomes: genitourinary diseases and diseases of the blood and blood-forming organs. The committee also used the term *multisymptom illness* to refer to a health outcome rather than the International Classification of Diseases, 9th revision, category of "signs, symptoms, and abnormal clinical and laboratory findings." Chronic fatigue syndrome and multiple chemical sensitivity were included in the section on multisymptom illnesses; hospitalization and mortality studies were discussed in the relevant health-outcome sections; and chronic widespread pain was included in the section on fibromyalgia.

All studies of each health outcome, including those originally cited in *Volume 4*, were reviewed and categorized as primary or secondary by the entire committee in plenary session before it came to a consensus on the appropriate category of association to be assigned to each health outcome. As in previous volumes of the *Gulf War and Health* series, the primary studies on which the committee based its conclusions are detailed in the evidence table at the end of each health-outcome section. Using the weight-of-the-evidence approach required that the Update committee be more rigorous in its review of the studies in *Volume 4*; as a result, some studies considered to be primary in *Volume 4* were recategorized as secondary for the present report and vice versa. Thus, the Update committee summarizes de novo the information from both *Volume 4* and any new publications to arrive at its conclusions on the strength of associations between deployment to the Gulf War and health outcomes. Box S-1 summaries the health outcomes assigned to each category of association by the Update committee.

QUALITY OF THE STUDIES

Many studies of Gulf War veterans have been conducted, but their quality is varied, and many have substantial limitations. As a result, there is still uncertainty about the relationship between deployment to the Gulf War and health outcomes. The limitations include

- Lack of representativeness of the entire Gulf War population in some studies, which affects external validity in such a way that what we learn from the population studied cannot be easily extrapolated to all Gulf War veterans.
- Low participation rates and differential participation rates in many studies, which affect internal validity because of selection bias (for example, significantly higher rate of response of deployed veterans than of nondeployed control groups and the possibility that deployed troops participated because they already experienced health problems).
- Narrowness of assessment of health status (for example, self-reported outcomes, such as hypertension, diabetes, and cardiovascular disease), or insufficient sensitivity or validity of instruments to detect abnormalities in deployed veterans (for example, death certificates or hospital discharge diagnoses); there is a particular problem with self-reported exposures, especially if respondents are aware of mass-media reports that link outcomes with putative exposures.

BOX S-1
Summary of Findings Regarding Associations Between Deployment to the Gulf War and Specific Health Outcomes

Sufficient Evidence of a Causal Relatioonship

- PTSD.

Sufficient Evidence of an Association

- Other psychiatric disorders, including generalized anxiety disorder, depression, and substance abuse, particularly alcohol abuse. These psychiatric disorders persist for at least 10 years after deployment.
- Gastrointestinal symptoms consistent with functional gastrointestinal disorders such as irritable bowel syndrome and functional dyspepsia.
- Multisymptom illness.
- Chronic fatigue syndrome.

Limited/Suggestive Evidence of an Association

- ALS.
- Fibromyalgia and chronic widespread pain.
- Self-reported sexual difficulties.
- Mortality from external causes, primarily motor-vehicle accidents, in the early years after deployment.

Inadequate/Insufficient Evidence to Determine Whether an Association Exists

- Any cancer.
- Diseases of the blood and blood-forming organs.
- Endocrine, nutritional, and metabolic diseases.
- Neurocognitive and neurobehavioral performance.
- Multiple sclerosis.
- Other neurologic outcomes, such as Parkinson's disease, dementia, and Alzheimer's disease.
- Incidence of cardiovascular diseases.
- Respiratory diseases.
- Structural gastrointestinal diseases.
- Skin diseases.
- Musculoskeletal system diseases.
- Specific conditions of the genitourinary system.
- Specific birth defects.
- Adverse pregnancy outcomes such as miscarriage, stillbirth, preterm birth, and low birth weight.
- Fertility problems.

Limited/Suggestive Evidence of No Association

- Peripheral neuropathy.
- Mortality from cardiovascular disease in the first 10 years after the war.
- Decreased lung function in the first 10 years after the war.
- Hospitalization for genitourinary diseases.

- Timing of investigations relative to the latency of some health outcomes (for example, cancer and some neurologic outcomes, such as multiple sclerosis [MS], ALS, and Parkinson's disease).

- Use of cross-sections, which limits assessment of symptom duration and chronicity, latency of onset, severity, and prognosis.

Virtually all the reports in the *Gulf War and Health* series have called for improved studies of Gulf War and other veterans. The Update committee reiterates that need but notes that it is difficult if not impossible 20 years after the war to reconstruct the exposures to which the veterans were subjected in theater or to establish years after deployment the predeployment physical and mental health status of the veterans for comparison purposes. Therefore, the committee believes that future studies of Gulf War veterans—and indeed any veteran population—need to be adequately designed to

- Provide sufficient statistical power (precision).
- Ensure validity, including the avoidance of such bias as response bias and recall bias, which lead deployed and nondeployed veterans to participate unequally, depending on general health and symptom presence and severity, or to report symptoms differently according to perceived exposures and health status.
- Improve disease measurement to avoid misclassification; for example, including information collected from non-DoD hospitals in studies of hospitalization, obtaining cancer incidence data from existing cancer registries, validating self-reports of health outcomes, and using the least error-prone measures of these outcomes.
- Characterize deployment and potential related adverse environmental influences better by, for example, collecting information on the length and location of deployment and on jobs and tasks.
- Measure and adjust for possible confounding factors by, for example, measuring and adjusting for lifestyle factors (such as smoking and risk-taking behaviors) and predeployment physical and psychologic health status.

RECOMMENDATIONS

After almost two decades of research on Gulf War veterans, important questions about their health remain unanswered. In particular, the nature and extent of the multisymptom illness reported in the veterans warrant further research to refine its diagnosis and develop effective treatments. The committee believes that the path forward for veterans has two branches. The first is continued surveillance of deployed and nondeployed Gulf War veterans.

- Although further investigations based solely on self-reporting are not likely to contribute substantially to the understanding of Gulf War illness, well-designed follow-up studies of mortality, cancer, neurologic, and psychiatric outcomes will continue to be valuable. Well-designed, adequately powered studies of MS and ALS incidence after deployment are also needed.
- Methodologically robust cohorts need to be assembled and followed carefully to track the development of ALS, MS, brain cancer, psychiatric conditions, and health problems that occur at a later age, such as other cancers, cardiovascular disease, and neurodegenerative diseases. Several well-characterized cohorts that could form the basis of future studies have already been established, such as the US cohort studied by VA, the two UK cohorts, and the

Canadian, Danish, and Australian cohorts. Relatively small cohorts, such as the Canadian and Australian veterans, might not be useful for outcomes of low incidence (for example, ALS and brain cancer), but they might be very useful for tracking frequent outcomes, for example, multisymptom illness, cardiovascular and respiratory diseases, other cancer types, such neurodegenerative conditions as dementia, and some psychiatric disorders.

- With regard to functional gastrointestinal disorders (irritable bowel syndrome and functional dyspepsia), recent evidence supports the need for two types of studies: to determine the role of prior acute gastroenteritis in the development of these disorders in deployed soldiers and to use symptom-specific criteria (for example, Rome criteria) to clarify the association of medical and psychosocial comorbidities with functional gastrointestinal disorders and their severity.
- Uncommon genetic variants and rare environmental events may not be recognized as associated with outcomes of interest unless very large numbers of people are studied or sophisticated capture methods are used to explore them. For example, new and objective information related to exposures that becomes available in the future might improve our ability to estimate individual exposures and to stratify groups of Gulf War veterans.

A second branch of inquiry is also important. It consists of a renewed research effort to identify and treat multisymptom illness in Gulf War veterans. Given the high prevalence of persistent symptoms and the steady advances in our understanding of genetics, molecular diagnostics, and imaging, it is now possible to plan and carry out adequately powered studies to identify inherited genetic variants, molecular profiles of gene expression, other epigenetic markers (for example, modifications of DNA structure related to environmental exposures), specific viral exposures, signatures of immune activation, and brain changes identified by sensitive imaging measures that distinguish Gulf War veterans who have persistent medical symptoms from healthy deployed or nondeployed veterans. The committee is optimistic that a rigorous, adequately powered study could identify useful biomarkers that are helpful for symptomatic veterans of the Gulf War and for nondeployed veterans and civilians who have a variety of medically unexplained symptoms, including chronic fatigue, muscle and joint pain, sleep disturbance, difficulty with concentration, and depression.

Finally, the committee notes that inadequate numbers of clinical trials have been undertaken to develop more effective and evidence-based treatments for multisystem illness. Aligned with efforts to improve care pathways for veterans suffering from multisymptom illness, a focused effort should be undertaken to support high-quality clinical trials informed by the best available biologic information related to the cause of multisystem illness. The committee believes that a continued and targeted research program is the most likely path to assist VA and other health-care providers in diagnosing and treating the health problems of Gulf War veterans and preventing illness in future veterans.

1

INTRODUCTION

On August 2, 1990, Iraq invaded Kuwait. Operation Desert Shield, the buildup of coalition forces in the Persian Gulf region led by the United States, began in response to that invasion. Operation Desert Storm began on January 16, 1991, with an air offensive, and the 4-day ground war was over by February 28; a ceasefire was signed in April 1991. During the war almost 700,000 US troops were deployed to the Persian Gulf region, although by June 1991 only about 50,000 US troops remained in the region. Although brief with relatively few injuries and deaths among the coalition, the legacy of the war has been a continuing plethora of health problems for many veterans even 20 years after the war. Numerous exposures have been implicated as the cause of these problems, ranging from oil-well fires to the use of the prophylactic antinerve agent pyridostigmine bromide (PB). These health problems, particularly a constellation of symptoms that have been termed multisymptom illness or Gulf War illness, continue to plague as many as a third of the veterans who were deployed to the Gulf War. Furthermore, these unexplained illnesses are seen in veterans from several of the countries that formed the coalition forces, including the United Kingdom (UK), Australia, Canada, and Denmark. Numerous researchers have studied the variety of health outcomes presented by Gulf War veterans and attempted to identify possible exposures that may have caused or contributed to those outcomes.

BACKGROUND

In 1998, in response to the growing concerns of Gulf War veterans, Congress passed two laws: PL 105-277, the Persian Gulf War Veterans Act, and PL 105-368, the Veterans Programs Enhancement Act. Those laws directed the secretary of veterans affairs to enter into a contract with the National Academy of Sciences (NAS) to review and evaluate the scientific and medical literature regarding associations between illness and exposure to toxic agents, environmental or wartime hazards, or preventive medicines or vaccines associated with Gulf War service and to consider the NAS conclusions when making decisions about compensation. The NAS assigned the study to the Institute of Medicine (IOM).

The Persian Gulf War legislation directs the IOM to study diverse biologic, chemical, and physical agents. Exposures to many of the Gulf War agents have been extensively studied and characterized, primarily in occupational settings (for example, exposure to pesticides, solvents, and fuels), but exposures to others have not been as well studied and characterized in human populations (for example, exposure to nerve agents and vaccines).

Given the large number of agents to study, IOM divided the task into several reviews, which are now complete: *Gulf War and Health, Volume 1: Depleted Uranium, Pyridostigmine Bromide, Sarin, Vaccines* (IOM, 2000); *Gulf War and Health, Volume 2: Insecticides and Solvents* (IOM, 2003); *Gulf War and Health: Updated Literature Review of Sarin* (IOM, 2004); *Gulf War and Health, Volume 3: Fuels, Combustion Products, and Propellants* (IOM, 2005); *Amyotrophic Lateral Sclerosis in Veterans: Review of the Scientific Literature* (IOM, 2006a); *Gulf War and Health, Volume 4: Health Effects of Serving in the Gulf War* (IOM, 2006b); *Gulf War and Health, Volume 5: Infectious Disease* (IOM, 2007); *Gulf War and Health, Volume 6: Physiologic, Psychologic, and Psychosocial Effects of Deployment-Related Stress* (IOM, 2008); and *Gulf War and Health, Volume 7: Long-Term Consequences of Traumatic Brain Injury* (IOM, 2009).

In 2005, the Department of Veterans Affairs (VA) requested that the IOM appoint a committee, the Committee on Gulf War and Health: A Review of the Medical Literature Relative to Gulf War Veterans' Health, to review that body of literature and to summarize what was known about the then current status of the veterans' health. In 2006 the committee produced a report, *Gulf War and Health, Volume 4: Health Effects of Serving in the Gulf War* that summarized the overall health effects in veterans and noted which health outcomes are more evident in Gulf War veterans than in their nondeployed counterparts, irrespective of the specific exposures experienced by the deployed veterans. This current report is an update of *Volume 4*, covering the literature published since 2006 on the health effects seen in veterans deployed to the Persian Gulf in 1990-1991.

THE GULF WAR SETTING[1]

In *Gulf War and Health, Volume 4,* that committee's charge was not to review the scientific evidence on the possible health effects of various agents to which Gulf War veterans were potentially exposed, but rather to look at the prevalence of the various health effects seen in Gulf War deployed veterans and to determine if that prevalence was greater than that seen in veterans who served in the military during the Gulf War but were not deployed. The current committee (the Update committee) is also not charged with looking at whether a specific exposure could cause a health effect, but like the Volume 4 committee, the Update committee recognized that its members needed to have an appreciation of the Gulf War experience, including the magnitudes of possible exposures for all the military forces that served in the gulf, including those deployed to the region after the war ended. Therefore, in addition to reviewing studies from the United States, the committee reviewed studies of Gulf War veterans from Australia, Canada, Denmark, the United Kingdom, Kuwait, and France.

The information in this section provides a context for the many scientific articles that the current committee reviewed and an appreciation (albeit limited) of the collective experience of Gulf War veterans. It is compiled from many sources including Gunby (1991), Hyams et al. (1995), IOM (1995, 1996, 1999), Joellenbeck et al. (1998), Lawler et al. (1997), NIH Technology Assessment Workshop Panel (1994), PAC (1996, 1997), Persian Gulf Veterans Coordinating Board (1995), Ursano and Norwood (1996), and VA (1998).

---

[1]This section is adapted from *Gulf War and Health, Volume 1* (IOM, 2000) and *Gulf War and Health, Volume 4* (IOM, 2006).

Deployment

The pace of the buildup for the Gulf War was unprecedented. Within 5 days after Iraq invaded Kuwait, the United States began moving troops into the region as part of Operation Desert Shield. By September 15, 1990, the number of American servicemembers reached 150,000 and included nearly 50,000 reservists. Within the next month, another 60,000 troops arrived in the Persian Gulf region; in November, an additional 135,000 reservists and National Guard members were called up. By February 24, 1991, more than 500,000 US troops had been deployed to the Persian Gulf region. In addition to the US troops, a coalition force of 34 member countries was eventually assembled.

The Gulf War reflected many changes from previous wars, particularly in the demographic composition of military personnel and the uncertainty of conditions for many reservists. Of the nearly 700,000 US troops who fought in Operation Desert Shield and Operation Desert Storm, almost 7% were women and about 17% (106,000) were from National Guard and reserve units. Military personnel were, overall, older than those who had participated in previous wars with a mean age of 28 years. Seventy percent of the troops were non-Hispanic/white; 23% were black, and 5% were Hispanic (Joseph, 1997). Rapid mobilization exerted substantial pressure on those who were deployed, disrupting lives, separating families, and, for reserve and National Guard units, creating uncertainty about whether jobs would be available when they returned to civilian life.

Living Conditions

Combat troops were crowded into warehouses and tents on arrival in the gulf region and then often moved to isolated desert locations. Most troops lived in tents and slept on cots lined up side by side, affording virtually no privacy or quiet. Sanitation was often primitive, with strains on latrines and communal washing facilities. Hot showers were infrequent, the interval between laundering uniforms was sometimes long, and desert flies were a constant nuisance, as were scorpions and snakes. Military personnel worked long hours and had narrowly restricted outlets for relaxation. Troops were ordered not to fraternize with local people, and alcoholic drinks were prohibited in deference to religious beliefs in the host countries. A mild, traveler's type of diarrhea affected more than half of the troops in some units. Fresh fruits and vegetables from neighboring countries were identified as the cause and were removed from the diet. Thereafter, the diet consisted mostly of packaged foods and bottled water.

For the first 2 months of troop deployment (August and September 1990) the weather was extremely hot, with air temperatures as high as 115°F and sand temperatures reaching 150°F. Except for coastal regions, the relative humidity was less than 40%. Troops had to drink large quantities of water to prevent dehydration. Although the summers were hot and dry, temperatures in winter (December-March) were low, with wind-chill temperatures at night dropping to well below freezing. Wind and blowing sand made protection of skin and eyes imperative. Goggles and sunglasses helped somewhat, but visibility was often poor.

Environmental and Chemical Exposures

The most visually dramatic environmental event of the Gulf War was the smoke from more than 750 oil-well fires in Kuwait. Smoke plumes from individual fires rose and combined to form giant plumes that could be seen for hundreds of kilometers. As noted in *Volume 4*, it has been difficult to correlate veterans' self-reports of exposure to the smoke with dispersion models based on troop location information (IOM, 2006b). There were additional potential sources of exposure to petroleum-based combustion products. Kerosene, diesel, and leaded gasoline were used in unvented tent heaters, cooking stoves, and portable generators. Exposures to tent-heater emissions were not specifically documented, but a simulation study was conducted after the war to determine exposure (Cheng et al., 2001). Petroleum products, including diesel fuels, were also used to suppress sand and dust, and petroleum fuels were used to aid in the burning of waste and trash.

Pesticides, including dog flea collars, were widely used by troops in the Persian Gulf to combat the region's ubiquitous insect and rodent populations, and although guidelines for use were strict, there were many reports of misuse. The pesticides used included methyl carbamates, organophosphates, pyrethroids, and chlorinated hydrocarbons. The use of those pesticides is covered in several reports (for example, DoD, 2001; RAND, 2000); however, objective information regarding individual levels of pesticide exposure is generally not available, and reports by individual veterans as to their use of and possible exposure to pesticides are subject to considerable recall bias.

Many exposures could have been related to particular occupational activities in the Gulf War. The majority of occupational chemical exposures appear to have been related to repair and maintenance activities, including battery repair (corrosive liquids), cleaning and degreasing (solvents, including chlorinated hydrocarbons), sandblasting (abrasive particles), vehicle repair (asbestos, carbon monoxide, and organic solvents), weapon repair (lead particles), and welding and cutting (chromates, nitrogen dioxide, and heated metal fumes). In addition, troops painted vehicles and other equipment used in the gulf with a chemical-agent-resistant coating either before being shipped to the gulf or at ports in Saudi Arabia. Working conditions in the field were not ideal and recommended occupational-hygiene standards might not have been followed at all times.

Exposure of US personnel to depleted uranium (DU) occurred as the result of friendly-fire incidents, cleanup operations, and accidents (including fires). Other personnel might have inhaled DU dust through contact with DU-contaminated tanks or munitions. Assessment of DU exposure, especially high exposure, is considered to be more accurate than assessment of exposure to most other agents because of the availability of biologic monitoring information.

Threat of Chemical and Biologic Warfare

When US troops arrived in the gulf, they had no way of knowing whether they would be exposed to biologic and chemical weapons. Iraq previously had used such weapons in fighting Iran and in attacks on the Kurdish minority in Iraq. Military leaders feared that the use of such weapons in the gulf could result in the deaths of tens of thousands of Americans. Therefore, in addition to the standard vaccinations before military deployment, about 150,000 troops received anthrax vaccine and about 8,000 troops received botulinum toxoid vaccine. In some cases, vaccination records were kept, and they provide an objective measure of exposure in addition to self-reporting by troops.

Troops were also given blister packs of 21 tablets of pyridostigmine bromide (PB) to protect against agents of chemical warfare, specifically nerve gas. Troops were to take PB on the orders of a commanding officer when a chemical-warfare attack was believed to be imminent. Chemical sensors and alarms were distributed throughout the region to warn of such attacks. The alarms were extremely sensitive and could be triggered by many substances, including some organic solvents, vehicle exhaust fumes, and insecticides. Alarms sounded often and troops responded by donning the confining protective gear and ingesting PB as an antidote to nerve gas. In addition to the alarms, there were widespread reports of dead sheep, goats, and camels, which troops were taught could be indication of the use of chemical or biologic weapons. The sounding of the alarms, the reports of dead animals, and rumors that other units had been hit by chemical warfare agents caused the troops to be concerned that they would be or had been exposed to such agents.

Despite the small numbers of US personnel injured or killed during combat in the Gulf War, the troops, as in any war, faced the fear of death, injury, or capture by the enemy. After the war, there was the potential for other exposures, including US demolition of a munitions storage complex at Khamisiyah, Iraq, which—unbeknownst to demolition troops at the time—contained stores of sarin and cyclosarin. The potential exposures to sarin and cyclosarin from the Khamisiyah incident have been the subject of specific modeling and health outcome studies. Depending on the dispersion model used to estimate the sarin and cyclosarin plume and troop unit locations, the number of Gulf War veterans who may have been exposed to the nerve agents ranged from an initial estimate of 10,000 troops within 25 km of Khamisiyah in 1997 to more than 100,000 troops using a 2000 model. However, more than 35,000 troops originally considered to have been exposed and notified that they may have been within the plume were subsequently considered to have been unexposed and 37,000 troops were newly identified as being in the hazard area (IOM, 2006b), adding to the confusion of how many troops were actually exposed to nerve agents and at what levels. As stated in *Volume 4*, "No medical reports by the US Army Medical Corps at the time of the release were consistent with signs and symptoms of acute exposure to sarin" (IOM, 2006b).

CHARGE TO THE COMMITTEE

The charge to the Volume 4 committee and to the current IOM committee (Update committee) is different from charges to other IOM Gulf War and Health committees in that the Volume 4 and Update committees were not asked to associate health outcomes with specific biologic, chemical, or other agents believed to have been present in the gulf, but rather to examine health outcomes related to deployment to the gulf region in general. The specific charge to the Update committee, as requested by the VA, was to review, evaluate, and summarize the literature on the following health outcomes noted in the 2006 report that seem to appear at higher incidence or prevalence in Gulf War-deployed veterans: cancer (particularly brain and testicular cancer), amyotrophic lateral sclerosis and other neurologic diseases (for example, Parkinson's disease and multiple sclerosis), birth defects and other adverse pregnancy outcomes, and postdeployment psychiatric conditions. The committee also was to review studies on cause-specific mortality in Gulf War veterans as recommended in the 2006 report. Finally, the committee was to examine the literature to identify any emerging health outcomes.

Thus, the current committee has limited its review to epidemiologic studies of health outcomes published since the last literature search conducted for *Volume 4* and those studies included in *Volume 4*. The studies must compare the health status of Gulf War veterans compared with nondeployed veterans or veterans deployed elsewhere such as Bosnia. Because the committee was not attempting to link health outcomes to any exposures other than deployment to a war zone, for which there is no known animal model, the committee did not review toxicologic, animal, or experimental studies. Where studies attempted to associate health effects with specific exposures, such as oil-well fire smoke or nerve gas agents, those studies were also considered.

COMMITTEE'S APPROACH TO ITS CHARGE

The committee began its evaluation by holding two public sessions. At those sessions, the committee heard from the VA and from Gulf War veterans about health outcomes that had been identified in Gulf War veterans during the past 20 years. During the second public session, the committee also heard presentations about health outcomes that were of particular concern to female veterans, a presentation from the chair of the IOM committee that had prepared *Gulf War and Health, Volume 4,* and from representatives of the VA Research Advisory Committee on Gulf War Veterans' Illnesses, who discussed that committee's findings and recommendations. Those sessions helped the committee to put its efforts in context and to clarify an approach to its task. The committee sought to characterize and weigh the strengths and limitations of the available evidence. It did not address policy issues, such as decisions regarding the potential costs of compensation.

Extensive searches of the epidemiologic literature published since 2005 were conducted using the same search strategy as that used for *Volume 4*; over 1000 potentially relevant references were retrieved. After an assessment of the titles and abstracts of the initial searches, the committee focused on some 400 potentially relevant epidemiologic studies for review and evaluation.

The committee adopted a policy of using only peer-reviewed published literature as the basis for its conclusions, with the exception of some government reports. The process of peer review by fellow professionals increases the likelihood of high quality but does not guarantee the validity of a study or the ability to generalize its findings. Accordingly, committee members read each study critically and considered its relevance and quality. The committee did not collect original data, nor did it perform any secondary data analysis.

To be comprehensive in its approach to the epidemiologic literature, the committee also reviewed the studies that had been included in *Volume 4* as primary or secondary studies. The Volume 4 committee did not draw conclusions as to the strength of association between an exposure, that is, deployment to the Gulf War, and a particular health effect. However, *Volume 4* did indicate what health outcomes had a greater prevalence in deployed veterans compared with nondeployed veterans. The Update committee has been asked to make a determination on the strength of the association between being deployed to the Gulf War and specific health effects. To make such a determination, the committee needed to review the studies cited in *Volume 4* to assess whether those studies would still be classified as primary or secondary. The committee then considered the epidemiologic studies identified in the updated literature search. These studies were also reviewed and classified as primary or secondary according to the criteria discussed below and in more detail in Chapter 2. Once the committee had assessed the studies cited in *Volume 4* and evaluated the new studies identified from the updated literature, it reviewed the entire body of relevant literature using a weight-of-the-evidence approach and determined the strength of the association between being deployed to the Gulf War and a specific health outcome based on the primary studies and supported by the secondary studies.

COMPLEXITIES IN RESOLVING GULF WAR AND HEALTH ISSUES

Investigations of the health effects of past wars have often focused on narrowly defined hazards or health outcomes, such as infectious diseases (for example, typhoid and malaria) during the Civil War, specific chemical hazards (for example, mustard gas in World War I and Agent Orange and other herbicides in Vietnam), and combat injuries. A discussion of the possible health effects of Gulf War service, however, involves many complex issues, some of which are explored below. They include exposure to multiple biologic and chemical agents as described above, limitations of exposure information collected during or modeled after deployment, individual variability factors, and illnesses that are often nonspecific and lack defined medical diagnoses or treatment protocols. The committee was not tasked with addressing those issues, but it presents them in this introductory chapter to acknowledge the difficulties faced by veterans, researchers, policymakers, and others in reaching an understanding about the veterans' ill health.

Multiple Exposures and Chemical Interactions

Although Operation Desert Shield and Operation Desert Storm were relatively brief, military personnel were potentially exposed to numerous harmful agents simultaneously. These include agents administered as preventive measures (such as PB, vaccines, pesticides, and insecticides), hazards of the natural environment (such as sand and endemic diseases), job-specific agents (such as paints, solvents, and diesel fumes), war-related agents (such as smoke from oil-well fires and DU), and hazards from cleanup operations (such as sarin and cyclosarin). Thus, military personnel might have been exposed to various agents at various doses for various periods. Many of the exposures are not specific to the Gulf War, but the number and combination of agents to which the veterans might have been exposed make it difficult to determine whether any agent or combination of agents is the cause of many Gulf War veterans' illnesses. The veterans also experienced numerous psychological stressors such as uncertainty about the presence of chemical and biological agents, seeing dead or wounded combatants and civilians, and anxiety about their families and jobs at home. The impacts of these psychologic stressors are discussed in more depth in *Gulf War and Health, Volume 6*.

Limitations of Exposure Information

Determining whether Gulf War veterans face an increased risk of illness because of their exposures during the war requires extensive information about each exposure, such as the actual agents, the duration of exposure, the route of entry, the internal dose, and documentation of adverse reactions. But very little is known about most Gulf War exposures. After the ground war, an environmental-monitoring effort was initiated primarily because of concerns related to smoke from oil-well fires and exposure to sarin and cyclosarin rather than for the other agents to which the troops might have been exposed. Consequently, exposure data on other agents are lacking or are severely limited. At the request of the DoD, the RAND Corporation conducted a postwar survey to assess possible exposures to pesticides (RAND, 2000).

Various exposure assessment tools have been used in research to fill gaps in exposure information, but there are problems in reconstruction of past exposure events. For example, veterans have been surveyed to obtain recollections about agents to which they might have been exposed, although survey results might be limited by recall bias. Models have been refined to estimate exposures to sarin and cyclosarin, but it is difficult to incorporate intelligence information, meteorologic data, transport and dispersion data, and troop-unit location information accurately (see *Volume 4, Chapter 2, Exposures in the Persian Gulf*). Extensive efforts have been made to model and obtain information on potential exposures to DU, smoke from oil-well fires, and other agents. Although modeling efforts are important for discerning the details of exposures of Gulf War veterans, they require external review and validation. Furthermore, even if there were accurate troop location data, the location of individual soldiers would be very uncertain. Because of the limitations in the exposure data, it is difficult to determine the likelihood of increased risk for disease or other adverse health effects in Gulf War veterans that are due specifically to biologic and chemical agents.

Although many studies have assessed military personnel exposures to various preventive agents including PB and pesticides during the Gulf War, these studies have been based on individuals' recall of the measures they received or took, frequently under stress situations, and have rarely been verified by in situ measurements or records. This potential for recall bias also contributes to the difficulty in identifying specific causes of the veterans' health problems.

Individual Variability

Differences among people in their genetic, biologic, psychologic, and social vulnerabilities add to the complexities in determining health outcomes related to specific agents. People with increased sensitivity to some agents will have different health outcomes than people who are less sensitive. For example, a person who is a poor metabolizer of a particular substance, depending on his or her genetic makeup, might be at higher or lower risk for specific health effects if exposed to the substance. For example, researchers are investigating the genotypes that code for two forms of an enzyme that differ in the rate at which they hydrolyze particular organophosphates (including sarin) (Costa et al., 1999). Lower hydrolyzing activity would mean that despite identical exposure to sarin, more sarin would be bioavailable in people who are poor metabolizers and could result in increased anticholinesterase effects. See Appendix A for a discussion of the metabolism of chemical agents.

VOLUME 4 CONCLUSIONS

In *Gulf War and Health, Volume 4* (IOM, 2006b), no associations were found between being deployed to the Gulf War and any health effects, nor were any associations found between specific exposures that may have occurred during deployment and health effects. The committee that prepared that volume, however, did report that Gulf War veterans, regardless of the country they served, consistently reported higher rates of nearly all symptoms examined than their nondeployed counterparts. This was true for veterans from the United States, the United Kingdom, Canada, Australia, and Denmark. The Volume 4 committee found that the majority of studies of Gulf War veterans relied on self-reports of symptoms and medical conditions. Fewer studies used objective measures or diagnostic medical tests to confirm the veterans' reports. The committee recognized that many of the veterans symptoms were subjective—for example, headache, joint pain—and could not be evaluated other than by self-report, but other symptoms and medical conditions—for example, fibromyalgia, irritable bowel syndrome—had diagnostic criteria or laboratory tests that could be used to make or verify a diagnosis. Therefore, the Volume 4 committee grouped the health effects in Gulf War veterans on the basis of whether the health effects were based primarily on symptoms and self-reports, or on objective measures and diagnostic medical tests. Box 1-1 summarizes of the *Volume 4* findings and recommendations.

BOX 1-1
Brief Summary of Findings and Recommendations

Outcomes Based Primarily on Symptoms or Self-Reports

- No unique syndrome, unique illness, or unique symptom complex in deployed Gulf War veterans was found. Veterans of the Gulf War report higher rates of nearly all symptoms or sets of symptoms than their nondeployed counterparts; 29% of veterans meet a case definition of "multisymptom illness," as compared with 16% of nondeployed veterans.
- Multisymptom-based medical conditions reported to occur more frequently among deployed Gulf War veterans include fibromyalgia, chronic fatigue syndrome, and multiple chemical sensitivity.
- Deployment places veterans at increased risk for symptoms that meet diagnostic criteria for a number of psychiatric illnesses, particularly posttraumatic stress disorder (PTSD), anxiety, depression, and substance abuse. In addition, co-morbidities were reported among a number of veterans, with PTSD, depression, anxiety, and/or substance abuse.
- Studies of Gulf War deployed veterans vs nondeployed have not demonstrated differences in cognitive and motor measures as determined through neurobehavioral testing.
- Studies of returning Gulf War veterans with at least one of the symptoms most commonly reported by Gulf War veterans (for example, fatigue, memory loss, confusion, inability to concentrate, mood swings, somnolence, gastrointestinal distress, muscle and joint pain, skin/mucous membrane complaints) found poorer performance on cognitive tests when compared to returning Gulf War veterans who did not report such symptoms.
- Other symptoms that appear to be self-reported more often by deployed veterans are gastrointestinal symptoms, particularly dyspepsia; dermatologic conditions, particularly atopic dermatitis and warts; and joint pains (arthralgias).

Outcomes with Objective Measures or Diagnostic Medical Tests

- Studies of mortality provide evidence for a modest increase in transportation-related injuries and mortalities among Gulf War deployed compared to nondeployed veterans in the decade immediately following deployment. However, studies with longer follow-up indicate that the increased injury rate was likely to have been restricted to the first several years after the war.
- With regard to all-causes of hospitalization, excess hospitalizations did not occur among veterans of the Gulf War who remained on active duty through 1994. However, Gulf War veterans who left the military reported worse health outcomes than those who remained.
- The studies do not demonstrate consistent evidence of increased overall cancer in the Gulf War veterans compared to nondeployed veterans. Studies of testicular cancer produced inconsistent results, but the latency period for many cancers may not have been reached among Gulf War veterans.
- Studies indicate that Gulf War veterans might be at increased risk for amyotrophic lateral sclerosis (ALS).
- There does not appear to be an increase in the prevalence of peripheral neuropathy in deployed versus non-deployed veterans, as defined by history, physical examination, and electrophysiologic studies.
- It does not appear that there is a difference in the prevalence of cardiovascular disease or diabetes between deployed and nondeployed veterans.
- Overall there is no consistent pattern of one or more birth defects with a higher prevalence for the offspring of male or female Gulf War veterans. Only one set of defects, urinary tract abnormalities, has been found to be increased in more than one well-designed study.
- Respiratory symptoms are strongly associated with Gulf War deployment when using comparison groups of non-deployed veterans in most studies addressing this question. However, studies with objective pulmonary function measures find no association between respiratory illnesses with Gulf War deployment across the four cohorts in which this has been investigated.

Outcomes with Objective Measures or Diagnostic Medical Tests Associated with Specific Gulf War Exposures

- Among studies that examined pulmonary outcomes in associations with specific exposures in the Gulf War Theater, exacerbation of asthma associated with oil-well fire smoke has been indicated.
- With respect to nerve agents at Khamisiyah, no study using objective estimates of exposure has found associations with pulmonary function measures or physician-diagnosed respiratory disease. Another study indicated that there might be an increase in brain cancer among such veterans; however, the exposure models are highly uncertain.

Recommendations

- Pre- and post-deployment screening of health status.
- Assessment of exposures.
- Surveillance for adverse health outcomes, specifically cancer, ALS, birth defects, adverse pregnancy outcomes, post-deployment psychiatric outcomes, and mortality.

Organization of the Report

Chapter 2 provides a brief background in epidemiology and describes the committee's methods for choosing the epidemiologic studies that are reviewed in later chapters. Chapter 3 describes the major Gulf War cohorts and provides information about the numerous studies that have been derived from them; the chapter includes a summary table that lists all the original cohorts and their derivative studies. The original table of studies was provided in *Volume 4* and has been updated here. Chapter 4 describes and analyzes the studies of health outcomes in Gulf War veterans; it also provides the basis for the committee's conclusions and recommendations, which are presented in Chapter 5. Appendix A briefly reviews the toxicity of cholinesterase inhibitors such as organophosphate pesticides and the adverse health outcomes that might result from exposure to them. Brief biographical sketches of the committee members are provided in Appendix B.

REFERENCES

Cheng, Y. S., Y. Zhou, J. Chow, J. Watson, and C. Frazier. 2001. Chemical composition of aerosols from kerosene heaters burning jet fuels. *Aerosol Science and Technology* 35(6):949-957.

Costa, L., W. Li, R. Richter, D. Shih, A. Lusis, and C. Furlong. 1999. The role of paraoxonase (PON1) in the detoxification of organophosphates and its human polymorphism. *Chemico-Biological Interactions* 119-120:429-438.

Department of Veterans Affairs. 1998. *Consolidation and Combined Analysis of the Databases of the Department of Veterans Affairs Persian Gulf Health Registry and the Department of Defense Comprehensive Clinical Evaluation Program.* Washington, DC: Environmental Epidemiology Service, Department of Veterans Affairs.

DoD (Department of Defense). 2001. *Environmental Exposure Report: Pesticides, Final Report.* Falls Church, VA: Department of Defense.

Gunby, P. 1991. Physicians provide continuum of care for Desert Storm fighting forces. *Journal of the American Medical Association* 265(5):557-559.

Hyams, K. C., K. Hanson, F. S. Wignall, J. Escamilla, and E. C. Oldfield, 3rd. 1995. The impact of infectious diseases on the health of U.S. troops deployed to the Persian Gulf during Operations Desert Shield and Desert Storm. *Clinical Infectious Diseases* 20(6):1497-1504.

IOM (Institute of Medicine). 1995. *Health Consequences of Service During the Persian Gulf War: Initial Findings and Recommendations for Immediate Action.* Washington, DC: National Academy Press.

IOM. 1996. *Health Consequences of Service During the Persian Gulf War: Recommendations for Research and Information Systems.* Washington, DC: National Academy Press.

IOM. 1999. *Gulf War Veterans: Measuring Health.* Washington, DC: National Academy Press.

IOM. 2000. *Gulf War and Health, Volume 1: Depleted Uranium Sarin, Pyridostigmine Bromide, Vaccines.* Washington, DC: National Academy Press.

IOM. 2003. *Gulf War and Health, Volume 2: Insecticides and Solvents.* Washington, DC: The National Academies Press.

IOM. 2004. *Gulf War and Health: Updated Literature Review of Sarin.* Washington, DC: The National Academies Press.

IOM. 2005. *Gulf War and Health, Volume 3: Fuels, Combustion Products, and Propellants.* Washington, DC: The National Academies Press.

IOM. 2006a. *Amyotrophic Lateral Sclerosis in Veterans: Review of the Scientific Literature.* Washington, DC: The National Academies Press.

IOM. 2006b. *Gulf War and Health, Volume 4: Health Effects of Serving in the Gulf War.* Washington, DC: The National Academies Press.

IOM. 2007. *Gulf War and Health, Volume 5: Infectious Diseases.* Washington, DC: The National Academies Press.

IOM. 2008. *Gulf War and Health, Volume 6: Physiologic, Psychologic, and Psychosocial Effects of Deployment-Related Stress.* Washington, DC: The National Academies Press.

IOM. 2009. *Gulf War and Health, Volume 7: Long-Term Consequences of Traumatic Brain Injury.* Washington, DC: The National Academies Press.

Joellenbeck, L. M., P. J. Landrigan, and E. L. Larson. 1998. Gulf War veterans' illnesses: A case study in causal inference. *Environmental Research* 79(2):71-81.

Joseph, S. C. 1997. A comprehensive clinical evaluation of 20,000 Persian Gulf War veterans. *Military Medicine* 162(3):149-155.

Lawler, M. K., D. E. Flori, R. J. Volk, and A. B. Davis. 1997. Family health status of National Guard personnel deployed during the Persian Gulf War. *Families, Systems, and Health* 15(1):65-73.

NIH Technology Assessment Workshop Panel. 1994. The Persian Gulf experience and health. *JAMA* 272(2):391-395.

PAC (Presidential Advisory Committee). 1996. *Presidential Advisory Committee on Gulf War Veteran' Illnesses: Final Report.* Washington, DC: US Government Printing Office.

PAC. 1997. *Presidential Advisory Committee on Gulf War Veterans' Illnesses: Special Report.* Washington, DC: Presidential Advisory Committee on Gulf War Veterans' Illnesses.

Persian Gulf Veterans Coordinating Board. 1995. Unexplained illnesses among Desert Storm veterans: A search for causes, treatment, and cooperation. *Archives of Internal Medicine* 155(3):262-268.

RAND. 2000. *Review of the scientific literature as it pertains to Gulf War illnesses. Volume 8: Pesticides.* Santa Monica, CA: RAND Corporation.

Ursano, R. J., and A. E. Norwood. 1996. *Emotional Aftermath of the Persian Gulf War: Veterans, Families, Communities, and Nations.* Washington, DC: American Psychiatric Publishing.

2

CONSIDERATIONS IN IDENTIFYING AND EVALUATING THE LITERATURE

This chapter presents the approach that the committee used to identify and evaluate the health and epidemiologic literature on Gulf War veterans. It provides information on how the committee searched the literature and discusses the major types of studies considered. The chapter also includes a discussion of the committee's evaluation criteria, the limitations of the studies reviewed, and the categories of association that the committee used in drawing conclusions about the possible health effects that might result from being deployed in the Gulf War.

Because the committee was tasked with determining the prevalence of diseases and symptoms in Gulf War veterans, the committee reviewed primarily observational studies that compared health outcomes seen in or reported by veterans deployed to the Gulf War with their nondeployed counterparts. The committee was not asked to associate diseases or health outcomes with exposures to specific biologic or chemical agents such as pesticides, nerve agents, or combustion products. The committee also did not concern itself with any policy issues, such as potential costs of compensation or policies regarding compensation. In *Volume 4* of the Gulf War and Health series, *Health Effects of Serving in the Gulf War*, that committee identified numerous cohort and case-control studies that it objectively reviewed without preconceived ideas about health outcomes. To assist it in its work, the committee developed criteria to determine which studies to include in its review. The Update committee reviewed and used those criteria to evaluate the studies that have been published since *Volume 4* but also used categories of association to determine the strength of the association between deployment to the Gulf War and health outcomes. The categories of association have been used by the other reports in the Gulf War and Health series, with the exception of *Volume 4*.

IDENTIFICATION OF THE LITERATURE

The committee began its work by overseeing extensive searches of the scientific literature, including published articles, other reports, and government documents that had been published after the last literature search for *Volume 4*, conducted in July 2005. The updated search retrieved over 1000 studies of potential pertinence to these analyses, and the titles and abstracts of those studies were reviewed. Studies that did not appear to have immediate relevance for this committee, based on an assessment of the title and abstract, were deleted from the search. Deleted studies included, but were not limited to, case studies, studies of civilians in the Persian

Gulf area, treatments, studies of short-term health outcomes only, rehabilitation, social outcomes (for example, employment), impacts on families, or studies of long-term outcomes from known physical events, such as gun-shot wounds. After the removal of these studies, approximately 400 potentially relevant epidemiologic studies were obtained for review and evaluation. The titles and abstracts of studies that had not been obtained as full text were available to the committee for review. The 400 studies that were obtained as full text were objectively evaluated by the committee members without preconceived ideas about what health outcomes might be seen and what, if any, associations might be found between being deployed to the Gulf War and any health outcomes.

The committee adopted a policy of using only published or unpublished literature that had undergone rigorous peer review as the basis of its conclusions. An exception to this policy was the inclusion of a few government reports. While the process of peer review by fellow professionals increases the likelihood that high-quality studies will appear in the literature, it does not guarantee the validity of any particular study or the ability to generalize its findings. Accordingly, committee members read each study critically and considered its relevance and quality. The committee did not collect original data, nor did they perform any secondary data analyses.

After securing the full text of the relevant studies, the committee determined which health conditions it would focus upon in the report. Initially, the health conditions listed in *Volume 4* were used but after reviewing numerous studies, new health outcomes were added, such as diseases of the blood and blood-forming organs and endocrine disorders. For each health outcome, one or more committee member with expertise or knowledge of a particular health outcome volunteered to screen all 400 studies in the database to identify all the epidemiologic studies that appeared to include information on that health outcome. The responsible committee member then conducted a preliminary review of the studies, including those cited in *Volume 4*, to determine what, if any, information the study had on the health outcome of interest and if an individual study met the inclusion criteria for a primary or secondary study (see below). The responsible committee member(s) then presented the information from the initial study screening and categorization to the full committee for discussion. Typically, the information presented included the populations used in the study, the methods for selecting and evaluating the populations, the study results, and the committee member's assessment of the strengths and limitations of the study. Each primary and secondary paper was discussed for each health outcome. Because of the variability in the description and diagnosis of the health conditions considered in this report, it was impossible for the committee to make a priori assumptions about the utility of any paper for a health outcome; each paper was discussed individually for each health outcome. After the studies had been discussed in plenary session, the responsible committee member drafted the text for that health outcome; the draft text was reviewed and discussed in further plenary sessions until all committee members reach a consensus on the description of the studies and the summary and conclusions. After this language was agreed upon, the full committee assigned a category of association based on the number and quality of the primary and secondary studies and expert judgment. It should be noted that the committee did not use a formulaic approach as to the number of primary and secondary studies that would be necessary to assign a specific category of association. Rather the committee found that each health outcome required a more considered and nuanced approach as described in the summary and conclusion section.

The following section briefly discusses types of evidence and the value of epidemiologic or clinical studies in determining whether an association exists. It is followed by a discussion of the committee's specific inclusion criteria that were developed to help decide whether a particular study would be included and evaluated for this report. The committee also notes the numerous factors that it considered in evaluating the evidence in a study and, finally, presents the categories of association used in drawing conclusions about the strength of associations.

TYPES OF EVIDENCE

The committee relied entirely on clinical and human epidemiologic studies to draw its conclusions about the strength of evidence regarding associations between deployment to the Gulf War and health outcomes seen in Gulf War veterans. The committee acknowledges, however, that animal studies might prove helpful in providing biologic understanding of many of the effects seen in humans from specific exposures, such as pesticides, solvents, and nerve agents, which have been reported by troops deployed in the Gulf War. Furthermore, information from molecular and cellular biology, neuroimaging, and other types of human studies can be used to understand the biological mechanisms and identification of biomarkers for clinical outcomes. Such studies, however, are not, in general, included in this review.

Epidemiologic Studies

In epidemiological research, analytical studies are designed to permit the examination of the association between two or more variables. *Predictor variable* or *independent variable* is a term used for an exposure to an agent of interest in a human population. *Outcome variable* or *dependent variable* is a term used to define a health or health-related event seen in a human population. Outcomes can also include a number of nonhealth results, such as use of medical services, social changes, and employment changes. One important goal of epidemiological research is to generate information that will help to understand whether exposure to a specific agent is associated with disease occurrence or other health outcomes. This goal is accomplished most straightforwardly in experimental studies in which the investigator controls the exposure (generally through random assignment) and the association between exposure and the subsequent occurrence of an outcome can be measured. Experimental studies are clearly not possible for studying the health effects of deployment to the Gulf War. Therefore, the studies included in this review are observational, not experimental, and compare health outcomes in those deployed to the Gulf with health outcomes seen in those who were in the military during the Gulf War but were not deployed to the Persian Gulf region. What is then assessed is the presence or absence of an association between the exposure and the outcomes.

Associations in Epidemiologic Studies

Association is primarily a statistical concept referring to the quantification of the relationship (positive, negative, or none) between two variables (e.g., independent and dependent). In the presence of association, additional considerations are required for causality to be judged as the reason behind the observed association. Apart from arising from a causal relationship between exposure and outcome, there may be other possible reasons for finding associations in observational studies including random error (chance), systematic error (bias), and reverse causality. Random error and systematic error can also be responsible for not observing an association when one truly does exist. It is essential to consider these alternative explanations in judging the findings of an epidemiological study.

Random error, sometimes referred to as "chance," is the statistical variation in a measurement of exposure, outcome, or both that arises from the fact that one cannot include an entire population in any study nor measure exposure or outcomes perfectly. The impact of random error can be mitigated through careful measurement and the inclusion of large samples, and it is quantified using statistical approaches including confidence intervals. For the most part, random error tends to result in an inability to find an association when one truly exists, that is, one is unable to separate out the signal from the noise. Systematic error or bias is the result of limitations in how the study was designed or conducted. Systematic error can cause an observed value to deviate from its true value and can falsely strengthen or weaken an association or generate a spurious association. Selection bias is one form of systematic error that occurs when the method of recruiting a study sample results in a sample that differs in some systematic way from the target population of the study. The findings of such a study are then potentially "biased" and may over- or underestimate the true association with the direction being dependent upon the form of selection bias. In addition, selection bias can also occur in a prospective study when there are losses to follow-up that differ between the exposed and unexposed group. Information bias relates to the way exposure or outcome factors are measured. If measurements are collected differently in groups that are to be compared then observed associations may be the result of these measurement differences rather than a true association.

Confounding bias occurs when a third variable, termed a confounding variable (or confounder), is associated with both the exposure and the outcome and mistakenly leads to the conclusion that the exposure is associated with the outcome. If the potential confounding variable is identified then statistical methods can be used to adjust for this form of bias.

Reverse causality bias may occur when the outcome actually precedes the exposure; for example, a study might suggest that a particular psychiatric outcome is a result of a traumatic brain injury. However, in reality, the psychiatric condition actually preceded the injury and the presence of the psychiatric condition placed individuals at increased risk of being injured.

Thus, the interpretation of the results of observational studies is complex. The committee reviewed the studies in this report with a view to considering the level of random error, the potential for bias, as well as the authors' strategies for examining and/or limiting the impact of each on the study findings.

To conclude that an association exists, it is necessary for the exposure to be followed by the outcome more often (or less often in the case of a protective exposure) than would be expected to occur by chance alone (that is, if no association actually existed). The strength of an association is typically expressed as a ratio of the frequency of an outcome in a group of participants who have a particular exposure to the frequency in a group without that same exposure. The strength of an association between exposure and outcome is generally estimated quantitatively by using prevalence ratios, relative risks (RRs, also called risk ratios), odds ratios (ORs), correlation coefficients, or hazard ratios (HRs) depending on the epidemiologic design used. A ratio greater than 1.0 indicates that the outcome variable has occurred more frequently in the exposed group, and a ratio less than 1.0 indicates that it has occurred less frequently. Ratios are typically reported with confidence intervals (CIs) to quantify random error. If a CI (for example, 95% CI) for a ratio measure includes 1.0, the observed association is said to be consistent with the null value (that is, no association). If the computed confidence interval does not include 1.0, the association is said to be consistent with a positive (or negative) association.

Inferring Causality

Determining whether an observed statistical association is causal requires additional considerations that must be examined carefully in the context of the particular relationship under study. Causality cannot be established directly through observational epidemiological studies for the reasons outlined above. The issue of causality is a major concern in epidemiology and in 1965, following the Surgeon General's report on the relationship between smoking and lung cancer, Sir Austin Bradford Hill, a British epidemiologist and statistician, described nine aspects that should be carefully considered when trying to come to a decision about whether an observed association might be causal (Hill, 1965). While all aspects are relevant in making inference about causality there is only one of the nine aspects that is truly necessary and that is temporality. The remaining eight aspects are neither necessary nor sufficient requirements for causation but do present a framework for consideration. While the committee was mindful of the Bradford Hill aspects when assigning the categories of association discussed later in the chapter, it did not use them as rigid criteria but rather guidelines to inform its conclusions about the association between deployment to the Gulf War and a particular health outcome. Aspects such as consistency, plausibility, and strength of association were discussed for each health outcome as the committee reached consensus on assigning a category of association but there was no requirement that all the aspects be met. The nine aspects are summarized below.

- *Strength of association.* Hill argues that a strong association is an important consideration and in the absence of other explanations would be a marker of causation. However he also points out that the absence of a strong association does not preclude a causal relationship.
- *Consistency.* If an association is observed in different studies, using different designs and in different settings then this would be supportive of a causal association.
- *Specificity.* If the association is specific to a particular exposure-disease outcome combination and there is no association between the exposure and other outcomes then such a finding would favor a causal association.
- *Temporality.* For an association to be causal it is essential that there be evidence that the exposure in question precedes the outcome of interest.
- *Biologic gradient.* Evidence of a biological gradient (also called a dose-response relationship) between increasing levels of the exposure and increasing frequency of the outcome supports a causal association.
- *Plausibility.* Hill suggested that if the observed association was biologically plausible this would add evidence for causality. He further noted, however, that if the observed association was new then biological plausibility might not be expected.
- *Coherence.* Following from biological plausibility, Hill suggested that at least the observed association should not contradict known facts.
- *Experiment.* An association would be judged more likely to be causal if evidence is based on randomized experiments.
- *Analogy.* Hill's final aspect for consideration was analogy: "In some circumstances it would be fair to judge by analogy." By this, Hill referred to the effect already having been shown for another similar exposure.

A strong association as measured by a high (or low) risk or ratio, an association that is found in a number of studies, and an increased risk of disease with increasing exposure or a decline in risk after cessation of exposure all strengthen the likelihood that an association seen in epidemiologic studies is causal. With deployment to a war-zone, there can be substantial uncertainty in the assessment of possible exposures in theater. To assess whether explanations other than causality (such as random or systematic error) are responsible for an observed association, one must bring together evidence from different studies and take into account the considerations presented by Hill and others (Evans, 1976; Hill, 1965; Susser, 1973, 1977, 1988, 1991; Wegman et al., 1997). For a recent review of those criteria, see the 2004 report of the US Surgeon General (Office of the Surgeon General, 2004).

TYPES OF EPIDEMIOLOGIC STUDIES

The committee focused on epidemiologic studies because epidemiology deals with the determinants, frequency, and distribution of disease in human populations. A focus on populations distinguishes epidemiology from medical disciplines that focus on the individual. Epidemiologic studies examine the relationship between exposures to agents of interest and health outcomes in a population (in this review, deployment is the exposure). Such studies can be used to generate hypotheses for study or to test hypotheses posed by investigators. This section describes the major types of epidemiologic studies considered by the committee.

Cohort Studies

A cohort study is an epidemiologic design that follows a defined group, or cohort, over a period of time. Using data from a cohort study, investigators can test hypotheses about whether exposure to a specific agent is related to the development of disease and can examine multiple health outcomes that might be associated with exposure to a given agent (for example, to deployment). A cohort study starts with people who are free of a disease (or other outcome) and classifies them according to whether they have been exposed to the agent of interest. It compares health outcomes in people who have been exposed to the agent in question with those who have not.

Cohort studies can collect data prospectively (such as in repeated follow-ups) or retrospectively (when exposure and outcome records exist). Generally, investigators select a group of subjects free of the health outcome at baseline (start of study follow-up) and determine who is exposed and not exposed to a given agent (independent variable) during follow-up while also determining the occurrence of the health outcome in both exposed and unexposed cohort members over time. In a retrospective (or historical) cohort study, investigators usually rely on records to determine past exposures for the cohort and another record system to ascertain the rate of disease. In a prospective cohort study both the exposure and disease assessment methods can be designed by the investigator rather than having to rely on existing records as is necessary for a retrospective cohort study. However, a prospective cohort study will not be able to provide sufficient data on chronic disease risk factors until a number of years, if not decades, of follow-up time have accrued. That is, many diseases have a lengthy latency period, for some health outcomes such as some cancers and cardiovascular disease, this can be 20 years or more.

Cohort studies can be used to estimate a risk difference or a relative risk, two statistics that measure association between the exposure groups. The risk difference, or attributable risk, is the rate of disease in exposed persons minus the rate in unexposed persons, representing the excess risk of disease possibly attributable to the exposure. The relative risk is determined by dividing the rate of disease in the exposed group (for example, the deployed group) by the rate of disease in the nonexposed group (for example, the nondeployed group). A relative risk greater than 1.0 suggests an association between exposure and disease onset; the higher the relative risk, the stronger the association. A relative risk of less than 1.0, on the other hand, suggests a protective role for the exposure under study.

Cohort studies have several advantages and disadvantages as described in detail in Chapter 3. Generally, the advantages outweigh the disadvantages if the study is well designed and conducted. The advantages of cohort studies include the following:

- The investigator knows that the predictor (exposure) variable preceded the outcome (disease) variable.
- Exposure can be defined and classified at the beginning of the study, and subjects can be selected based on exposure definition.
- Information on potential confounding variables can be collected in a prospective cohort study so that they may be taken into account in the analysis.
- Rare or unique exposures (such as Gulf War exposures) can be studied, and the investigators can study multiple health outcomes.
- Absolute rates or risk of disease incidence and prevalence can be estimated.[1]

Disadvantages of cohort studies include the following:

- They are often expensive because of the long periods of follow-up required to accrue sufficient number of disease outcomes for analysis.
- Long follow-up periods result in attrition of study subjects and delay in obtaining results.
- They are inefficient for the study of rare diseases or diseases of long latency.
- There is a possibility of the "healthy-worker effect"[2] (Monson, 1990), which might introduce bias and can diminish the true exposure-disease relationship.

Case-Control Studies

In a case-control study, subjects (cases) are selected on the basis of having a disease; controls are selected on the basis of not having the disease. Cases and controls are asked about their exposures to specific agents. Cases and controls can be matched on characteristics such as age, sex, and socioeconomic status as a method of increasing efficiency and controlling for

---

[1]Incidence is the occurrence of new cases of an illness or disease in a given population during a specified period. Incidence rate uses person-time in the denominator and cumulative incidence uses number of people at risk in the denominator. Prevalence is the number of cases of an illness or disease existing in a given population at a specific time.

[2]The healthy-worker effect may arise when an employed population is examined and mortality/morbidity rates are compared to those in the general population. The concern is that an employed population may be healthier by virtue of remaining employed and would experience lower mortality/morbidity than the general population, which consists of a mix of healthy and unhealthy people. In the context of this report the concern is the healthy-warrior effect where personnel who were deployed to the Persian Gulf region may have been in better health than military personnel who were not deployed.

confounders. The odds of exposure to the agent among the cases is then compared with the odds of exposure among controls. The comparison generates an OR, which is a statistic that depicts the odds of having a disease among those exposed to the agent of concern relative to the odds of having the disease among an unexposed comparison group. An OR of greater than 1 indicates that there is a potential association between exposure to the agent and the disease; the further from 1.0 the OR ratio, the stronger the association. The OR is a measure of association that is interpreted in the same way as a relative risk or a risk ratio.

Case-control studies are especially useful and efficient for studying the etiology of rare diseases, having the advantages of ease, speed, and relatively low cost. They are also valuable for probing multiple exposures or risk factors. However, case-control studies are vulnerable to several types of bias, such as recall bias, which can enhance (or dilute) apparent associations between disease and exposure. Other problems include identifying representative groups of cases, choosing suitable controls, and collecting comparable information about exposures on both cases and controls. Those problems might lead to unidentified confounding variables that differentially influence the selection of cases or control subjects or the detection of exposure. Case-control studies are often the first approach to testing a hypothesis, especially one related to a rare outcome.

A nested case-control study draws cases and controls from a previously defined cohort. Thus, it is said to be "nested" inside a cohort study. Baseline data are collected at the time that the cohort is identified, and this ensures more uniform data collection on both cases and controls. Within the cohort, individuals identified with disease serve as cases, and a sample of those who are disease-free serve as controls. Using baseline data, exposure in cases and controls is compared, as in a regular case-control study. Using particular statistical approaches, changes in exposures over time can also be incorporated in the analysis. Nested case-control studies are efficient in terms of time and cost in reconstructing exposure histories on cases and on only a sample of controls rather than the entire cohort. Additionally, because the cases and controls come from the same previously established cohort, concerns about unmeasured confounders and selection bias are decreased.

Cross-Sectional Studies

The main differentiating feature of a cross-sectional study is that exposure and disease information is collected at the same point (period) of time. The selection of people for the study—unlike selection for cohort and case-control studies—is independent of both the exposure to the agent under study and disease characteristics. In a cross-sectional study, effect size is measured as prevalence ratio, or prevalence OR. In such studies disease or symptom prevalence between groups with and without exposure to the specific agent are compared. Several health studies of Gulf War veterans are cross-sectional studies that compare a sample of veterans who were deployed to the Gulf War with a sample of veterans who served during the same period but were not deployed to the Gulf War.

Cross-sectional studies are easier and less expensive to perform than cohort studies and can identify the prevalence of diseases and exposures in a defined population. They are useful for generating hypotheses, but they are much less useful for determining cause and effect relationships, because disease and exposure data are collected simultaneously (Monson, 1990); for this reason it may be difficult to determine the temporal sequence of exposures and symptoms or disease.

Standardized Mortality Studies

For comparison purposes, some cohort studies use mortality or morbidity rates in the general population rather than from within the same cohort since in some cases it might be difficult to identify a suitable group of unexposed people. One statistic that is used in such a comparison is the standardized mortality ratio (SMR), which is the ratio of the observed number of deaths in a cohort (from a specific cause, such as traumatic brain injury [TBI], for example) to the number of deaths from TBI expected in a carefully chosen reference population. An SMR greater than 1.0 generally suggests an increased risk of death in the exposed group. The standardization refers to the methodology used to ensure that any differences in observed and expected numbers of death are not due to differences in the age (or sex) distribution of the study cohort and the comparison cohort. Such measures can also be used to examine morbidity, such as cancer.

The major problem in comparing rates in the general population with rates in military cohorts is the so-called healthy-warrior effect described earlier. That effect arises when a military population experiences a lower mortality or morbidity rate than the general population. Inasmuch as military personnel must meet physical-health criteria when they enter the military and while they are on active duty, the group's health status is usually better than that of the general population of the same age and sex. Since military personnel are at overall lower risk of adverse health outcomes compared to the general population, any excess risk associated with an exposure they experience must be large enough to overcome their inherent advantage in order to be detectable by such methods as SMR.

INCLUSION CRITERIA

The Update committee included studies that would answer the question, "What does the literature tell us about the health status of Gulf War veterans?" To that end, the committee searched the literature and included descriptive epidemiologic studies of health outcomes in military personnel that served in the Gulf War theater. The studies were not restricted to US personnel only. The Volume 4 committee developed inclusion criteria for studies; the Update committee reviewed those criteria and found them to be appropriate for this update. Primary studies provide the basis for the committee's findings. For a study to be included in the committee's review as a primary study it had to meet specified criteria. A study needed to demonstrate rigorous methods (for example, was published in a peer-reviewed journal, included details of methods, had a control or reference group, and included adjustments for confounders when needed), include information regarding a persistent health outcome, have a medical evaluation conducted by a health professional, and use appropriate laboratory testing. Those types of studies constituted the committee's primary literature. The committee did not evaluate studies of acute trauma, rehabilitation, medical treatment, or transient illness, nor did the committee consider health outcomes seen in veterans of conflicts other than the Gulf War unless those veterans formed an appropriate control group (for example, veterans who had served in Bosnia). Although the responsible committee member initially presented his or her determination of whether a study met the criteria, the committee discussed the study's methods and results using the inclusion criteria at some length before agreeing as to whether the study should be classified as primary.

Studies reviewed by the committee that did not necessarily meet all the criteria of a primary study were considered secondary studies. Secondary studies are typically not as methodologically rigorous as primary studies and might present subclinical findings, that is, studies of altered functioning consistent with later development of a diagnosis but without clear predictive value.

Another step that the committee took in organizing its literature was to determine how all the study cohorts were related to one another. Numerous Gulf War cohorts have been assembled from several different countries, and it is from those original cohorts that many derivative studies have been conducted and published. The committee organized the literature into the major cohorts and derivative studies because they did not want to interpret the findings of the same cohorts as though they were results from unique groups (Chapter 3). The report excludes studies of participants in Gulf War registries established by the Department of Veterans Affairs (VA) or the Department of Defense (DoD), such as the DoD's Comprehensive Clinical Evaluation Program. Registry participants can not be considered representative of all Gulf War veterans in that they are self-selected subjects, many of whom have joined the registries because they believe that they have symptoms of a new medical syndrome; they were not randomly selected from all Gulf War military personnel, and there is no nondeployed control group.

Finally, in assessing the descriptive studies, the committee was especially attentive to potential sources of bias, confounding, chance, and multiple comparisons, as discussed in the following sections.

Methodologic Rigor

A study had to be published in a peer-reviewed journal or other rigorously peer-reviewed publication, such as a government report, dissertation, or monograph; include sufficient methodologic details to allow the committee to judge whether it met inclusion criteria; include an unexposed control or reference group; and use reasonable methods to control for confounders.

Exposure Assessment

In *Volume 4*, Chapter 3 describes the possible exposures Gulf War military personnel might have experienced. It also details the exposure modeling and biological monitoring that was conducted by the DoD and others to estimate troop exposures to some chemical agents such as depleted uranium, sarin and cyclosarin, and oil-well fire smoke. As noted in that chapter, there is poor agreement between subjective and objective measurements of exposures to depleted uranium and oil-well fire smoke. Some studies also show evidence of reporting bias regarding vaccinations and ingestion of pyridostigmine bromide tablets. The modeling of the possible exposures to sarin and cyclosarin from the demolition of the Khamisiyah complex has also been criticized. The committee did consider studies that compared health outcomes seen in deployed veterans who may or may not have been exposed to nerve agents as a result of the Khamisiyah detonation and to oil-well fire smoke; some of these studies also included nondeployed control groups.

Health Outcome Assessment

For medical conditions that have no morphological features, the use of validated symptom criteria, such as those of the Rome Foundation for irritable bowel syndrome, are preferred over reports of medical symptoms or group of symptoms. For a study to be considered primary, the committee preferred studies that had an independent assessment of an outcome rather than self-reports of an outcome or reports by family members. It was preferable to have the health effect diagnosed or confirmed by a clinical evaluation, imaging, hospital record, or other medical record. For psychiatric outcomes, standardized interviews were preferred, such as the Structured Clinical Interview for the DSM-IV-TR (*Diagnostic and Statistical Manual of Mental Disorders-IV-TR*), the Diagnostic Interview Schedule, and the Composite International Diagnostic Interview. Similarly, for neurocognitive outcomes, standardized and validated tests were preferred. Additionally, the outcome had to be diagnosed after deployment. However, as self-reports of health outcomes and exposures account for the bulk of the Gulf War and health literature, the committee decided that it would not exclude such studies but rather considered them to be secondary. The committee recognized the potential for misclassification of a health outcome due to inaccurate recall in such studies.

CONSIDERATIONS IN ASSESSING THE STRENGTH OF EVIDENCE

The committee's process for reaching conclusions about deployment during the Gulf War and its potential for adverse health outcomes was collective and interactive. Once a study was included in the review because it met the committee's criteria, there were several considerations in assessing causality, including strength of the association, presence of a dose-response relationship, presence of a temporal relationship, consistency of the association, and biologic plausibility. The committee as a group reviewed the primary and secondary studies identified by the committee member responsible for each health outcome. The strengths and limitations of each study and its categorization as primary and secondary were discussed in plenary session and all committee members agreed on its contribution to the evidence base for each category of association for each health outcome. Because many of the studies were cited for more than one health outcome, committee members evaluated each study with equal vigor for every health outcome. The evidence tables were refined to include study limitations for the primary studies and to present the pertinent results; secondary studies were not included in the evidence tables. It should be noted that some of the larger cohort studies used a variety of methods and instruments to assess the health status of Gulf War veterans and it is for this reason that the committee discussed at some length the diagnostic approaches and use of self-reports for each paper. The assignment of a category of association was reached by committee consensus based on the weight of the evidence, including the studies cited in *Volume 4*, as well as any new studies. Those aspects of the committee's review required thoughtful consideration of all the studies as well as expert judgment and could not be accomplished by adherence to a narrowly prescribed formula of what data would be required for each category of association or for a particular health outcome.

Categories of Association

The committee attempted to express its judgment of the available data clearly and precisely in the Summary and Conclusion section for each health outcome. It agreed to use the categories of association that have been established and used by previous Committees on Gulf War and Health and other Institute of Medicine committees that have evaluated vaccine safety, effects of herbicides used in Vietnam, and indoor pollutants related to asthma (IOM, 2000, 2003,

2005, 2006, 2007). Those categories of association have gained wide acceptance for more than a decade by Congress, government agencies (particularly the VA), researchers, and veterans groups.

The five categories below describe different levels of association and present a common message: the validity of an association is likely to vary to the extent to which common sources of spurious associations could be ruled out as the reason for the observed association. Accordingly, the criteria for each category express a degree of confidence based on the extent to which sources of error were reduced. The committee discussed the evidence and reached consensus on the categorization of the evidence for each health outcome in Chapter 4.

Sufficient Evidence of a Causal Relationship

Evidence is sufficient to conclude that a causal relationship exists between being deployed to the Gulf War and a health outcome. The evidence fulfills the criteria for sufficient evidence of a causal association in which chance, bias, and confounding can be ruled out with reasonable confidence. The association is supported by several of the other considerations used to assess causality: strength of association, dose-response relationship, consistency of association, temporal relationship, specificity of association, and biologic plausibility.

Sufficient Evidence of an Association

Evidence suggests an association, in that a positive association has been observed between deployment to the Gulf War and a health outcome in humans; however, there is some doubt as to the influence of chance, bias, and confounding.

Limited/Suggestive Evidence of an Association

Some evidence of an association between deployment to the Gulf War and a health outcome in humans exists, but this is limited by the presence of substantial doubt regarding chance, bias, and confounding.

Inadequate/Insufficient Evidence to Determine Whether an Association Exists

The available studies are of insufficient quality, validity, consistency, or statistical power to permit a conclusion regarding the presence or absence of an association between deployment to the Gulf War and a health outcome in humans.

Limited/Suggestive Evidence of No Association

There are several adequate studies, covering the full range of levels of exposure that humans are known to encounter, that are consistent in not showing an association between deployment to the Gulf War and a health outcome. A conclusion of no association is inevitably limited to the conditions, levels of exposure, and length of observation covered by the available studies. In addition, the possibility of a very small increase in risk at the levels of exposure studied can never be excluded.

ADDITIONAL CONSIDERATIONS

The Bradford Hill aspects to consider when evaluating evidence to assess whether an association is causal have important exceptions and qualifications; therefore, the aspects, however useful, are neither criteria nor hard and fast rules for assessing causality (Rothman and Greenland, 2005). The validity of data and individual studies that may contribute evidence as to whether an association is causal must also be considered. Although strict rules are not available, design flaws that threaten the validity of a study often fall into one of three major categories: selection bias, confounding, and misclassification or information bias. Of particular relevance here is the healthy warrior effect described earlier. Failure to account for such differences can lead to biased estimates of an effect. These factors were all considered by the committee in evaluating the quality of data and individual studies, in determining the primary and secondary literature that would be used to draw conclusions, and in evaluating how those studies contribute to the body of evidence concerning health effects seen in Gulf War veterans.

Bias

Bias refers to systematic, or nonrandom, error. Bias causes an observed value to deviate from the true value, and can weaken an association, strengthen an association or generate a spurious association. Because all studies are susceptible to bias, a primary goal of the research design is to minimize bias or to adjust the observed value of an association by correcting for bias if the sources are known. There are different types of bias, such as selection bias. Selection bias refers to a systematic error in the way subjects are identified, recruited, included, excluded, or the way they participate in the study that leads to a distortion of the true association.

Information bias results from the manner in which data are collected and can result in measurement errors, imprecise measurement, and misdiagnosis. Those types of errors might be uniform in an entire study population or might affect some parts of the population more than others. Information bias might result from misclassification of study subjects with respect to the outcome variable or from misclassification of exposure. Other common sources of information bias are the inability of study subjects to recall the circumstances of their exposure accurately (recall bias) and the likelihood that one group more frequently reports what it remembers than another group (reporting bias). Information bias is especially harmful in interpreting study results when it affects one comparison group more than another.

Confounding

Confounding occurs when a variable or characteristic otherwise known to be predictive of an outcome and associated with the exposure (and not on the causal pathway under consideration) can account for part or all of an apparent association. A confounding variable is an uncontrolled variable that influences the outcome of a study to an unknown extent, and makes precise evaluation of its effects impossible. Carefully applied statistical adjustments can often control for or reduce the influence of a confounder.

Sampling Error

Sampling error (sometimes referred to as chance or random error) is a type of error that can lead to an apparent association between an exposure to an agent and a health effect when no association is present or to a finding of no association when in fact one exists. An apparent effect of deployment on a health outcome might be the result of random variation due to sampling of the study population rather than the result of exposure to the agent. Standard methods that use confidence intervals, for example, allow one to assess the role of chance variation due to sampling.

Multiple Comparisons

When an investigator initiates a large number of analyses simultaneously on the same dataset, multiple comparisons pose a problem. When looking at so many different comparisons, the investigator is bound to find something of note by chance alone. For example, in many Gulf War veteran studies, the investigators are comparing multiple outcomes and multiple exposures. There are, however, ways to correct for multiple comparisons in studies. One way is to use a Bonferroni correction, a statistical adjustment for multiple comparisons. It effectively raises the standard of proof needed when an investigator looks at a wide array of hypotheses simultaneously.

LIMITATIONS OF GULF WAR VETERAN STUDIES

The epidemiologic and clinical studies to date have provided valuable information regarding the health of Gulf War veterans; however, many of the studies have limitations that hinder accurate assessment of the veterans' health status. The limitations include the possibility that study samples do not represent the entire Gulf War population, the relatively young age of the exposed population, low rates of participation in studies, reinforcement of self-reporting of symptoms and exposures, insensitivity of instruments for detecting abnormalities in deployed veterans, and a period of investigation that is too brief to detect health outcomes that have long latency, such as cancer. In addition, many of the US studies are cross-sectional and this limits the opportunity to learn about symptom duration and chronicity, latency of onset, and prognosis. Finally, the problem of multiple comparisons that is common in many of the Gulf War studies results in confusion over whether the effect is real or occurring by chance. Those limitations make it difficult to interpret the results of the findings, particularly when several well-conducted studies produce inconsistent results.

REFERENCES

Evans, A. S. 1976. Causation and disease: The Henle-Koch postulates revisited. *Yale Journal of Biology and Medicine* 49(2):175-195.

Hill, A. B. 1965. The environment and disease: Association or causation? *Proceedings of the Royal Society of Medicine* 58:295-300.

IOM (Institute of Medicine). 2000. *Gulf War and Health, Volume 1: Depleted Uranium, Sarin, Pyridostigmine Bromide, Vaccines.* Washington, DC: National Academy Press.

IOM. 2003. *Gulf War and Health, Volume 2: Insecticides and Solvents.* Washington, DC: The National Academies Press.

IOM. 2005. *Gulf War and Health, Volume 3: Fuels, Combustion Products, and Propellants.* Washington, DC: The National Academies Press.

IOM. 2006. *Gulf War and Health, Volume 4: Health Effects of Serving in the Gulf War.* Washington, DC: The National Academies Press.

IOM. 2007. *Gulf War and Health, Volume 5: Infectious Diseases.* Washington, DC: The National Academies Press.

Monson, R. 1990. *Occupational Epidemiology.* 2nd ed. Boca Ration, FL: CRC Press.

Office of the Surgeon General. 2004. *The Health Consequences of Smoking: A Report of the Surgeon General.* http://www.surgeongeneral.gov/library/smokingconsequences (accessed July 31, 2008).

Rothman, K. J., and S. Greenland. 2005. Causality and causal inference in epidemiology. *American Journal of Public Health* 95:S144-S150.

Susser, M. 1973. *Casual Thinking in the Health Sciences: Concepts and Strategies of Epidemiology.* New York: Oxford University Press.

Susser, M. 1977. Judgment and causal inference: Criteria in epidemiologic studies. *American Journal of Epidemiology* 105(1):1-15.

Susser, M. 1988. Falsification, verification, and causal inference in epidemiology: Reconsideration in the light of Sir Karl Popper's philosophy. In *Causal Inference*, edited by K. J. Rothman. Chestnut Hill, MA: Epidemiology Resources. Pp. 33-58.

Susser, M. 1991. What is a cause and how do we know one? A grammar for pragmatic epidemiology. *American Journal of Epidemiology* 133(7):635-648.

Wegman, D. H., N. F. Woods, and J. C. Bailar. 1997. Invited commentary: How would we know a Gulf War syndrome if we saw one? *American Journal of Epidemiology* 146(9):704-711.

3

MAJOR COHORT STUDIES

This chapter provides an overview of the major cohort studies of Gulf War veterans, and describes in detail the populations studied, the methods used to select those populations, and the approaches used to identify the health status of the veterans—including questionnaires, examinations, and laboratory tests. The findings from the studies described in this chapter are reviewed and evaluated in Chapter 4.

The major cohort studies are important for understanding the health of Gulf War veterans. Some of these cohorts were brought together in the first few years after the Gulf War; others were assembled more recently. The largest studies of Gulf War veterans have been conducted in countries that were members of the Gulf War coalition, including the United States, the United Kingdom (UK), Denmark, and Australia. Most of the studies compare sizable groups of deployed veterans with groups of nondeployed veterans or with veterans who were deployed to locations other than the Persian Gulf (for example, Bosnia or Germany).

Most major cohorts, once established, led to numerous studies that examined more detailed questions about Gulf War veterans' health; the committee refers to those studies as derivatives. A derivative study is included and summarized under the original cohort from which the study population was drawn. This organization helped the committee identify populations that have been studied and understand which studies were independent of one another; establishing which studies rely on the same population sample is important because it helped the committee avoid double counting when weighing the evidence.

GENERAL LIMITATIONS OF GULF WAR COHORT STUDIES AND DERIVATIVE STUDIES

The cohort studies of Gulf War veterans and their derivative studies have contributed greatly to our understanding of veterans' health, but they are beset by limitations that are commonly encountered in epidemiologic studies (see Chapter 2), including lack of representativeness, selection bias, lack of control for potential confounding factors, self-reports of exposures, lack of a diagnosis by a health professional for some health effects, and outcome misclassification.

The foremost limitation is lack of representativeness, which limits one's ability to generalize results to the entire population of interest; for example, about half the cohorts focus on groups of veterans that are selected for study according to where they served in the military, that is, a military-unit-based study. Military-unit studies are not representative of all Gulf War veterans with respect to their duties and location during deployment, their military status during the war (active duty, reserves, or National Guard), their military status after the war (active duty, reserves, or discharged), their branch of service (Army, Navy, Air Force, or Marines), or ease of ascertainment (IOM, 1999). The most representative studies are population-based: the cohorts are selected on the basis of where their members reside. In population-based studies of Gulf War veterans, the cohort might be the entire deployed population, as in studies of Canadian and Australian veterans, or a random selection from the population of interest, as in several studies of US and UK veterans. The committee, in evaluating major cohort studies, gave greater weight to Gulf War studies that were population based.

A study's representativeness, even if it is population based, can be compromised by low participation rates. Low participation rates can introduce selection bias, such as when Gulf War veterans who are symptomatic choose to participate more frequently than those who are not symptomatic. Nondeployed veterans, who might be healthier, may be less inclined to participate. In some studies, researchers not only try to assess the potential for selection bias by comparing participants with nonparticipants from both deployed and nondeployed populations, but also implement strategies to reduce the impact of selection bias, such as by oversampling nondeployed populations as in the study by Eisen and colleagues (2005).

Selection bias might also occur through the so-called healthy warrior effect. That form of bias has the potential to occur in most of the major cohorts that compare deployed veterans with nondeployed personnel. The healthy warrior effect is a form of selection bias insofar as chronically ill or less fit members of the armed forces might be less likely to have been deployed than more fit members. Some of the best studies attempt to measure the potential for selection bias and adjust for it in the analysis.

Many cohort studies rely on self-reports of symptoms and medical conditions. This may introduce reporting bias, which occurs when the study population (in this case the deployed veterans) over- or underreports symptoms or medical conditions relative to a comparison group (in this case the nondeployed veterans). This over- or underreporting may be related to beliefs about the effect of deployment on health, especially among deployed veterans who, if they are experiencing health problems, may have already formed an opinion on the cause of their malady. Comparison groups, in contrast, may have little reason to conjecture possible links between past exposures and any current health conditions they may be experiencing. In most cases, reporting bias leads to an overestimation of the prevalence of symptoms or diagnoses in the deployed population.

Self-reports of symptoms or medical conditions might sometimes introduce another type of bias known as outcome misclassification, in which there are errors in how symptoms or medical conditions are classified into outcomes and analyzed. One Gulf War study sought to document outcome misclassification by comparing veterans' symptom reporting on questionnaires with clinical examination about 3 months later (McCauley et al., 1999a). The study found that the extent of misclassification depended on the type of symptom being reported; agreement between questionnaire and clinical examination ranged from 4% to 79%. The overall problem led the investigators to caution that questionnaire data, in the absence of clinical evaluation or adjustment, might lead to outcome misclassification (McCauley et al., 1999b). Another study also found poor reliability and validity of self-reported medical diagnoses when compared with medical records (Gray et al., 1999). In contrast, a study by the Department of Veterans Affairs (VA) (Kang et al., 2000), which verified a random subset of self-reported conditions (n = 4200) against medical records, found a strong correlation between the two (above

93%). Those data, however, were available only for the 45.2% who signed consent forms that allowed researchers to verify records.

The concerns relating to symptom self-reporting are best addressed through medical evaluations in which the veterans' reports of symptoms can be further explored with a health professional. This was done by VA researchers (for example, Eisen et al., 2005) and by several other investigators with the resources to conduct medical evaluations (for example, Sim et al., 2003). The committee acknowledges that many medical conditions, such as chronic fatigue syndrome (CFS) and fibromyalgia, are diagnosed solely on the basis of symptom reports, but where possible these symptoms should be evaluated by a medical professional.

Another limitation of most major cohort studies is self-reporting of exposures, often years after the exposure had occurred. Self-reporting of exposures, as with self-reporting of symptoms, introduces the possibility of recall bias, the tendency for participants who are symptomatic to overestimate (or underestimate) their exposures compared with those who are not symptomatic. Indeed, a major study from the United Kingdom found that Gulf War veterans with more symptoms were likely to report more exposures than those not deployed to the gulf (Unwin et al., 1999). Exposures often cannot be validated by objective means, may have occurred years earlier, and might have been perceived rather than actual (Fricker et al., 2000). For example, the high sensitivity of chemical-warfare monitors used in the Persian Gulf War to warn of impending attacks led to many false alarms, which might have been perceived by veterans as actual exposures. Enhanced recordkeeping and monitoring of environmental exposures during and after the Gulf War would have averted this exposure reporting problem. Indeed, many expert panels have recommended improved recordkeeping and environmental monitoring in future deployments (for example, IOM, 1999; NRC, 2000a,b,c).

Other limitations of the body of evidence are that studies might be too narrow in their assessment of health status, the measurement instruments might have been too insensitive to detect health problems that affect deployed veterans, and the period of investigation has been too brief to detect health outcomes that have a long latency or require many years to progress to the point where disability, hospitalization, or death occurs. Virtually all US studies are cross-sectional, and this limits the opportunity to learn about symptom duration and chronicity, latency of onset (especially for health conditions with a long latency, such as cancer), and prognosis.

ORGANIZATION OF THIS CHAPTER

This chapter describes the major cohort studies and their derivative studies used by the Update committee to provide the evidence for the conclusions presented in Chapter 4. For each separately assembled cohort, the reference study is described first, followed by a summary of any derivative studies cited in Chapter 4 or Appendix A. The majority of the cohort studies are population-based, although some military-unit-based studies are described later in the chapter. Table 3-1 lists the reference and derivative studies of each cohort cited in this chapter and Chapter 4.

The committee did not identify any new major cohort studies for this report. Furthermore, not all derivative studies for a particular cohort study are included in this chapter or in Chapter 4. In many cases, the derivative studies identified by the committee from the literature searches were highly specialized; for example, they reported on family issues, pathologic changes in a subgroup of veterans, or treatment outcomes. Such studies are not included in this chapter or in Chapter 4.

TABLE 3-1 Reference and Derivative Studies for the Major Gulf War Cohorts

Cohort/Reference Study	Derivatives	Purpose/Outcome
VA National Health Survey of Gulf War Veterans and Their Families/Kang et al., 2000		
Volume 4	Davis et al., 2004	Presence of distal symmetric polyneuropathy
	Eisen et al., 2005	Numerous health outcomes and general health assessment
	Kang et al., 2001	Self-reported birth defects
	Kang et al., 2002	Association of symptom clusters with self-reported exposures
	Kang et al., 2003	Prevalence of PTSD and chronic fatigue syndrome
	Kang et al., 2005	Role of sexual assault and harassment on the risk of PTSD
	Karlinsky et al., 2004	Pulmonary function and self-reported respiratory symptoms
New	Kang et al., 2009	Self-reported general health status
	Page et al., 2005a,b	Possible exposure at Khamisiyah and self-reported morbidity
	Blanchard et al., 2005	Prevalence of chronic multisymptom illness
	Toomey et al., 2007	Prevalence of psychiatric disorders, symptom self-report, and quality of life status
	Toomey et al., 2009	Neuropsychological functioning
Iowa Veterans/Iowa Persian Gulf Study Group, 1997		
Volume 4	Barrett et al., 2002	Association between PTSD and self-reported physical health status
	Black et al., 1999	Impact of multiple chemical sensitivity on quality of life and utilization of health services
	Black et al., 2000	Risk factors and prevalence of multiple chemical sensitivity
	Black et al., 2004a	Prevalence of psychiatric disorders
	Black et al., 2004b	Prevalence and risk factors for anxiety disorders
	Doebbling et al., 2000	Factor analysis of self-reported symptoms (Definition of Persian Gulf War Syndrome)
	Lange et al., 2002	Exposure to Kuwait oil fires and risk of asthma and bronchitis
New	Ang et al., 2006	Identification of predictors of chronic widespread pain
	Black et al., 2006	Prevalence of borderline personality disorder
	Forman-Hoffman et al., 2007	Prevalence of self-reports of symptoms of chronic widespread pain
UK Veterans: University of London/Unwin et al., 1999		
Volume 4	Hotopf et al., 2003a,b	Neurologic assessments
	Macfarlane et al., 2000	Self-reported exposure and mortality
	Macfarlane et al., 2003	Incidence of cancer
	Reid et al., 2001	Self-reported exposure and multiple chemical sensitivity and chronic fatigue syndrome

Cohort/Reference Study	Derivatives	Purpose/Outcome
	Rose et al., 2004	Neuromuscular symptoms evaluated through objective tests
	Sharief et al., 2002	Neuromuscular symptoms evaluated by objective tests
	Nisenbaum et al., 2004	Factor analysis of self-reported symptoms
	Macfarlane et al., 2005	Self-reported exposure and mortality
New	Stimpson et al., 2006	Self-report of chronic widespread pain
	Ismail et al., 2008	Prevalence of chronic fatigue and related disorders through assessment
UK Veterans: University of Manchester/Cherry et al., 2001a,b		
Volume 4	None	
New	None	
UK Veterans: London School of Hygiene and Tropical Medicine/Maconochie et al., 2003		
Volume 4	Doyle et al., 2004	Prevalence of miscarriage, stillbirth, and congenital malformations
	Maconochie et al., 2004	Self-report of fertility problems
	Simmons et al., 2004	Self-report of medical symptoms or disease
New	None	
Danish Peacekeepers/Ishoy et al., 1999b		
Volume 4	Proctor et al., 2003	Prevalence of neuropsychologic symptoms and neurobehavioral performance
	Ishoy et al., 1999a	Prevalence of gastrointestinal symptoms and diseases, skin disease, and respiratory symptoms and function
	Ishoy et al., 2001a,b	Self-report of sexual dysfunction and birth defects
New	None	
Australian Veterans/Sim et al., 2003		
Volume 4	Kelsall et al., 2004a	Association between self-reported exposures with numerous symptoms and medical conditions
	Ikin et al., 2004	Prevalence of psychiatric disorders
	McKenzie et al., 2004	Psychological health and functioning
	Kelsall et al., 2004b	Self-reported exposure and respiratory health status
	Kelsall et al., 2005	Self-report of exposures and neurological symptoms
	Forbes et al., 2004	Factor analysis of self-reported symptoms
New	Kelsall et al., 2006	Self-reported exposure and prevalence of chronic fatigue syndrome
	Kelsall et al., 2007	Self-reported birth defects and other pregnancy outcomes
Oregon and Washington Veterans/McCauley et al., 1999a		
Volume 4	Bourdette et al., 2001	Prevalence of unexplained illness

Cohort/Reference Study	Derivatives	Purpose/Outcome
	Spencer et al., 2001	Self-reported exposure and unexplained illness
New	None	
Canadian Veterans/Goss Gilroy, 1998		
Volume 4	Statistics Canada, 2005	Mortality rate and cancer incidence
New	None	
Kansas Veterans Study/Steele et al., 2000		
Volume 4	None	
New	None	
Fort Devens and New Orleans Cohorts/Proctor et al., 1998		
Volume 4	White et al., 2001	Self-reported exposure and neuropsychological functioning
	Proctor et al., 2001a	Assessment of health-related quality of life
	Proctor et al., 2001b	Overlap between symptoms of chronic fatigue and chemical sensitivity, and the case definition for chronic multisymptom illness
New	Proctor et al., 2006	Possible exposure at Khamisiyah and neuropsychological functioning
Seabee Veterans/Haley et al., 1997b		
Volume 4	Haley and Kurt, 1997; Haley et al., 1997a	Self-reported exposure to neurotoxicants and nervous system-based syndromes
	Haley et al., 1999	Genetic susceptibility and risk of neurologic damage
New	Haley et al., 2009	
Gray et al., 1999		
Volume 4	Gray et al., 2002	Self-report of symptoms and general health status
	Knoke et al., 2000	Self-report of symptoms
New	Phillips et al., 2009	Exposure to vaccines and chronic multisymptom illness
Pennsylvania Air National Guard Veterans/Fukuda et al., 1998		
Volume 4	Nisenbaum et al., 2000	Self-reported exposures and chronic multisymptom illness
	Nisenbaum et al., 2004	Factor analysis of self-reported symptoms
New	None	
Hawaii and Pennsylvania Active-Duty and Reserve/Stretch et al., 1995		
Volume 4	Stretch et al., 1996a	Prevalence of psychiatric disorders
	Stretch et al., 1996b	Prevalence of PTSD

Cohort/Reference Study	Derivatives	Purpose/Outcome
New	None	
New Orleans Reservists/Sutker et al., 1995		
Volume 4	Brailey et al., 1998	Prevalence of psychiatric disorders
	Sutker et al., 1995	Prevalence of psychologic disorders
New	None	

Department of Veterans Affairs Study

Volume 4 described seven derivative studies of the National Health Survey of Gulf War Veterans and Their Families, conducted by the VA (Kang et al., 2000). The Update committee identified six additional derivative studies of this cohort that examine specific health outcomes or conducted a follow-up survey and analysis.

Reference Study

A major population-based study of US veterans was mandated by PL 103-446, with the purpose of estimating the prevalence of symptoms and other health outcomes (including reproductive outcomes in spouses and birth defects in children) in Gulf War deployed versus nondeployed veterans. This three-phase retrospective study, the National Health Survey of Gulf War Veterans and Their Families, was designed to be representative of the nearly 700,000 US veterans sent to the Persian Gulf and 800,680 veterans who were not deployed but who were in the military between September 1990 and May 1991.

In the first phase, begun in 1995, the VA mailed questionnaires to a stratified random sample of 15,000 Gulf War and 15,000 veterans not deployed to the Gulf War identified by the Defense Manpower Data Center (DMDC) (Kang et al., 2000). Women and those serving in the National Guard and reserves were oversampled, resulting in a study population that was approximately 20% women, 25% National Guard, and 33% reservists. The controls were stratified by gender, unit, and branch of service to mirror the population of deployed veterans. The self-administered structured health questionnaire contained a 48-symptom inventory (somatic and psychological symptoms) and questions about chronic medical conditions, functional limitations, use of medical services, and environmental exposures (for example, immunizations, use of the prophylactic antinerve agent pyridostigmine bromide [PB], smoke from oil-well fires, pesticides, and insecticides).

Phase II used telephone interview software in an attempt to capture those who did not respond to the mailed questionnaire. In addition, medical records were obtained for a random sample of 4200 respondents (either phase I or II) to validate self-reports of clinic visits or hospitalizations within the last year. Of the 2233 veterans with at least one clinic visit, 43.2% provided medical record release consent; of the 310 with at least one hospitalization, 45.2% provided medical record release consent. A total of 11,441 (75%) deployed and 9476 (64%) nondeployed veterans participated in the study; 15,817 veterans responded to phase I, and 5100 responded to the telephone portion of phase II (Kang and Bullman, 2001; Kang et al., 2000). Gulf War veterans reported significantly higher rates of functional impairment (27.8% vs 14.2%), limitations of employment (17.2% vs 11.6%), and health-care use as assessed by clinic visits (50.8% vs 40.5%) or hospitalizations (7.8% vs 6.4%) compared with nondeployed veterans. In a randomly selected subset of veterans, medical record reviews verified more than 90% of self-reported reasons for clinic visits or hospitalizations (Kang et al., 2000).

Kang et al. (2000) did not assess exposure–symptom relationships but rather noted the percentage of veterans who reported each of 23 environmental exposures and nine vaccine or prophylactic exposures (such as to PB). The five most common environmental exposures reported by more than 60% of survey participants were to the following: diesel, kerosene, or other petrochemical fumes; local food other than that provided by the armed forces; chemical protective gear; smoke from oil-well fires; and burning trash or feces.

Derivative Studies

In *Volume 4*, seven derivative studies were identified: Davis et al. (2004), Eisen et al. (2005), Kang et al. (2001, 2002, 2003, 2005), and Karlinsky et al. (2004).

Davis et al. (2004) studied the presence of distal symmetric polyneuropathy (DSP) determined by medical history, physical examination by a neurologist, blood tests, and standardized electrophysiologic assessment of motor and sensory nerves in the cohort of 1061 deployed veterans and 1128 nondeployed veterans from the National Health Survey of Gulf War Veterans and Their Families. Spouses of deployed (n = 484) and nondeployed (n = 533) veterans were studied to evaluate whether an infectious agent or environmental contaminant brought back from the gulf could be responsible for any adverse health outcomes. Evaluations of 244 Khamisiyah-exposed (data provided by the DoD) versus 817 nonexposed deployed veterans for the presence of DSP were conducted. See Chapter 4 for more details.

In the third phase of the National Health Survey of Gulf War Veterans and Their Families, conducted 10 years after the Gulf War, Eisen and colleagues (2005) performed a cross-sectional study on numerous health outcomes of veterans 10 years after the Gulf War. The study population consisted of a stratified random sample of the 11,441 deployed and 9476 nondeployed veterans who participated in the above described phase I or II. This phase included a comprehensive medical examination and laboratory testing. Of the 1996 eligible deployed veterans, 1061 (53.1%) were examined; 680 (34.1%) declined and 255 (12.8%) were not located. Of the 2883 eligible nondeployed veterans, 1128 (39.1%) were examined; 1316 (45.7%) declined and 439 (15.2%) were not located. Despite three waves of recruitment into the study, the participation rate was low—60.9% of Gulf War deployed veterans and 46.2% of the nondeployed.

Study participants were assigned a medical center closest to their residence where physicians and nurses performed medical, neurologic, psychiatric, and gynecologic histories and examinations; laboratory, nerve conduction, pulmonary function, and neuropsychological tests were also performed. Twelve primary health outcome measures and physical functioning on SF-36 were examined.[1] Outcome measures were chosen by the authors to cover the most common symptoms reported by veterans, such as musculoskeletal pain, fatigue, rashes, and neuropathy (Kang et al., 2000). Gulf War veterans reported worse physical health on the SF-36 (49.3 vs 50.8) but the magnitude of the difference, although statistically significant, was not clinically meaningful. Four of 12 conditions were more prevalent among Gulf War veterans: fibromyalgia (2.0% vs 1.2%), CFS (1.6% vs 0.1%), dermatologic conditions (34.6% vs 26.8 %), and dyspepsia (9.1% vs 6.0%). Further details are discussed in Chapter 4.

[1]The SF-36 is a standardized instrument instrument to measure physical and mental health, physical and social functioning, and general well-being. It is the Medical Outcome Study's 36-item questionnaire known as the Short Form-36, or SF-36.

Kang and colleagues (2001) assessed the association between self-reported adverse pregnancy outcomes and deployment to the gulf using data from the phase I questionnaire. Results are based on the 3397 (2761 males, 636 females) deployed and 2645 (1951 males, 695 females) nondeployed veterans who reported their or their partner's first pregnancy ending after June 30, 1991. See Chapter 4 for discussion of reproductive outcomes.

A nested case-control analysis was performed on the 277 (2.4%) deployed veterans from Phases 1 and 2 who met the case definition for a possible neurological cluster of symptoms including blurred vision, loss of balance or dizziness, tremors or shaking, speech difficulty, concentration or memory problems, and irregular heartbeat, to determine which of 23 self-reported exposures were more common among cases than among the controls (6730 Gulf War veteran respondents who lacked symptoms) (Kang et al., 2002). Exposure to a variety of chemical agents were reported to be higher among cases than controls, specifically to chemical-agent-resistant compound paint, depleted uranium, nerve gas, food contaminated with oil or smoke, and bathing in or drinking water contaminated with oil or smoke. Further details on results from this study are found in Chapter 4 in the section on Multisymptom Illness.

Kang et al. (2003) used the Kang et al. (2000) cohorts to assess the prevalence of PTSD and CFS in Gulf War veterans. The questionnaire administered to the veterans in Phases 1 and 2 described above included eight symptoms to be used to diagnose CFS, the PTSD Checklist was used to identify symptoms of PTSD. Assessment of CFS was based on the CDC case definition after exclusion of alternate medical causes of the symptoms. Further details on results from this study are found in Chapter 4 in the section on Mental and Behavioral Disorders.

Kang and colleagues (2005) conducted a nested case-control study evaluating the role of sexual assault on the risk of PTSD from the 11,441 Gulf War veteran respondents of the 1995 questionnaire described above. A score of 50 or higher on the PTSD checklist (PCL) was necessary to have met the criteria for PTSD; 1381 (12.1%) Gulf War veterans (336 females and 1045 males) screened positive for PTSD, while 10,060 (1795 females and 8265 males) screened negative and were used as a comparison group. Adjustments for age, race, branch, combat, rank, and unit type, and self-report of sexual harassment and assault were made. Further details on results described above are found in Chapter 4 in the section on Female Veterans' Health.

Karlinsky and colleagues (2004) examined pulmonary function and self-reported respiratory symptoms in the deployed (n = 1036) versus nondeployed (n = 1103) veterans drawn from the National Health Survey of Gulf War Veterans and Their Families. Results of pulmonary function tests were classified into five categories: normal pulmonary function, nonreversible airway obstruction, reversible airway obstruction, restrictive lung physiology, and small-airway obstruction. The authors also reported on the pattern of pulmonary function test results in those exposed (n = 159) and those not exposed (n = 877) (according to DoD exposure estimates developed in 2002) to nerve agents from destruction of munitions at the storage site at Khamisiyah in 1991. See Chapter 4 for more details.

The Update committee identified six studies (Blanchard et al., 2005; Kang et al., 2009; Page et al., 2005a,b; Toomey et al., 2007, 2009) published after *Volume 4* that used data from the VA National Health Survey of Gulf War Veterans and Their Families. Findings from those studies are described in Chapter 4.

Page and colleagues (2005a) assessed the possible health effects of Khamisiyah exposure (determined from models developed by the Department of Defense [DoD] and Central Intelligence Agency) in 5555 deployed army veterans drawn from the 11,441 deployed cohort who responded to either phase I or II (postal or telephone questionnaire). When the survey was completed in 1995, veterans were not yet notified of possible chemical agent exposure in Khamisiyah. No difference in self-perception of health status was found between the exposed (n = 1898) and unexposed (n = 3336) groups.

Page and colleagues (2005b) also examined the association between notification of possible exposure at Khamisiyah and self-reported morbidity. In 2000, a subsample of 1056 deployed army veterans was surveyed; of the 600 notified subjects, 438 (73%) responded, and of the 456 nonnotified subjects, 318 (70%) responded. Results indicate no significant difference in activity limitations, bed days, or number of clinic or hospital visits among the groups.

Blanchard and colleagues (2005) assessed the prevalence and severity of chronic multisymptom illness (CMI) in the same cohort of deployed (n = 1061) and nondeployed (1128) veterans as described by Eisen and colleagues (2005). Combat exposure was significantly associated with CMI. The prevalence of CMI in the nondeployed population has remained relatively constant at 4, 7, and 10 years postwar. Among the deployed veterans, CMI prevalence has decreased from 44.7% at 4 years to 28.9% after 10 years (Fukuda et al., 1998; Steele, 2000). Blanchard et al. (2005) also assessed for the presence of CMI based on the possible exposure of deployed veterans to nerve agents as a result of the Khamisiyah demolition. Based on DoD modeling, 236 (22.2%) of the deployed veterans were exposed; 92 (39.0%) had CMI, and 144 (61.0%) did not. See Chapter 4 for more details.

Toomey and colleagues (2007) examined the prevalence of mental health disorders, self-report of symptoms, and quality of life in the same cohort of 1061 Gulf War deployed versus 1128 nondeployed veterans 10 years postconflict as that of Eisen et al. (2005). Deployed veterans self-reported lower levels of life satisfaction and their SF-36 scores were significantly lower than the nondeployed veterans. See Chapter 4 for more details.

Toomey and colleagues (2009) also evaluated neuropsychologic functioning 10 years postconflict in the same population as the study described above (Toomey et al., 2007). The measures assessed were based on those previously found to be different between the deployed and nondeployed groups in earlier studies of the same cohort; examples include measures of general intelligence, attention or executive functioning, motor ability, visuospatial processing, and verbal and visual memory. Further details can be found in Chapter 4.

Kang and colleagues (2009) conducted a 10-year follow-up general health assessment using the population of the National Health Survey of Gulf War Veterans and Their Families (15,000 Gulf War deployed and 15,000 nondeployed). In phase I of the follow-up, VA and Social Security records through December 2002 were used to identify and mail health questionnaires to the 29,607 living participants. Phase II consisted of telephone interviews with 2000 nonresponsive participants and a sample of 1000 participants who had indicated a clinic visit or hospitalization within the previous 12 months in order to obtain permission for medical record retrieval. After phases I and II, 6111 (40%) deployed and 3859 (27%) nondeployed participants responded to the survey; overall response rate was low, only 34%. The administered questionnaire was a modified version of that used in the 1995 survey and included the Psychopathy Check List (PCL), the Patient Health Questionnaire (PHQ), and the SF-12[2] in addition to other items used to assess general health status. See Chapter 4 for more details.

[2] "The 12-Item Short Form Health Survey (SF-12) was developed for the Medical Outcomes Study, a multiyear study of patients with chronic conditions. The instrument was designed to reduce respondent burden while achieving minimum standards of precision for purposes of group comparisons involving multiple health dimensions" (RAND Corporation, 2010).

The Iowa Persian Gulf Study

In *Volume 4*, the Iowa Persian Gulf Study was presented as the reference study with eight derivative studies. The Update committee identified three new studies derived from the original Iowa cohort.

Reference Study

The Iowa study was a cross-sectional survey of a representative sample of 4886 military personnel who listed Iowa as their home of record at the time of enlistment and served between August 2, 1990, and July 31, 1991 (Iowa Persian Gulf Study Group, 1997). The DMDC identified 29,010 potentially eligible military personnel; 42 records were not included for a variety of reasons including incomplete data or duplicate records, leaving a representative sample of 28,968.

Study subjects were divided into four groups: Gulf War-deployed active duty, Gulf War-deployed National Guard or reserve, Gulf War nondeployed active duty, and Gulf War nondeployed National Guard or reserve; samples were evenly selected from each of the four domains. A total of 4886 study subjects were randomly selected from the four groups; of the study subjects who were contacted, 3695 (76%) completed a telephone interview. Trained examiners used standardized questionnaires, instruments, and scales to collect information from the subjects. Sources of questions included the National Health Interview Survey, the Behavioral Risk Factor Surveillance Survey, the National Medical Expenditures Survey, the Primary Care Evaluation of Mental Disorders, the Brief Symptom Inventory, the CAGE questionnaire (for alcoholism),[3] the PTSD (Posttraumatic Stress Disorder) Checklist—Military, the Centers for Disease Control and Prevention Chronic Fatigue Syndrome Questionnaire, the Chalder Fatigue Scale, the American Thoracic Society questionnaire, and the Sickness Impact Profile. The conditions listed were not diagnosed, because no clinical examinations were performed. Rather, before conducting their telephone survey, researchers grouped sets of symptoms from their symptom checklists into a priori categories of diseases or disorders. After a veteran identified himself or herself as having the requisite set of symptoms, researchers analyzing responses considered the veteran as having symptoms "suggestive" of or consistent with a particular disorder but not as having a formal diagnosis of the disorder.

Gulf War veterans scored significantly lower on all eight subscales for physical and mental health on the SF-36. The subscales for bodily pain, general health, and vitality showed the greatest absolute differences between deployed and nondeployed veterans. The Iowa study assessed exposure–symptom relationships by asking veterans to report on their deployment exposures including to solvents or petrochemicals, smoke or combustion products, lead from fuels, pesticides, ionizing or nonionizing radiation, chemical warfare agents, PB use, infectious agents, and physical trauma. The authors concluded that no exposure to any single agent was related to the medical conditions found to be more prevalent in Gulf War veterans (Iowa Persian Gulf Study Group, 1997).

[3]The CAGE is a four-item scale to assess cutting down (C), feeling annoyed by people criticizing your drinking (A), feeling guilty about drinking (G), and using alcohol as an eye-opener in the morning (E).

Derivative Studies

Eight derivative studies of the Iowa cohort were described in *Volume 4* (Barrett et al., 2002; Black et al., 1999, 2000, 2004a,b; Doebbling et al., 2000; Lange et al., 2002). The Update committee identified three new studies of this cohort.

Subsequent cross-sectional studies of the Iowa cohort examined the presence of possible multiple chemical sensitivity (MCS) in these veterans, including the impact of MCS on quality of life and utilization of health services (Black et al., 1999) and the prevalence of and risk factors the development of MCS (Black et al., 2000).

Doebbling et al. (2000) used factor analysis to attempt to determine if the symptoms reported by Gulf War veterans after their deployment were different than those reported by nondeployed veterans and if the symptoms seen in the deployed veterans could possibly constitute a unique Gulf War syndrome.

Three studies assess the prevalence of psychiatric disorders in Gulf War deployed and nondeployed veterans. Barrett et al. (2002) examined the association between PTSD and self-reported physical health status. The prevalence of and risk factors for current anxiety disorder was studied by Black et al. (2004b) who used the PRIME-MD in a structured telephone interview to identify symptoms of anxiety. In a case-control study, however, Black et al. (2004a) used the SCID-IV to diagnose current or lifetime depression in 608 of the Iowa veterans, of whom 192 met the case definition for lifetime depressive disorder (132 deployed and 60 nondeployed). The prevalence of comorbid psychiatric diagnoses was determined. The findings of these studies are discussed in more detail in Chapter 4.

Lange et al. (2002) examined the impact of exposure of deployed Gulf War veterans to Kuwaiti oil-well fire and the prevalence of asthma and bronchitis 5 years after the war. Modeled exposures were developed using a geographic information system to integrate spatial and temporal records of smoke concentrations with troop movements ascertained from global positioning systems records. Results for modeled exposures were compared with self-reported exposures. More details are presented in Chapter 4.

The Update committee identified three new studies based on the Iowa cohort: Ang et al. (2006) and Forman-Hoffman et al. (2007) that both looked at the presence of chronic widespread pain in Iowa Gulf War veterans and Black et al. (2006) who assessed the prevalence of borderline personality disorder in the Iowa veterans.

Approximately 5 years after the initial survey described above, Ang and colleagues (2006) designed a follow-up evaluation to determine predictive factors for development of chronic widespread pain (CWP) in Gulf War veterans. A sample of 1040 veterans who previously met the criteria for cognitive dysfunction, CWP, and a control group was evaluated. Fifty-eight percent (n = 602) of the targeted population completed the assessment. Results indicated that deployment was not significantly associated with development of CWP; however, the association with combat exposure was significant. See Chapter 4 for more details.

Forman-Hoffman et al. (2007) also conducted a cross-sectional survey 5 years postconflict to determine the effect of deployment on the development of CWP in the Iowa cohort. The authors used the same 3695 participants as sampled in Black et al. (2006) below. Findings from this study are discussed further in Chapter 4.

Black and colleagues (2006) assessed the prevalence of borderline personality disorder (BPD) traits in a sample of the Iowa Persian Gulf War veterans using the Schedule for Adaptive and Nonadaptive Personality. The population was drawn from the initial 3695 surveyed individuals; a second assessment (in-person interviews and medical examinations) was administered to 602 individuals who previously met the criteria for one or more of the following: depression, chronic widespread pain, and cognitive dysfunction. The overall response rate was 95.7% (n = 576). See Chapter 4 for further detail.

United Kingdom Veteran Studies

Three reference studies of UK Gulf War veterans were identified in *Volume* 4: Cherry et al. (2001a,b); Maconochie et al. (2003); and Unwin et al. (1999). Two teams of researchers in the UK studied separate, nonoverlapping, stratified random samples of the over 53,000 military personnel sent to the Gulf War. The first team was from the University of London (Guy's, King's, and St. Thomas Medical Schools); the second team was from the University of Manchester. In addition, a third team of researchers from the London School of Hygiene and Tropical Medicine surveyed the entire cohort of 53,000 veterans examining birth defects and other reproductive outcomes. The Update committee identified only one new derivative study which was based on the University of London cohort study.

University of London Veteran Studies

Reference Study

At the University of London, Unwin and colleagues (1999) studied the health effects of deployment by randomly sampling the entire UK contingent deployed to the Gulf War (n = 53,462)[4]; the control groups consisted of those deployed to the conflict in Bosnia (n = 39,217) and servicemembers who were deployed in the same period to noncombat locations outside the United Kingdom (n = 250,000). The nondeployed control group was recruited from among the subset of nondeployed servicemembers who were fit for combat duty, thus avoiding selection bias related to the healthy warrior effect. Investigators distributed a mailed questionnaire that asked about symptoms (50 items), medical disorders (39 items), exposure history (29 items), functional capacity, and other topics. Potential confounding factors (including sociodemographic and lifestyle factors) were controlled for in multiple logistic regression analysis. Response rates were as follows: 70.4% Gulf War deployed; 61.9% Bosnia cohort; and 62.9% era cohort. The Gulf War deployed veterans reported a higher prevalence of symptoms and diminished functioning than did either comparison group.

The two UK Gulf War cohorts completed a second questionnaire with details of the dates they were deployed to each location and the exposures they had experienced. The questionnaire listed 14 exposures, such as combat exposure, number of inoculations, number of days handling pesticides, days exposed to smoke from oil fires, and duration of stay in the gulf. The main analysis involved a multiple regression of each of the seven factors identified through factor analysis on all exposures and other potential confounders. Many of the reported exposures correlated with one another. In the multivariate regression analysis, the number of days veterans handled pesticides was related to the overall severity score and to the peripheral and neurologic factors; the number of days they applied insecticide to their skin was related to severity and to the peripheral, respiratory, and appetite factors. The number of inoculations was associated with skin and musculoskeletal symptoms. Further results are discussed in detail in Chapter 4.

---

[4]UK military personnel in the Gulf War were somewhat different from US personnel in demographics, combat experience, and exposures to particular agents (United Kingdom Ministry of Defence, 2000).

Derivative Studies

Nine derivative studies of this cohort were described in *Volume 4* (Hotopf et al., 2003a,b; Macfarlane et al., 2000, 2003, 2005; Nisenbaum et al., 2004; Reid et al., 2001; Rose et al., 2004; Sharief et al., 2002). The Update committee identified two new studies of this cohort (Stimpson et al., 2006; Ismail et al., 2008).

A follow-up study using a postal survey was sent 11 years after the war to a stratified random sample of 3305 participants (1472 Gulf War deployed, 909 Bosnian deployed, 924 era veterans) from the total who completed the first study described above. The response rates were as follows: 74.0% Gulf War deployed; 70.2% Bosnia deployed; 69.7% era veterans. To assess physical symptoms, respondents completed the SF-36. Receiving multiple vaccinations during deployment was weakly associated with five of the six health outcomes examined, including chronic multisymptom illness (as defined by the CDC) (Hotopf et al., 2003a). Hotopf et al. (2003b) studied a subset of these veterans assess PON1 activity and genotype for PON1–55 and PON1–192. Four groups were selected: deployed veterans who reported physical symptoms after the war (n = 115); healthy deployed veterans (n = 95); symptomatic Bosnia peacekeeping veterans (n = 52); and symptomatic nondeployed military controls (n = 85).

Macfarlane and colleagues (2000) assessed mortality among the entire UK cohort of deployed veterans (n = 53,462) compared with frequency matched controls; the follow-up period was from the end of the Gulf War (April 1, 1991) to March 31, 1999. Results from a 13-year follow-up (ending June 30, 2004) of the same cohort remained consistent (Macfarlane et al., 2005). See Chapter 4 for more details.

Incidence of cancer, as identified on the National Health Service register, was followed from the end of the Gulf War until July 31, 2002, in all deployed UK servicemembers compared with nondeployed matched controls (era veterans). Of the 51,721 Gulf War veterans, 270 were diagnosed with cancer; of the 50,755 era veterans, 269 were diagnosed (Macfarlane et al., 2003). Additional discussion of the findings is provided in Chapter 4.

Another separate analysis of a subgroup of veterans meeting case criteria for MCS symptoms found that they were significantly more likely to report several types of pesticide exposures. Veterans meeting case criteria for CFS were not more likely to report pesticide exposure; a strong association was found between CFS and reporting of combat-related injury in the deployed veterans (Reid et al., 2001).

Rose et al. (2004) and Sharief et al. (2002) conducted a case-control study examining neuromuscular symptoms in 49 Gulf War veterans with more than four neuromuscular symptoms and lower functioning according to the SF-36 compared with 26 healthy Gulf War-deployed veterans, 13 symptomatic Bosnian veterans, and 22 symptomatic nondeployed controls. Testing of peripheral nerves, skeletal muscles, or neuromuscular junctions found no statistically significant differences between deployed and nondeployed veterans who had symptoms of Gulf War illness. See Chapter 4 for further details.

Nisenbaum et al. (2004) used a factor analysis on symptom data from both the UK reference study and the Pennsylvania Air Force unit study (Fukuda et al., 1998; discussed later in this chapter) to look at the interrelationships between symptoms. Each sample was split in half to provide an exploratory and a confirmatory sample. Four correlated factors were identified in each of the samples: respiratory, mood-cognition, peripheral nervous, and gastrointestinal/urogenital. Further detail is discussed in Chapter 4.

Macfarlane et al. (2005) examined self-reported exposures and mortality in the population of Gulf War deployed described above. No difference in mortality was found between those who reported exposure to antibiologic warfare prophylaxis, pesticide handling, smoke from oil-well fires, or Scud missiles, versus the self-reported unexposed. Results also indicate that those who handled pesticides and those exposed to depleted uranium were at higher risk of death due to external causes and death due to disease-related causes, respectively; however, neither of these was statistically significant. See Chapter 4 for additional detail.

The Update committee identified two new studies based on the University of London study. Stimpson and colleagues (2006) used the same population and methods described in Unwin et al. (1999) to specifically examine the prevalence of reported pain and its association with deployment status. Ismail and colleagues (2008) assessed the prevalence of chronic fatigue syndrome by implementing a two-phase study approach that was a continuum of the Unwin et al. (1999) (phase I) cohort above. Phase II consisted of a random sampling of the 244 veterans (Gulf War and Bosnia deployed, and era veterans) who screened positive for a physical disability (score less than or equal to 72.2 on the SF-36) in the Unwin study; 111 (45.5%) were Gulf War deployed and 133 (54.5%) were non-Gulf veterans (Bosnia: n = 54, era: n = 79). See Chapter 4 for more detail.

University of Manchester Veteran Study

Seven years after the Gulf War, the University of Manchester study surveyed a random sample of all UK veterans, distinct from that of Unwin et al. (1999), who deployed between September 1990 and June 1991, as indentified by the Ministry of Defense (Cherry et al., 2001a,b). Eligible deployed veterans (n = 9505) were divided into two groups—main cohort (n = 4755) and validation cohort (n = 4750) to permit replication of analysis and to assess consistency. The control population (n = 4749) was nondeployed veterans in good general health. Veterans were sent a questionnaire about the extent to which they were burdened, within the last month, by any of 95 symptoms. By asking them to mark their answers on a visual analogue scale, investigators sought to determine the degree of symptom severity. Investigators also sought to determine areas of peripheral neuropathy by asking veterans to shade body areas on two mannequins in which they were experiencing pain or numbness and tingling. Deployed veterans reported greater symptom severity on almost all symptoms. Findings from this reference study are discussed in Chapter 4.

No derivative studies were identified for this UK cohort in *Volume 4* or by the Update committee.

London School of Hygiene and Tropical Medicine Veteran Study

Reference Study

The third United Kingdom study was a very large mail survey that began in August 1998 (with reminders until 2001). It was conducted by researchers from the London School of Hygiene and Tropical Medicine (Maconochie et al., 2003). The study was designed to assess reproductive outcomes among Gulf War veterans and also contained open-ended questions regarding general health. The exposed cohort consisted of all UK Gulf War veterans, and the unexposed cohort consisted of a random sample of nondeployed UK military personnel from the same period. The number of surveys returned in the study was large (25,084 from Gulf War veterans and 19,003 from non-Gulf War veterans); however, the participation rates were low (47.3% and 37.5% of male and female Gulf War veterans, respectively, and 57.3% and 45.6% of male and female nondeployed veterans). The survey included items on reproductive and child health, exposure history, current health, and health of sexual partners; it was supplemented by examination of medical records for pregnancies, live births, and outcomes. Male participants (n = 42,818) reported 27,929 pregnancies in their partners and female participants (n = 1269) reported 861 pregnancies. Reports of miscarriages and congenital malformation were clinically validated.

Derivative Studies

Three derivative studies were described in *Volume 4*; no new derivative studies were identified by the Update committee. Based on results of Maconochie et al. (2003), Doyle et al. (2004) examined the associations between risk of miscarriage, stillbirth, or congenital malformations for deployed and nondeployed women. Maconochie et al. (2004) assessed the risk of infertility male Gulf War veterans (females not included in study); self-reports were validated with clinical diagnosis. Findings from the 2004 study by Maconochie and colleagues are discussed in Chapter 4.

In a subanalysis of the population described by Maconochie et al. (2004) above, Simmons et al. (2004) indicated that 61% of Gulf War veterans reported at least one new medical symptom or disease since 1990 compared with 37% of nondeployed veterans. Further details regarding outcomes are described in Chapter 4.

Australian Veteran Studies

In *Volume 4*, the reference study for evaluations of the Australian Gulf War veterans was cited as Kelsall et al. (2004a) but the Update committee identified the original report of the study methods and initial findings (Sim et al., 2003). Sim et al. (2003) is considered to be the reference study in this report. Six derivative studies were described in *Volume 4* (Forbes et al., 2004; Ikin et al., 2004; Kelsall et al., 2004a,b, 2005; McKenzie et al., 2004) and the Update committee identified two new derivative studies (Kelsall et al., 2006, 2007) based on the Sim et al. cohort. All of these studies are discussed in Chapter 4.

Reference Study

Investigators from Monash University in Australia conducted a study examining the health of all 1871 Australian veterans deployed to the Gulf War region from August 2, 1990, to September 4, 1991; members of the navy were overrepresented (86.5%) in this cohort (Sim et al. 2003). The control group consisted of 2924 nondeployed Australian Defence Force personnel matched by service type, sex, age, and military status. Participation rates were 81% (n = 1456) for the deployed and 57% (n = 1588) for the control group.

A postal questionnaire was distributed, which included the SF-12, GHQ-12, and questions regarding physical and psychological health, military service history, and exposures during deployment. In addition, participants were asked to attend one of 10 Health Services Australia medical clinics to undergo a comprehensive health assessment, a full physical examination, blood work, and fitness tests. Interview-administered questionnaires such as the Composite International Diagnostic Interview (CIDI) were given to all participants (Sim et al., 2003). Gulf War veterans reported more general health symptoms and ones more severe in nature than the nondeployed controls. Chapter 4 discusses the findings of this reference study in greater detail.

Derivative Studies

Kelsall et al. (2004a) reported the results of the Sim et al. (2003) report. They stated that participants in the exposed cohort reported a higher prevalence of all symptoms and reported more severe symptoms. Ikin et al. (2004) used responses to the CIDI and a service experience questionnaire to assess the relationship between the presence of a psychiatric disorder and the veterans' perceptions of stressors during deployment. Very few personnel experienced direct combat; however, despite their lack of combat exposure, deployment was a stressful event with veterans experiencing higher rates of fear and threat of entrapment, attack (including nerve agent warfare), and death or injury. In a follow-up study, Ikin et al. (2005) found that reporting of stressful experiences was associated with younger age, lower rank, and deployment at the height of the conflict. Findings from Ikin et al. (2004) and Kelsall et al. (2004a) are discussed in Chapter 4.

McKenzie et al. (2004) reported that Gulf War veterans had poorer psychological health and that the number of stressful exposures correlated with poorer scores on three standard instruments used to measure functioning and psychological health. Greater symptom severity was seen in Australian veterans who received 10 or more immunizations; used PB, pesticides, or insect repellents; were present in a chemical weapons area; or reported stressful military service (Kelsall et al., 2004a). Kelsall et al. (2004b) also assessed the respiratory health status of a random sample of the Australian Gulf War veterans via questionnaire, spirometric testing, and a physical examination. Health status was assessed in relation to reported exposure to Kuwaiti oil-well fire smoke and dust storms. See Chapter 4 for more details.

In 2005, Kelsall and colleagues studied the neurological status of the Australian cohort. Of the 1424 deployed veterans who completed the postal questionnaire, 1382 undertook the neurological examination; 1376 of the 1548 controls completed both the questionnaire and neurological examination (described in Sim et al., 2003, above). The authors found an increase in the reporting of neurological symptoms associated with self-reports of immunizations and exposure to various chemical agents including PB and pesticides. Details regarding results are found in Chapter 4.

Forbes et al. (2004) used factor analysis to attempt to group symptom complexes for this cohort. This well-designed study confirms the extent and greater severity of symptoms in Gulf War veterans, even in a predominantly naval population with few direct military attacks, no deaths, and few casualties. The results suggest a deployment effect in the absence of actual combat.

The Update committee identified two new derivative studies of the Australian Gulf War veterans. Kelsall et al. (2006) also conducted a study on the prevalence of chronic fatigue syndrome (CFS) from August 2000 to April 2002 in the Australian veterans. The participation rates were as follows: 1456 (80.5%) of the 1808 eligible veterans and 1588 (56.8%) of 2796 controls. Of those, 1384 deployed veterans and 1379 controls completed both the postal questionnaire and medical assessment. In addition to questions on general health, fitness tests, laboratory work, and pulmonary function, clinical examiners specifically inquired about any tiredness or fatigue following normal activities and its duration within the last 12 months. The odds of general fatigue increased with self-report of more PB tablets used, exposure to pesticides, belief in being near chemical weapons, and being in the gulf during air war. Findings are discussed in Chapter 4.

Male reproductive health in the deployed versus nondeployed population was also assessed. The study population consisted of the 1424 deployed veterans and 1548 controls who completed the postal questionnaire; response rates were 80.5% among eligible deployed veterans and 56.8% of eligible nondeployed, as stated above. Questions of interest included those related to pregnancy outcomes (live birth, miscarriage, stillbirth), and for live births, participants were asked about date, weight, gestation, and birth defects (Kelsall et al., 2007). Detailed results regarding all outcomes for this study are found in Chapter 4.

Danish Peacekeeper Studies

One reference study was conducted on the Danish peacekeepers sent to the Persian Gulf at the end of the war (Ishoy et al., 1999b). *Volume 4* cited four derivative studies based on the initial cohort. The Update committee did not identify any additional derivative studies on the Danish Gulf War veterans.

Reference Study

Military personnel from Denmark were involved in peacekeeping or humanitarian missions occurring predominantly after the Gulf War ceasefire, but were located in the same areas as other coalition forces who served in Gulf War combat (Ishoy et al., 1999b). A total of 821 Danes, deployed between August 1990 to December 1997, were eligible for inclusion in this population-based cohort; 686 (83.6%) agreed to participate in the study. The deployed veterans were matched by age, sex, and profession to 400 members of the Danish armed forces who were not deployed to the Gulf War; the participation rate was 57.8% (n = 231). Participants completed a detailed questionnaire, including 22 neuropsychologic symptoms, and then received detailed clinical health and laboratory examinations (e.g., height, weight, blood pressure, battery of urinary and blood work, battery of neuropsychologic tests) and physician interviews about their medical history and symptoms. Gulf War participants were also asked about their exposures while in the gulf. The examinations were conducted between 1997 and 1998. Further discussion of the findings is provided in Chapter 4.

Derivative Studies

Proctor et al. (2003) assessed neuropsychologic symptoms in the Danish Gulf War veterans. Gastrointestinal symptoms and diseases and symptoms related to the skin or allergies were evaluated by Ishoy et al. (1999a). Gastrointestinal symptoms were associated with two exposures: burning of waste or manure and exposure to insecticide against cockroaches (Ishoy et al., 1999a).

The investigators also examined male participants for sexual dysfunction and reproductive health. Self-reports of sexual problems were validated with medical examinations and laboratory testing, such as reproductive hormone parameters (Ishoy et al., 2001a,b). Further details can be found in Chapter 4.

One analysis investigated whether 22 neuropsychologic symptoms were associated with 18 self-reported environmental exposures[5] (physical, chemical, biologic exposures, and psychological stressors) (Suadicani et al., 1999). Most exposures were significantly associated with three to five relevant neuropsychologic symptoms in bivariate analyses. One psychologic exposure ("having watched colleagues or friends threatened or shot at") and environmental

---

[5]Exposures did not include pyridostigmine bromide or vaccinations against chemical or biologic warfare agents, because Danish veterans had a peacekeeping role and thus were not at risk for chemical or biologic warfare.

exposures, especially "bathing in or drinking contaminated water (fumes, oil, chemicals)," remained significant after adjustment for associations of exposures with one another in a multiple logistic regression model.

Oregon and Washington Veteran Studies

One reference study discussed in *Volume* 4 examined Gulf War veterans who listed Oregon or Washington as their residence at the time of their deployment (McCauley et al., 1999a); two derivative studies were also described in that volume (Bourdette et al., 2001; Spencer et al., 2001). The Update committee did not identify any new studies that used this data set.

Investigators from the Portland Environmental Hazards Research Center examined numerous health outcomes in Gulf War veterans who were deployed between August 1, 1990, and July 31, 1991, and listed Oregon or Washington as their home state of record at the time of deployment; data was obtained from the DMDC (McCauley et al., 1999a).

Beginning November 1995 and ending in June 1998, a mailed questionnaire aimed to assess general health through symptom self-reports was distributed to a representative and random sample (n = 2343) of the total eligible 8603 Gulf War veterans mentioned above; the response rate was 48.4%. The study did not include a nondeployed comparison group. The next phase consisted of a clinical examination of the first 225 participants who showed differences between the symptoms they reported on questionnaires and the symptoms they reported at time of clinical examination. The greatest differences were in rash or lesions (4% agreement between questionnaire and clinical examination), gastrointestinal complaints (20% agreement), and musculoskeletal pain (35% agreement). The authors interpreted those findings as suggesting the likelihood of outcome misclassification due to reliance on self-administered questionnaires (McCauley et al., 1999a).

Derivative Studies

In *Volume* 4, Bourdette et al. (2001) was considered a reference study although it used the same data set as McCauley et al. (1999a). Bourdette and colleagues (2001) compared 244 potential cases of unexplained illness as evaluated through clinical examination with 113 potential controls from 799 of those eligible for the clinical study, and located participants who had completed the questionnaire described above. Findings from this study are discussed in Chapter 4.

A nested case-control analysis of the cohort examined 142 items related to Gulf War self-reported exposure that might account for cases of unexplained illness (Spencer et al., 2001). The sample consisted of 241 veterans with unexplained illness and 113 healthy controls (drawn from those who completed the 1995-1998 questionnaire above). According to multivariate analysis, exposures most highly associated with unexplained illness were combat conditions, heat stress, and having sought medical attention during the Gulf War. When controlled for multiple simultaneous exposures, PB exposure, insecticides and repellents, and stress were not statistically significantly associated with unexplained illness leading investigators to conclude that unexplained illnesses were not associated with cholinesterase-inhibiting neurotoxic chemicals. One strength of this study was its elimination of numerous self-reported exposures (such as anthrax and botulinum toxoid vaccines) with questionable validity as determined by lack of test-retest reliability or time-dependent information (for example, chemical weapon exposure reported by precombat veterans or postcombat veterans who could not have been so exposed) (McCauley et al., 1999b).

Canadian Gulf War Veterans Study

In *Volume 4* the Canadian Gulf War Veterans Study was not included in the presentation of major cohort studies. The Canadian study (Goss Gilroy, 1998) was considered to be a secondary study in *Volume 4* and the Update committee agreed because the study relied on self-reports gathered through a mailed questionnaire. The Update committee identified one new study based on the Canadian Gulf War veterans (Statistics Canada, 2005), although it is unclear if the cohort in the new study was the same as that studied by Goss Gilroy, Inc. Findings from both studies are discussed in Chapter 4.

Reference Study

The Canadian Department of National Defence tasked Goss Gilroy (1998) to study the overall health status and prevalence of symptoms in all Canadian Forces personnel who were deployed to the Gulf War conflict compared to a representative sample of Canadian personnel who served in the military at the same time but who had not been deployed to the Persian Gulf. Military personnel were also compared to the general population as represented by the 1990 Ontario Health Survey. A survey questionnaire was mailed out to 9947 participants in 1997 and included information on sociodemographic factors, medical history and current status, and Gulf War deployment and exposure. Response rates were as follows: 73% (n = 3113) for the Gulf War deployed and 60.3% (n = 3439) for the deployed elsewhere controls. Income was the most important confounding factor, followed by rank. Lower income and lower rank personnel had a higher prevalence of adverse health outcomes than higher income and upper rank personnel. Psychological stressors, physical trauma, while in theater, and self-reported exposure to chemical warfare agents, such as PB, diesel or gasoline fumes, and infectious agents, was associated with adverse health outcomes (Goss Gilroy, 1998).

Derivative Study

A 9-year follow-up study was conducted on mortality and cancer incidence in the cohort of deployed Canadian personnel (n = 5117) compared to Canadian Forces who were eligible but not deployed to the gulf (n = 6093). The national mortality database and national cancer registry provided the information necessary for record linkage. No significant difference in risk of death was found between the two groups—42 deaths in the deployed cohort and 54 deaths in the nondeployed. No significant difference in risk of cancer diagnosis was observed—29 cases were diagnosed in the deployed and 42 cases were diagnosed in the nondeployed (Statistics Canada, 2005). Further details are found in Chapter 4.

Kansas Veteran Study

In *Volume 4*, the study of Kansas Gulf War veterans (Steele, 2000) was considered to be a secondary study for most health outcomes. No derivative studies using the Kansas cohort were identified in that volume, or by the Update committee.

Using lists of eligible veterans from the DMDC, Steele (2000) conducted a population-based survey to determine health problems of veterans who listed Kansas as their home state of record. A stratified random sample of 3138 veterans was selected; 2396 (76%) were located with instate contact information and 2211 met further eligibility requirements. Of those, 2030 agreed to be interviewed; the response rate was 92%. The sample included 1548 Gulf War deployed veterans and 482 nondeployed veterans.

The survey, mailed out in 1998, inquired about 16 specific physician-diagnosed or physician-treated medical or psychiatric conditions; 37 symptoms; service branch and locations during the Gulf War (including whether the veterans were notified about the Khamisiyah demolitions); and vaccinations. Using her own definition of Gulf War illness, which was similar to that used by the Centers for Disease Control and Prevention (CDC) (Fukuda et al., 1998), Steele found the prevalence of Gulf War illness to be associated with the period and location in the gulf in which veterans served. Findings from this study are discussed further in Chapter 4.

Fort Devens and New Orleans Cohort Studies

Gulf War veterans from military units stationed in Fort Devens, Massachusetts and New Orleans are among the most studied. The reference study is Proctor et al. (1998) which was described in *Volume 4*. Three derivative studies (Proctor et al., 2001a,b; White et al., 2001) from the cohort were described in *Volume 4*. The Update committee identified one additional study (Proctor et al., 2006), which is described in Chapter 4.

Reference Study

The symptom experience of two deployed cohorts of Gulf War veterans was studied by Boston-based researchers. The first, an army cohort based in Fort Devens, Massachusetts, was surveyed longitudinally at three time points (1991, 1993-1994, and 1997). From 1994 to 1996, Proctor (1998) surveyed the deployed cohorts (Fort Devens and New Orleans) with a medical and occupational history questionnaire, an environmental interview, a battery of neuropsychological tests, scales assessing psychological symptoms. Psychological symptoms were assessed with the Brief Symptom Interview and the Mississippi Scale for PTSD; psychiatric disorders were diagnosed using the Clinician Administered Scale for PTSD and the Structured Clinical Interview for DSM-IIIR Axis I Disorders, and structured interviews assessing psychological outcomes. A second deployed cohort from New Orleans and a unit deployed to Germany during the Gulf War were studied only at the second time period. The Germany deployed unit, serving as the controls (n = 47), was an air ambulance company of National Guard from Maine that handled wounded personnel evacuated from the gulf. The study's nearly 300 subjects were a stratified random sample of 2949 troops (n = 220) from Fort Devens and 928 (n = 73) from New Orleans; both groups consisted of active duty, reserve, and National Guard troops. See Chapter 4 for more detail.

Derivative Studies

Psychiatric interviews and other clinical evaluations were administered between 1993 and 1994 to all three cohorts. White et al. (2001) assessed neuropsychological functioning the cohorts and examined whether any links could be made between performance on a battery of tests and self-reported exposure to a variety of toxicants experienced during deployment. The neuropsychological test battery was designed to assess abilities across the following functional domains: general intelligence, attention/executive function, motor ability, visuospatial processing, verbal and visual memory, mood, and motivation. In addition, eight exposures were surveyed, and respondents were asked to rate each on a scale of 0-2, (0 = no exposure; 1 = exposed; 2 = exposed and felt sick at the time). Using standardized regression, the authors found the strongest associations between musculoskeletal, neurologic, neuropsychologic, and psychologic symptoms and several exposures—debris from Scuds and chemical and biologic warfare agents. Findings from this study are discussed in Chapter 4.

The health-related quality of life among the Fort Devens cohort (n = 141) and the Germany deployed cohort (n = 46) was evaluated by Proctor et al. (2001a). The SF-36 was administered to a stratified, random sample of the original cohort, approximately 4 years after the war. Proctor et al. (2001b) assessed 180 deployed veterans from the Fort Devens cohort and 46 Germany deployed veterans for symptoms of chronic fatigue and chemical sensitivity to assess the prevalence of the symptoms and whether there was an overlap between these symptoms and the case definition of chronic multisymptom illness.

The Update committee identified one new derivative study. Proctor et al. (2006) assessed neurobehavioral functioning in relationship to potential exposure to sarin and cyclosarin as a result of the demolition of the Khamisiyah munitions dump. Data had been collected in 1994 to 1996, before veterans had been notified about their potential exposure to the nerve agents. The neurobehavioral tests included those for attention, executive function, psychomotor function, visuospatial abilities, and short-term memory. See Chapter 4 for further details.

Seabee Studies

Numerous studies have been conducted on the Seabees, members of the reserve naval construction battalions. Two reference studies were included in *Volume 4*. Haley et al. (1997b) began a study on one cohort of Seabees and Gray et al. (1999a) surveyed a subset of the Haley cohort that excluded Gulf War veterans who were no longer in the service at the time of their study. Three derivative studies for Haley et al. (1997b) are presented in *Volume 4* along with two derivative studies for Gray et al. (1999a). The Update committee identified one new derivative study of the Haley et al. (1997b) cohort; none were identified for the Gray et al. (1999a) cohort.

Reference Study

Haley et al. (1997b) studied members of the Twenty-Fourth Reserve Naval Construction Battalion living in five southern states who were called to active duty for the Gulf War. More than half the battalion had left the military by the time of the study. Participants were recruited from those that investigators had addresses for and from veterans' meetings; 58.0% (n = 606) were located, and 41.1% (n = 249) agreed to participate in the study; there was no comparison cohort of nondeployed veterans. Of those participating, 70% reported having had a serious health problem since returning from the Gulf War. A telephone survey of a random sample of nonparticipants found that, while they were demographically similar to participants, 43% reported having serious health problems since the war. Eleven percent of participants and 3% of nonparticipants were unemployed.

Derivative Studies

The three syndromes identified by Haley and colleagues (1997a) were the focus of another case-control study that examined their relationship to self-reported exposures to neurotoxicants. The study tested the hypothesis that exposure to organophosphates and related chemicals that inhibit cholinesterase are responsible for the three nervous system-based syndromes (Haley and Kurt, 1997). Results of this study are discussed in Appendix A.

Another study by Haley and collaborators (1999) examined whether genetic susceptibility could play a role in placing some veterans at risk for neurologic damage by organophosphate chemicals. The investigators studied 45 veterans: 25 with chronic neurologic symptoms identified through their earlier factor analysis study and 20 healthy controls from the same battalion. Investigators measured blood butyrylcholinesterase and two types, or allozymes, of paraoxonase/arylesterase-1 (PON1). The genotypes encoding the allozymes were also studied. Results of this study are also discussed in Appendix A.

The Update committee identified one new study by Haley et al. (2009) that looked at abnormal brain response to cholinergic challenge in a small group of Gulf War veterans. Twenty-one Gulf War veterans with symptom complexes used by Haley to define three forms of Gulf War illness and 17 age-, sex- and education-matched controls, underwent a 99mTc-HMPAO-SPECT brain scan with and without an infusion of PB.

Reference Study

The first in a series of studies by Gray et al. (1999) surveyed Seabees who remained on active duty for at least 3 years after the Gulf War. The Seabees were from 14 commands at two locations (Port Hueneme, California, and Gulfport, Mississippi). Those who were deployed to the Gulf War were in mobile construction battalions serving in the same tasks and at the same sites as did the reserve Seabee battalion studied by Haley et al. (1997b), Gray et al. (1999) excluded Gulf War veterans who were no longer on active duty at the time of study.

In 1994, 1497 study subjects were enrolled: 527 Gulf War veterans and 970 nondeployed veterans. The participation rate of eligible Seabees was 53%. The following were administered to the study participants: eight-page questionnaire regarding medical history, Gulf War exposures, postwar symptoms, hospitalization, and pregnancy outcomes; questions regarding the presence of chronic fatigue syndrome and PTSD; laboratory testing—sera, blood, urine; and pulmonary function and handgrip strength tests. Findings of this study can be found in Chapter 4.

Derivative Studies

Beginning in May 1997, Gray et al. (2002) distributed a postal questionnaire to all regular and reserve navy personnel (n = 18,945) who served on active-duty Seabee command during the Gulf War period. The questionnaire collected information regarding medical history, current health status, symptoms, and environmental exposures (for example, PB). Of the 17,559 located participants, 11,868 completed and returned the survey: 3831 Gulf War deployed, 4933 deployed elsewhere, and 4933 nondeployed. Compared with the two control groups, the deployed were more likely to report having more symptoms and being in fair or poor health. Outcome specific results are found in Chapter 4.

Knoke et al. (2000) used the same Seabee cohort to conduct a factor analysis of the symptoms reported by the veterans on the Hopkins Symptom Checklist to determine whether there was a unique Gulf War syndrome.

Pennsylvania Air National Guard Study

Reference Study

In response to requests from the DoD, the VA, and the Commonwealth of Pennsylvania, Fukuda and colleagues (1998) conducted a factor analysis study in 1995 to assess health status and prevalence and causes of an unexplained illness in Gulf War deployed and nondeployed members of a currently active Air National Guard unit (n = 667). Three demographically similar air force units were used as comparison groups (n = 538, 838, and 1680). Questionnaires regarding military characteristics, demographics, health status, and 35 specific symptoms previously identified to be of concern were distributed and completed by 3723 participants (1163 Gulf War deployed, 2560 nondeployed). Participation rates were as follows: 62% index unit; 35% unit A; 73% unit B; and 70% unit C. To assess symptom prevalence, investigators combined the four units and compared questionnaire responses of deployed and nondeployed. The authors further studied health outcomes in a subset of participants from the index unit of the Pennsylvania Air Force National Guard. Of the 490 (45%) deployed members of this unit, 173 (35%) volunteered to participate in the clinical evaluation and completed a mailed clinical questionnaire and the SF-36. This study is discussed in Chapter 4.

Derivative Studies

A nested case-control study of the same cohort (n = 1002) sought to identify self-reported exposures associated with cases of chronic multisymptom illness (Nisenbaum et al., 2000). Results indicate that meeting the case definition of severe and mild-to-moderate illness was associated with use of PB, use of insect repellent, and belief in a threat from biologic or chemical weapons. Having an injury requiring medical attention was also associated with having a severe case of chronic multisymptom illness. Nisenbaum et al. (2004) conducted a factor analysis of the symptoms reported by the UK Gulf War veterans combined with those reported by the Pennsylvania Air Force veterans. Further details from these studies are discussed in Chapter 4.

Hawaii and Pennsylvania Active Duty and Reserve Study

Reference Study

One of the first epidemiologic studies of US Gulf War veterans was a congressionally mandated study evaluating the psychologic and physical health of active-duty and reserve army, navy, air force, and marine personnel from bases in Pennsylvania and Hawaii (Stretch et al., 1995). Self-reported questionnaires were mailed to 16,167 potential study participants and inquired about the following: demographics; physical, psychological, and psychosocial symptoms; deployment type; and perceived sources of stress prior to, during, and after combat or deployment. A total of 4334 veterans returned the questionnaires for a response rate of 31%. Of those, 715 active duty and 766 reserves were deployed to the Gulf War; 1576 active duty and 948 reserves were not deployed. Findings are discussed in Chapter 4.

Derivative Studies

Two derivative studies of Stretch et al. (1995) were identified. In response to a questionnaire, deployed veterans commonly reported significant levels of stress during deployment, including operating in desert climates, long duty days, extended periods in chemical-protective clothing, lack of sleep, crowding, lack of private time, physical workload, and boredom. Significant levels of stress continued postdeployment (Stretch et al., 1996a). Another publication examined PTSD in this cohort (Stretch et al., 1996b). The prevalence of PTSD symptoms was measured by the Impact of Event Scale and the Brief Symptom Inventory.

New Orleans Reservist Studies

Reference Study

A study by Sutker et al. (1995) and colleagues analyzed psychologic outcomes in a cohort of New Orleans reservists (n = 1520). The cohort consisted of Louisiana National Guard and reservists from the army, air force, and navy who had been deployed to combat. Of the 1272 who responded (overall response rate of 83.7%), 876 had been deployed and 396 had not been deployed. A discriminant function model was used to assess the relationship between personal and environmental resources and psychological outcomes. Low personality hardiness, high avoidance coping, and low perceived family cohesion were the personality and coping factors found to increase the likelihood of PTSD (Sutker et al., 1995).

Derivative Studies

One derivative study of Sutker et al. (1995) was identified. Assessed by survey at an average of 9 months (time 1) after the war, veterans completed the Beck Depression Inventory, the Brief Symptom Inventory for Anxiety and Depression, the PTSD checklist, and the Mississippi Scale for PTSD (Brailey et al., 1998). See Chapter 4 for more detail.

REFERENCES

Ang, D. C., P. M. Peloso, R. F. Woolson, K. Kroenke, and B. N. Doebbeling. 2006. Predictors of incident chronic widespread pain among veterans following the first Gulf War. *Clinical Journal of Pain* 22(6):554-563.

Barrett, D. H., C. C. Doebbeling, D. A. Schwartz, M. D. Voelker, K. H. Falter, R. F. Woolson, and B. N. Doebbeling. 2002. Posttraumatic stress disorder and self-reported physical health status among U.S. Military personnel serving during the gulf war period: A population-based study. *Psychosomatics* 43(3):195-205.

Black, D. W., B. N. Doebbeling, M. D. Voelker, W. R. Clarke, R. F. Woolson, D. H. Barrett, and D. A. Schwartz. 1999. Quality of life and health-services utilization in a population-based sample of military personnel reporting multiple chemical sensitivities. *Journal of Occupational and Environmental Medicine* 41(10):928-933.

Black, D. W., B. N. Doebbeling, M. D. Voelker, W. R. Clarke, R. F. Woolson, D. H. Barrett, and D. A. Schwartz. 2000. Multiple chemical sensitivity syndrome: Symptom prevalence and risk factors in a military population. *Archives of Internal Medicine* 160(8):1169-1176.

Black, D. W., C. P. Carney, V. L. Forman-Hoffman, E. Letuchy, P. Peloso, R. F. Woolson, and B. N. Doebbeling. 2004a. Depression in veterans of the first Gulf War and comparable military controls. *Annals of Clinical Psychiatry* 16(2):53-61.

Black, D. W., C. P. Carney, P. M. Peloso, R. F. Woolson, D. A. Schwartz, M. D. Voelker, D. H. Barrett, and B. N. Doebbeling. 2004b. Gulf War veterans with anxiety: Prevalence, comorbidity, and risk factors. *Epidemiology* 15(2):135-142.

Black, D. W., N. Blum, E. Letuchy, C. Carney Doebbeling, V. L. Forman-Hoffman, and B. N. Doebbeling. 2006. Borderline personality disorder and traits in veterans: Psychiatric comorbidity, healthcare utilization, and quality of life along a continuum of severity. *CNS Spectrums* 11(9):680-689; quiz 719.

Blanchard, M. S., S. A. Eisen, R. Alpern, J. Karlinsky, R. Toomey, D. J. Reda, F. M. Murphy, L. W. Jackson, and H. K. Kang. 2005. Chronic multisymptom illness complex in Gulf War I veterans 10 years later. *American Journal of Epidemiology* 163(1):66-75.

Bourdette, D. N., L. A. McCauley, A. Barkhuizen, W. Johnston, M. Wynn, S. K. Joos, D. Storzbach, T. Shuell, and D. Sticker. 2001. Symptom factor analysis, clinical findings, and functional status in a population-based case control study of Gulf War unexplained illness. *Journal of Occupational and Environmental Medicine* 43(12):1026-1040.

Brailey, K., J. J. Vasterling, and P. B. Sutker. 1998. Psychological aftermath of participation in the Persian Gulf War. In *The Environment and Mental Health: A Guide for Clinicians*, edited by A. Lundberg. London, UK: Lawrence Erlbaum Associates. Pp. 83-101.

Cherry, N., F. Creed, A. Silman, G. Dunn, D. Baxter, J. Smedley, S. Taylor, and G. J. Macfarlane. 2001a. Health and exposures of United Kingdom Gulf War veterans. Part I: The pattern and extent of ill health. *Occupational and Environmental Medicine* 58(5):291-298.

Cherry, N., F. Creed, A. Silman, G. Dunn, D. Baxter, J. Smedley, S. Taylor, and G. J. Macfarlane. 2001b. Health and exposures of United Kingdom Gulf War veterans. Part II: The relation of health to exposure. *Occupational and Environmental Medicine* 58(5):299-306.

Davis, L. E., S. A. Eisen, F. M. Murphy, R. Alpern, B. J. Parks, M. Blanchard, D. J. Reda, M. K. King, F. A. Mithen, and H. K. Kang. 2004. Clinical and laboratory assessment of distal peripheral nerves in Gulf War veterans and spouses. *Neurology* 63(6):1070-1077.

Doebbeling, B. N., W. R. Clarke, D. Watson, J. C. Torner, R. F. Woolson, M. D. Voelker, D. H. Barrett, and D. A. Schwartz. 2000. Is there a Persian Gulf War syndrome? Evidence from a large population-based survey of veterans and nondeployed controls. *American Journal of Medicine* 108(9):695-704.

Doyle, P., N. Maconochie, G. Davies, I. Maconochie, M. Pelerin, S. Prior, and S. Lewis. 2004. Miscarriage, stillbirth and congenital malformation in the offspring of UK veterans of the first Gulf War. *International Journal of Epidemiology* 33(1):74-86.

Eisen, S. A., H. K. Kang, F. M. Murphy, M. S. Blanchard, D. J. Reda, W. G. Henderson, R. Toomey, L. W. Jackson, R. Alpern, B. J. Parks, N. Klimas, C. Hall, H. S. Pak, J. Hunter, J. Karlinsky, M. J. Battistone, M. J. Lyons, and Gulf War Study Participating Investigators. 2005. Gulf War veterans' health: Medical evaluation of a U.S. cohort. *Annals of Internal Medicine* 142(11):881-890.

Forbes, A. B., D. P. McKenzie, A. J. Mackinnon, H. L. Kelsall, A. C. McFarlane, J. F. Ikin, D. C. Glass, and M. R. Sim. 2004. The health of Australian veterans of the 1991 Gulf War: Factor analysis of self-reported symptoms. *Occupational and Environmental Medicine* 61(12):1014-1020.

Forman-Hoffman, V. L., P. M. Peloso, D. W. Black, R. F. Woolson, E. M. Letuchy, and B. N. Doebbeling. 2007. Chronic widespread pain in veterans of the first Gulf War: Impact of deployment status and associated health effects. *Journal of Pain* 8(12):954-961.

Fricker, R. D., E. Reardon, D. M. Spektor, S. K. Cotton, J. Hawes-Dawson, J. E. Pace, and S. D. Hosek. 2000. *Pesticide Use During the Gulf War: A Survey of Gulf War Veterans*. Santa Monica, CA: RAND Corporation.

Fukuda, K., R. Nisenbaum, G. Stewart, W. W. Thompson, L. Robin, R. M. Washko, D. L. Noah, D. H. Barrett, B. Randall, B. L. Herwaldt, A. C. Mawle, and W. C. Reeves. 1998. Chronic multisymptom illness affecting Air Force veterans of the Gulf War. *JAMA* 280(11):981-988.

Goss Gilroy Inc. 1998. *Health study of Canadian forces personnel involved in the 1991 conflict in the Persian Gulf*. Ottawa, Canada: Goss Gilroy Inc. and Department of National Defence.

Gray, G. C., K. S. Kaiser, A. W. Hawksworth, F. W. Hall, and E. Barrett-Connor. 1999. Increased postwar symptoms and psychological morbidity among U.S. Navy Gulf War veterans. *American Journal of Tropical Medicine and Hygiene* 60(5):758-766.

Gray, G. C., R. J. Reed, K. S. Kaiser, T. C. Smith, and V. M. Gastanaga. 2002. Self-reported symptoms and medical conditions among 11,868 Gulf War-era veterans: The Seabee Health Study. *American Journal of Epidemiology* 155(11):1033-1044.

Haley, R. W., and T. L. Kurt. 1997. Self-reported exposure to neurotoxic chemical combinations in the Gulf War: A cross-sectional epidemiologic study. *JAMA* 277(3):231-237.

Haley, R. W., J. Hom, P. S. Roland, W. W. Bryan, P. C. Van Ness, F. J. Bonte, M. D. S. Devous, D. Mathews, J. L. Fleckenstein, F. H. J. Wians, G. I. Wolfe, and T. L. Kurt. 1997a. Evaluation of neurologic function in Gulf War veterans. A blinded case-control study. *JAMA* 277(3):223-230.

Haley, R. W., T. L. Kurt, and J. Hom. 1997b. Is there a Gulf War syndrome? Searching for syndromes by factor analysis of symptoms. *JAMA* 277(3):215-222.

Haley, R. W., S. Billecke, and B. N. La Du. 1999. Association of low PON1 type Q (type A) arylesterase activity with neurologic symptom complexes in Gulf War veterans. *Toxicology and Applied Pharmacology* 157(3):227-233.

Haley, R. W., J. S. Spence, P. S. Carmack, R. F. Gunst, W. R. Schucany, F. Petty, M. D. Devous, Sr., F. J. Bonte, and M. H. Trivedi. 2009. Abnormal brain response to cholinergic challenge in chronic encephalopathy from the 1991 Gulf War. *Psychiatry Research: Neuroimaging* 171(3):207-220.

Hotopf, M., A. S. David, L. Hull, V. Nikalaou, C. Unwin, and S. Wessely. 2003a. Gulf War illness—Better, worse, or just the same? A cohort study. *British Medical Journal* 327(7428):1370-1372.

Hotopf, M., M. I. Mackness, V. Nikolaou, D. A. Collier, C. Curtis, A. David, P. Durrington, L. Hull, K. Ismail, M. Peakman, C. Unwin, S. Wessely, and B. Mackness. 2003b. Paraoxonase in Persian Gulf War veterans. *Journal of Occupational and Environmental Medicine* 45(7):668-675.

Ikin, J. F., M. R. Sim, M. C. Creamer, A. B. Forbes, D. P. McKenzie, H. L. Kelsall, D. C. Glass, A. C. McFarlane, M. J. Abramson, P. Ittak, T. Dwyer, L. Blizzard, K. R. Delaney, K. W. A. Horsley, W. K. Harrex, and H. Schwarz. 2004. War-related psychological stressors and risk of psychological disorders in Australian veterans of the 1991 Gulf War. *British Journal of Psychiatry* 185(2):116-126.

Ikin, J. F., D. P. McKenzie, M. C. Creamer, A. C. McFarlane, H. L. Kelsall, D. C. Glass, A. B. Forbes, K. W. A. Horsley, W. K. Harrex, and M. R. Sim. 2005. War zone stress without direct combat: The Australian naval experience of the Gulf War. *Journal of Traumatic Stress* 18(3):193-204.

IOM (Institute of Medicine). 1999. *Strategies to Protect the Health of Deployed US Forces: Medical Surveillance, Record Keeping, and Risk Reduction.* Washington, DC: National Academy Press.

Iowa Persian Gulf Study Group. 1997. Self-reported illness and health status among Gulf War veterans: A population-based study. *JAMA* 277(3):238-245.

Ishoy, T., P. Suadicani, B. Guldager, M. Appleyard, and F. Gyntelberg. 1999a. Risk factors for gastrointestinal symptoms. The Danish Gulf War Study. *Danish Medical Bulletin* 46(5):420-423.

Ishoy, T., P. Suadicani, B. Guldager, M. Appleyard, H. O. Hein, and F. Gyntelberg. 1999b. State of health after deployment in the Persian Gulf. The Danish Gulf War Study. *Danish Medical Bulletin* 46(5):416-419.

Ishoy, T., A. M. Andersson, P. Suadicani, B. Guldager, M. Appleyard, F. Gyntelberg, and N. E. Skakkebaek. 2001a. Major reproductive health characteristics in male Gulf War veterans. The Danish Gulf War Study. *Danish Medical Bulletin* 48(1):29-32.

Ishoy, T., P. Suadicani, A.-M. Andersson, B. Guldager, M. Appleyard, N. Skakkebaek, and F. Gyntelberg. 2001b. Prevalence of male sexual problems in the Danish Gulf War Study. *Scandinavian Journal of Sexology* 4(1):43-55.

Ismail, K., K. Kent, R. Sherwood, L. Hull, P. Seed, A. S. David, and S. Wessely. 2008. Chronic fatigue syndrome and related disorders in UK veterans of the Gulf War 1990-1991: Results from a two-phase cohort study. *Psychological Medicine* 38(7):953-961.

Kang, H. K., and T. A. Bullman. 2001. Mortality among US veterans of the Persian Gulf War: 7-year follow-up. *American Journal of Epidemiology* 154(5):399-405.

Kang, H. K., C. M. Mahan, K. Y. Lee, C. A. Magee, and F. M. Murphy. 2000. Illnesses among United States veterans of the Gulf War: A population-based survey of 30,000 veterans. *Journal of Occupational and Environmental Medicine* 42(5):491-501.

Kang, H., C. Magee, C. Mahan, K. Lee, F. Murphy, L. Jackson, and G. Matanoski. 2001. Pregnancy outcomes among U.S. Gulf War veterans: A population-based survey of 30,000 veterans. *Annals of Epidemiology*. 11(7):504-511.

Kang, H. K., C. M. Mahan, K. Y. Lee, F. M. Murphy, S. J. Simmens, H. A. Young, and P. H. Levine. 2002. Evidence for a deployment-related Gulf War syndrome by factor analysis. *Archives of Environmental Health* 57(1):61-68.

Kang, H. K., B. H. Natelson, C. M. Mahan, K. Y. Lee, and F. M. Murphy. 2003. Post-traumatic stress disorder and chronic fatigue syndrome-like illness among Gulf War veterans: A population-based survey of 30,000 veterans. *American Journal of Epidemiology* 157(2):141-148.

Kang, H., N. Dalager, C. Mahan, and E. Ishii. 2005. The role of sexual assault on the risk of PTSD among Gulf War veterans. *Annals of Epidemiology* 15(3):191-195.

Kang, H. K., B. Li, C. M. Mahan, S. A. Eisen, and C. C. Engel. 2009. Health of U.S. veterans of 1991 Gulf War: A follow-up survey in 10 years. *Journal of Occupational and Environmental Medicine* 51(4):401-410.

Karlinsky, J. B., M. Blanchard, R. Alpern, S. A. Eisen, H. Kang, F. M. Murphy, and D. J. Reda. 2004. Late prevalence of respiratory symptoms and pulmonary function abnormalities in Gulf War I veterans. *Archives of Internal Medicine* 164(22):2488-2491.

Kelsall, H. L., M. R. Sim, A. B. Forbes, D. C. Glass, D. P. McKenzie, J. F. Ikin, M. J. Abramson, L. Blizzard, and P. Ittak. 2004a. Symptoms and medical conditions in Australian veterans of the 1991 Gulf War: Relation to immunisations and other Gulf War exposures. *Occupational and Environmental Medicine* 61(12):1006-1013.

Kelsall, H. L., M. R. Sim, A. B. Forbes, D. P. McKenzie, D. C. Glass, J. F. Ikin, P. Ittak, and M. J. Abramson. 2004b. Respiratory health status of Australian veterans of the 1991 Gulf War and the effects of exposure to oil fire smoke and dust storms. *Thorax* 59(10):897-903.

Kelsall, H., R. Macdonell, M. Sim, A. Forbes, D. McKenzie, D. Glass, J. Ikin, and P. Ittak. 2005. Neurological status of Australian veterans of the 1991 Gulf War and the effect of medical and chemical exposures. *International Journal of Epidemiology* 34(4):810-819.

Kelsall, H., M. Sim, D. McKenzie, A. Forbes, K. Leder, D. Glass, J. Ikin, and A. McFarlane. 2006. Medically evaluated psychological and physical health of Australian Gulf War veterans with chronic fatigue. *Journal of Psychosomatic Research* 60(6):575-584.

Kelsall, H. L., M. R. Sim, J. F. Ikin, A. B. Forbes, D. P. McKenzie, D. C. Glass, and P. Ittak. 2007. Reproductive health of male Australian veterans of the 1991 Gulf War. *BMC Public Health* 7:79.

Knoke, J. D., T. C. Smith, G. C. Gray, K. S. Kaiser, and A. W. Hawksworth. 2000. Factor analysis of self-reported symptoms: Does it identify a Gulf War syndrome? *American Journal of Epidemiology* 152(4):379-388.

Lange, J. L., D. A. Schwartz, B. N. Doebbeling, J. M. Heller, and P. S. Thorne. 2002. Exposures to the Kuwait oil fires and their association with asthma and bronchitis among gulf war veterans. *Environmental Health Perspectives* 110(11):1141-1146.

Macfarlane, G. J., E. Thomas, and N. Cherry. 2000. Mortality among UK Gulf War veterans. *Lancet* 356(9223):17-21.

Macfarlane, G. J., A.-M. Biggs, N. Maconochie, M. Hotopf, P. Doyle, and M. Lunt. 2003. Incidence of cancer among UK Gulf War veterans: Cohort study. *British Medical Journal* 327(7428):1373-1375.

Macfarlane, G. J., M. Hotopf, N. Maconochie, N. Blatchley, A. Richards, and M. Lunt. 2005. Long-term mortality amongst Gulf War Veterans: Is there a relationship with experiences during deployment and subsequent morbidity? *International Journal of Epidemiology* 34(6):1403-1408.

Maconochie, N., P. Doyle, G. Davies, S. Lewis, M. Pelerin, S. Prior, and P. Sampson. 2003. The study of reproductive outcome and the health of offspring of UK veterans of the Gulf War: Methods and description of the study population. *BMC Public Health* 3(1):4.

Maconochie, N., P. Doyle, and C. Carson. 2004. Infertility among male UK veterans of the 1990-1 Gulf War: Reproductive cohort study. *British Medical Journal* 329(7459):196-201.

McCauley, L. A., S. K. Joos, M. R. Lasarev, D. Storzbach, and D. N. Bourdette. 1999a. Gulf War unexplained illnesses: Persistence and unexplained nature of self-reported symptoms. *Environmental Research* 81(3):215-223.

McCauley, L. A., S. K. Joos, P. S. Spencer, M. Lasarev, and T. Shuell. 1999b. Strategies to assess validity of self-reported exposures during the Persian Gulf War. *Environmental Research* 81(3):195-205.

McKenzie, D. P., J. F. Ikin, A. C. McFarlane, M. Creamer, A. B. Forbes, H. L. Kelsall, D. C. Glass, P. Ittak, and M. R. Sim. 2004. Psychological health of Australian veterans of the 1991 Gulf War: An assessment using the SF-12, GHQ-12 and PCL-S. *Psychological Medicine* 34(8):1419-1430.

Nisenbaum, R., D. H. Barrett, M. Reyes, and W. C. Reeves. 2000. Deployment stressors and a chronic multisymptom illness among Gulf War veterans. *Journal of Nervous and Mental Disease* 188(5):259-266.

Nisenbaum, R., K. Ismail, S., Wessely, C. Unwin, L. Hull, and W. C. Reeves. 2004. Dichotomous factor analysis of symptoms reported by UK and US veterans of the 1991 Gulf War. *Population Health Metrics* 2(1):8.

NRC (National Research Council). 2000a. *Strategies to Protect the Health of Deployed US Forces: Analytical Framework for Assessing Risks.* Washington, DC: National Academy Press.

NRC. 2000b. *Strategies to Protect the Health of Deployed US Forces: Detecting, Characterizing, and Documenting Exposures.* Washington, DC: National Academy Press.

NRC. 2000c. *Strategies to Protect the Health of Deployed US Forces: Force Protection and Decontamination.* Washington, DC: National Academy Press.

Page, W. F., C. M. Mahan, T. A. Bullman, and H. K. Kang. 2005a. Health effects in Army Gulf War veterans possibly exposed to chemical munitions destruction at Khamisiyah, Iraq: Part I. Morbidity associated with potential exposure. *Military Medicine* 170(11):935-944.

Page, W. F., C. M. Mahan, H. K. Kang, and T. A. Bullman. 2005b. Health effects in Army Gulf War veterans possibly exposed to chemical munitions destruction at Khamisiyah, Iraq: Part II. Morbidity associated with notification of potential exposure. *Military Medicine* 170(11):945-951.

Phillips, C. J., G. R. Matyas, C. J. Hansen, C. R. Alving, T. C. Smith, and M. A. K. Ryan. 2009. Antibodies to squalene in US Navy Persian Gulf War veterans with chronic multisymptom illness. *Vaccine* 27(29):3921-3926.

Proctor, S. P., T. Heeren, R. F. White, J. Wolfe, M. S. Borgos, J. D. Davis, L. Pepper, R. Clapp, P. B. Sutker, J. J. Vasterling, and D. Ozonoff. 1998. Health status of Persian Gulf War veterans: Self-reported symptoms, environmental exposures and the effect of stress. *International Journal of Epidemiology* 27(6):1000-1010.

Proctor, S. P., R. Harley, J. Wolfe, T. Heeren, and R. F. White. 2001a. Health-related quality of life in Persian Gulf War veterans. *Military Medicine* 166(6):510-519.

Proctor, S. P., K. J. Heaton, R. F. White, and J. Wolfe. 2001b. Chemical sensitivity and chronic fatigue in Gulf War veterans: A brief report. *Journal of Occupational and Environmental Medicine* 43(3):259-264.

Proctor, S. P., R. F. White, T. Heeren, F. Debes, B. Gloerfelt-Tarp, M. Appleyard, T. Ishoy, B. Guldager, P. Suadicani, F. Gyntelberg, and D. M. Ozonoff. 2003. Neuropsychological functioning in Danish Gulf War veterans. *Journal of Psychopathology and Behavioral Assessment* 25(2):85-93.

Proctor, S. P., K. J. Heaton, T. Heeren, and R. F. White. 2006. Effects of sarin and cyclosarin exposure during the 1991 Gulf War on neurobehavioral functioning in US Army veterans. *Neurotoxicology* 27(6):931-939.

RAND Corporation. 2010. *12-Item Short Form Health Survey (SF-12).* http://www.rand.org/health/surveys_tools/mos/mos_core_12item.html (accessed January 5, 2010).

Reid, S., M. Hotopf, L. Hull, K. Ismail, C. Unwin, and S. Wessely. 2001. Multiple chemical sensitivity and chronic fatigue syndrome in British Gulf War veterans. *American Journal of Epidemiology* 153(6):604-609.

Rose, M. R., M. K. Sharief, J. Priddin, V. Nikolaou, L. Hull, C. Unwin, R. Ajmal-Ali, R. A. Sherwood, A. Spellman, A. David, and S. Wessely. 2004. Evaluation of neuromuscular symptoms in UK Gulf War veterans: A controlled study. *Neurology* 63(9):1681-1687.

Sharief, M. K., J. Priddin, R. S. Delamont, C. Unwin, M. R. Rose, A. David, and S. Wessely. 2002. Neurophysiologic analysis of neuromuscular symptoms in UK Gulf War veterans: A controlled study. *Neurology* 59(10):1518-1525.

Sim, M., M. Abramson, P. A. Forbes, D. Glass, J. Ikin, P. Ittak, H. Kelsall, K. Leder, D. McKenzie, and J. McNeil. 2003. *Australian Gulf War Veterans' Health Study.* Canberra, Australia: Department of Veterans' Affairs.

Simmons, R., N. Maconochie, and P. Doyle. 2004. Self-reported ill health in male UK Gulf War veterans: A retrospective cohort study. *BMC Public Health* 4(1):27.

Spencer, P. S., L. A. McCauley, J. A. Lapidus, M. Lasarev, S. K. Joos, and D. Storzbach. 2001. Self-reported exposures and their association with unexplained illness in a population-based case-control study of Gulf War veterans. *Journal of Occupational and Environmental Medicine* 43(12):1041-1056.

Statistics Canada. 2005. *The Canadian Persian Gulf Cohort Study: Detailed Report.* Ottawa, Ontario: Minister of Industry.

Steele, L. 2000. Prevalence and patterns of Gulf War illness in Kansas veterans: Association of symptoms with characteristics of person, place, and time of military service. *American Journal of Epidemiology* 152(10):992-1002.

Stimpson, N. J., C. Unwin, L. Hull, T. David, S. Wessely, and G. Lewis. 2006. Prevalence of reported pain, widespread pain, and pain symmetry in veterans of the Persian Gulf War (1990-1991): The use of pain manikins in Persian Gulf War health research. *Military Medicine* 171(12):1181-1186.

Stretch, R. H., P. D. Bliese, D. H. Marlowe, K. M. Wright, K. H. Knudson, and C. H. Hoover. 1995. Physical health symptomatology of Gulf War-era service personnel from the states of Pennsylvania and Hawaii. *Military Medicine* 160(3):131-136.

Stretch, R. H., P. D. Bliese, D. H. Marlowe, K. M. Wright, K. H. Knudson, and C. H. Hoover. 1996a. Psychological health of Gulf War-era military personnel. *Military Medicine* 161(5):257-261.

Stretch, R. H., D. H. Marlowe, K. M. Wright, P. D. Bliese, K. H. Knudson, and C. H. Hoover. 1996b. Post-traumatic stress disorder symptoms among Gulf War veterans. *Military Medicine* 161(7):407-410.

Suadicani, P., T. Ishoy, B. Guldager, M. Appleyard, and F. Gyntelberg. 1999. Determinants of long-term neuropsychological symptoms. *Danish Medical Bulletin* 46(5):423-427.

Sutker, P. B., J. M. Davis, M. Uddo, and S. R. Ditta. 1995. War zone stress, personal resources, and PTSD in Persian Gulf War returnees. *Journal of Abnormal Psychology* 104(3):444-452.

Toomey, R., H. K. Kang, J. Karlinsky, D. G. Baker, J. J. Vasterling, R. Alpern, D. J. Reda, W. G. Henderson, F. M. Murphy, and S. A. Eisen. 2007. Mental health of US Gulf War veterans 10 years after the war. *British Journal of Psychiatry* 190:385-393.

Toomey, R., R. Alpern, J. J. Vasterling, D. G. Baker, D. J. Reda, M. J. Lyons, W. G. Henderson, H. K. Kang, S. A. Eisen, and F. M. Murphy. 2009. Neuropsychological functioning of US Gulf War veterans 10 years after the war. *Journal of the International Neuropsychological Society* 15(5):717-729.

United Kingdom Ministry of Defence. 2000. *Background to the Use of Medical Countermeasures to Protect British Forces During the Gulf War (Operation Granby).* http://www.mod.uk/issues/gulfwar/info/medical/ukchemical.htm (accessed September 26, 2003).

Unwin, C., N. Blatchley, W. Coker, S. Ferry, M. Hotopf, L. Hull, K. Ismail, I. Palmer, A. David, and S. Wessely. 1999. Health of UK servicemen who served in Persian Gulf War. *Lancet* 353(9148):169-178.

White, R. F., S. P. Proctor, T. Heeren, J. Wolfe, M. Krengel, J. Vasterling, K. Lindem, K. J. Heaton, P. Sutker, and D. M. Ozonoff. 2001. Neuropsychological function in Gulf War veterans: Relationships to self-reported toxicant exposures. *American Journal of Industrial Medicine* 40(1):42-54.

4

HEALTH OUTCOMES

Veterans who were deployed to the Persian Gulf War have reported a constellation of symptoms and medical conditions during their deployment and since their return home. Epidemiologic studies comparing veterans who were deployed to the Gulf War with veterans who were in the military during the Gulf War but were not deployed have confirmed that deployed veterans have a greater prevalence of a number of medical conditions, illnesses, and symptoms. This increased reporting of symptoms and prevalence of medical conditions has also been seen in deployed veterans from many of the countries that formed the coalition forces, including the United States, the United Kingdom (UK), Australia, Canada, and Denmark. Recently, French forces deployed to the Gulf War have also been under study, but as yet few results have been published on this cohort.

In this chapter, the studies that have examined the health outcomes that have been reported or diagnosed in Gulf War veterans are presented. In the majority of studies, the prevalence of each medical condition or symptom seen in the deployed veterans is compared with the prevalence seen in nondeployed veterans. Where the prevalence of a symptom or condition has been linked by the study authors to any specific exposures experienced during deployment such as vaccines, oil-well fire smoke, anti-nerve-gas agents, or combat, the committee reviewed those associations as well.

ORGANIZATION OF THE CHAPTER

The committee presents the health outcomes in the order they appear in the *International Statistical Classification of Diseases and Related Health Problems, 10th Edition* (ICD-10),[1] except for the last section, which examines the health status of female Gulf War veterans. The committee considered all possible health effects identified in the studies it reviewed, regardless of the potential cause of the health effect, with the exception of health effects related to or resulting from infectious and parasitic diseases as those outcomes were examined in *Gulf War and Health, Volume 5: Infectious Diseases* (IOM, 2007). The committee considered studies that attempted to link health effects seen in Gulf War veterans to specific deployment exposures such as nerve gas and oil-well fire smoke, but an exhaustive search of the toxicologic and

[1]The *International Statistical Classification of Diseases and Related Health Problems* (ICD) provides a detailed description of known diseases and injuries. Every disease (or group of related diseases) is given a unique code. ICD is periodically revised and is currently in its 10th edition (ICD-10) and available at http://www.who.int/classifications/apps/icd/icd10online/.

epidemiologic literature on all the possible environmental agents to which Gulf War veterans might have been exposed was not conducted.

For each health effect presented in this chapter, the committee first summarizes the primary studies and secondary or supporting studies that were included in *Gulf War and Health, Volume 4: Health Effects of Serving in the Gulf War* (referred to as *Volume 4*). The committee then identifies additional primary and secondary studies from its updated literature searches and reconsiders the studies described in *Volume 4* taking into account these updates. Although many of the studies are new and were published after *Volume 4* was completed in 2006, some of the additional studies cited by the Update committee were published before or during 2006 but were not discussed in *Volume 4*. Because the Volume 4 committee was tasked with identifying those health effects seen at greater prevalence in deployed versus nondeployed Gulf War veterans and not with determining the strength of the association between deployment and the development of a particular health effect, not every study that examined an association between a health effect and Gulf War exposures was included in *Volume 4*. Therefore, the Update committee reviewed the categorization (primary or secondary) of all of the studies considered for *Volume 4* as well as any new studies identified from an updated literature search. All studies for each health outcome, including those originally cited in *Volume 4*, were reviewed and categorized as primary or secondary by the entire committee in plenary session, before it came to a consensus on the appropriate category of association to be assigned to each health outcome. Consistent with previous volumes of the *Gulf War and Health* series, the primary studies on which the committee based its conclusions are detailed in the evidence table at the end of each health outcome section. Using this weight-of-the-evidence approach required that the Update committee be more rigorous in its review of the studies in *Volume 4*; as a result some studies considered to be primary in *Volume 4* were recategorized as secondary for this report and vice versa. Thus, the Update committee summarizes de novo the information from both *Volume 4* and any new literature to arrive at its conclusions on the strength of the association between deployment to the Gulf War and a health outcome.

As described in Chapter 2, a primary study had to include information about the putative exposure (generally deployment) and specific health outcomes, demonstrate rigorous methods, include adequate details of its methods to allow a thorough assessment, include an appropriate control or reference group, and provide appropriate adjustment for confounders. It is of note that many of the large cohort studies examined multiple outcomes and so might be referred to in more than one place in this report. A given study might be deemed a primary study for one or more health outcome and be a secondary study for another outcome, based on how each health outcome was defined and measured. For example, a particular study might be well designed for assessing diabetes because the authors used a strong indicator such as blood glucose levels to identify this disorder, but the same study might not be well designed for assessing a psychiatric disorder because the authors used only a screening instrument to identify the disorder. In general, only primary studies appear in the evidence tables that accompany the discussion of each health outcome.

A secondary study typically had methodological limitations, such as not including a rigorous or well-defined method of diagnosis, or a lack of an appropriate control group. The secondary studies were reviewed and included in the discussion because they evaluated the same health outcomes and in some cases provided useful information on veteran populations from the same conflicts as the primary studies. For this reason it was felt that secondary studies add information that might modify (increase or decrease) confidence in the conclusions, which are made based on review of primary studies. Confidence in a secondary study is substantially reduced if the statistical analysis did not include adjustment for confounders, if the data were obtained from self-reported cross-sectional surveys or from screening instruments that relied solely on self-reports of diagnoses, or if response rates were unacceptably low. Without supportive evidence from primary studies, the potential for unreliable findings due to bias, chance, or multiple comparisons may outweigh the extent to which secondary studies may contribute, even collectively, to the overall conclusion of the committee about an association between deployment and any specific health outcome. Understanding the relationship between a health outcome and deployment may also be hampered by attempts to identify specific harmful exposures based on recall many years after the war. Virtually none of the studies verified veterans' reported exposures against military records.

This chapter excludes studies of participants in Gulf War registries established by the Department of Veterans Affairs (VA) or the Department of Defense (DoD), which were not intended to be representative of the population of Gulf War veterans. Registry participants cannot be considered representative of all Gulf War veterans in that they are self-selected, and many may have joined the registries because they believed that they have symptoms of a new medical syndrome; they were not a random sample of Gulf War military personnel, and there is no nondeployed comparison group.

CANCER

Cancer can develop at any age but about 77% of cancers are diagnosed in people aged 55 and older. Furthermore, cancer is a disease of long latency, meaning that often the diagnosis of a cancer does not occur until 15 to 20 years or longer after the exposure that caused it (Cogliano et al., 2004). Therefore, many veterans are still young for cancer diagnoses (the mean age of military personnel during the Gulf War was 28), and for most cancers, the time since the Gulf War is probably too short to expect to observe the onset of cancer. Cancers with younger average age at onset, and also possible shorter latency periods, can include testicular cancer, skin cancer, leukemias and lymphomas, and brain cancer.

The majority of observations on the association of overall and cause-specific cancers (that is, malignant neoplasms) with Gulf War deployment are discussed in studies of general mortality and hospitalizations, rather than in reports focused specifically on cancer. However, a few studies on brain and testicular cancer in Gulf War veterans have been published. All studies in which malignant neoplasms, as a group or at particular sites, are specifically identified are reviewed here and summarized in Table 4-1.

Summary of *Volume 4*

Brain Cancer

The Volume 4 committee identified one cohort mortality study assessing the relationship between nerve-agent exposure caused by weapons demolition at Khamisiyah with brain cancer deaths in US Gulf War veterans. Bullman et al. (2005) explored the relationship between estimated exposure to chemical munitions destruction (sarin gas) at Khamisiyah in 1991 with cause-specific mortality of Gulf War veterans through December 31, 2000. Using the DoD's 2000 sarin plume exposure model (Rostker, 2000), 100,487 military personnel were identified as potentially exposed and 224,980 similarly deployed military personnel were considered unexposed. The study reported an increased risk of brain cancer deaths in the exposed population (relative risk [RR] 1.94, 95% confidence interval [CI] 1.12-3.34; 25 exposed cases vs 27 unexposed cases) and there was a suggestion of a dose-response relationship with increased risk among those who were considered exposed for 2 days (6 cases) relative to 1 day (19 cases) (RR 3.26, 95% CI 1.33-7.96 and RR 1.72, 95% CI 0.95-3.10, respectively). The authors also discussed modeling exposure to smoke from oil-well fires as a confounder, and the effect estimates for exposure to Khamisiyah nerve agents remained elevated. There was no significant elevation in risk associated with exposure to oil-well fires as a main effect. Because brain cancer likely has a latent period of 10-20 years and Bullman et al. (2005) had fewer than 9 years of follow-up, the Volume 4 committee concluded that additional follow-up is needed to draw any definitive conclusions concerning the association between deployment to the Gulf War and the development of brain cancer.

Testicular Cancer

The Volume 4 committee identified two studies that specifically examined testicular cancer among US servicemen during the Gulf War: Knoke et al. (1998) and Levine et al. (2005), and one study of military hospitalizations where a positive association for testicular cancer was observed (Gray et al., 1996). Gray and colleagues (1996) examined all-cause hospitalizations in DoD hospitals from August 1, 1991, through September 30, 1993, for 517,223 deployed and 1,291,323 nondeployed Gulf War servicemen. They observed an increased risk of hospitalization for testicular cancer among the deployed (standardized rate ratio 2.12, 95% CI 1.11-4.02) in the last 5 months of 1991, the period immediately after the end of deployment. However, the increased risk did not carry over into 1992 or into the first 9 months of 1993. Knoke et al. (1998) focused on the cases of first diagnosis of testicular cancer in this cohort, continuing follow-up until March 31, 1996. They observed no association with deployment status (standardized rate ratio 1.05, 95% CI 0.86-1.29). This pattern of increased incidence immediately after the war with a tapering off with time likely demonstrates a healthy warrior effect. In other words, the peak probably represented a regression to the mean after healthier people were selected for deployment and there was deferment of care during deployment. The limitations of these studies are that they were restricted to active-duty military personnel and did not include veterans who may have left the service because of poor health or those who sought treatment elsewhere.

Levine et al. (2005) conducted a pilot study matching data from the District of Columbia and New Jersey cancer-registry cases with the records of 621,902 deployed Gulf War veterans and 746,248 veterans serving at the same time as the Gulf War but not deployed. Testicular cancer cases yielded a crude proportional incidence rate (PIR) of 3.05 (95% CI 1.47-6.35) that was attenuated after adjustment for state of residence, deployment status, race, and age (PIR 2.33; 95% CI 0.95-5.70). No definitive conclusions could be made until additional registries are added.

All Cancers

The Volume 4 committee included results from two primary mortality studies. Kang and Bullman (2001) compared cause-specific mortality rates in the same database of Gulf War deployed veterans and nondeployed veterans used for the Levine et al. (2005) study described above. Vital status was determined using databases of the VA and the Social Security Administration (SSA). Over the follow-up period of 1991 to 1997, there were no significant excesses of overall cancer deaths or deaths from cancer at any specific site among deployed veterans compared with the controls (total cancers: males, OR 0.90, 95% CI 0.81-1.01; females, OR 1.11, 95% CI 0.78-1.57).

Macfarlane et al. (2003) conducted a cohort study among 51,721 UK servicemembers deployed to the Persian Gulf and 50,755 nondeployed servicemembers using the National Health Service Cancer Register to identify first diagnoses of malignant cancer through July 31, 2002. The rate ratio for unspecified cancer was 0.99 (95% CI 0.83-1.17), after adjusting for sex, age, service branch, and rank. In subgroups of the cohort who participated in morbidity surveys and provided information on smoking and alcohol use, the adjusted rate ratio for all cancers was 1.12 (95% CI 0.86-1.45).

Updated and Supplemental Literature

Primary Studies

The Update committee identified one new primary study of brain cancer mortality. It also identified three studies of hospitalization or incidence, one mortality study, and one combined study where cancer was specifically assessed.

Brain Cancer

In continued mortality follow-up through 2004 of the 621,902 Gulf War deployed veterans and 746,248 nondeployed veterans originally studied by Kang and Bullman (2001), Barth et al. (2009) focused on mortality from neurological causes, that is, amyotrophic lateral sclerosis (ALS), multiple sclerosis (MS), Parkinson's disease, and primary brain cancer. The cases included in the Bullman et al. study (2005) described above, also were identified from this cohort and were included in the Barth et al. study. A total of 144 cases of brain cancer were identified among the deployed veterans and 228 among the nondeployed for a mortality rate ratio (RR) of 0.90 (95% CI 0.73-1.11), adjusted for race, branch of service, type of unit, age, marital status at entry to follow-up, and sex. Within the Gulf War cohort, exposure to nerve agents from the Khamisiyah explosion for 2 or more days (Winkenwerder, 2002) and exposure to oil-well fire smoke (Rostker, 2000) were both positively associated with risk of brain cancer mortality when modeled simultaneously (adjusted rate ratios 2.71, 95% CI 1.25-5.87 and 1.81, 95% CI 1.00-3.27, respectively). Of the 43 brain cancer cases exposed to oil-well fires, 20 were also exposed for at least 1 day at Khamisiyah (S. Barth, Department of Veterans Affairs, personal communication, November 30, 2009).

Medical records were obtained for 236 of the 372 cases of brain cancer (63%). The record review resulted in 204 confirmed cases, 13 probable cases, and 19 misclassified cancers. The risk of dying from brain cancer did not change with the removal of the 19 misclassified cancers.

Hospitalization Studies

Gray et al. (2000) conducted an expanded analysis of their original 1996 study of hospitalizations to include US Gulf War veterans (n = 652,979) and nondeployed veterans (random selection of n = 652,922 from 2,912,737 total) who had separated from the armed services and those who served in the National Guard or reserve. Hospitalization data from the DoD, the VA, and California Office of Statewide Health Planning and Development over the period August 1, 1991, through December 31, 1994, were assessed separately. There was no evidence of increased hospitalization from neoplasms among the Gulf War veterans compared to the nondeployed veterans in any of the three hospital systems.

Smith et al. (2006) compared cause-specific postdeployment hospitalization in DoD military treatment facilities during the period October 1, 1988, through December 31, 2000, among US active-duty servicemembers who served in the Gulf War (n = 455,465), Southwest Asia following the Gulf War (n = 249,047), or Bosnia, also following the Gulf War (n = 44,341). After adjusting for age, sex, marital status, pay grade, race/ethnicity, service branch, occupation, and predeployment hospitalization, the hazard ratio (HR) for nondefined neoplasms was 1.03 (95% CI 0.93-1.15) for the Gulf War deployed veterans compared to the Southwest Asia cohort and 0.61 (95% CI 0.50-0.76) compared to the Bosnia group. The adjusted HR for testicular cancer in Gulf War veterans was 0.64 (95% CI 0.32-1.28) and 0.80 (95% CI 0.27-2.39) compared to the Southwest Asia and Bosnia groups, respectively.

Mortality Studies

The UK Defence Analytical Service Agency (DASA, 2009) published summary statistics comparing mortality rates of 53,409 UK Gulf War veterans with those of 53,143 UK armed forces personnel of similar age, sex, service status, and rank who were in service at the same time, but not deployed to the gulf (era cohort). It reported 209 and 228 malignant neoplasms among the gulf and era cohorts, respectively (age-adjusted mortality RR 0.97, 95% CI 0.81-1.18). They did not observe any significant associations for specific neoplasms.

The Canadian Department of National Defense used the national mortality database and the national cancer registry to examine mortality rates and cancer incidence among Canadian Gulf War veterans from 1991 through 1999 (Statistics Canada, 2005). Two cohorts were established—the deployed cohort consisting of 5117 servicemembers sent to the gulf between August 1990 and October 1991, and the nondeployed cohort of 6093 servicemembers who were eligible for deployment but were not deployed. During the follow-up period, 10 deaths from cancer were identified in the deployed cohort and 15 in the nondeployed. The age-adjusted HR was 0.85 (95% CI 0.38-1.90). Among the deployed and nondeployed cohorts 29 and 42 incident cancers, respectively, were identified (age-adjusted HR 0.86, 95% CI 0.54-1.39). The largest number of the cases were cancers of the digestive tract (n = 15). There were also 8 testicular cancers and 4 brain cancers (all among the nondeployed). There was no evidence of an association between deployment and these specific cancers.

In continued follow-up of the study by Macfarlane et al. (2003) (discussed above), there was still no excess risk of mortality from malignant neoplasms with 2 more years of data (RR 1.01, 95% CI 0.79-1.30) (Macfarlane et al., 2005).

Secondary Studies

The Update committee identified eight secondary studies of multiple outcomes that had been included in *Volume 4*, but had not been considered in that review of malignant neoplasms (Goss Gilroy, 1998; Iowa Persian Gulf Study Group, 1997; Ishoy et al., 1999a; Kang et al., 2000; Kelsall et al., 2004a; McCauley et al., 2002; Simmons et al., 2004; Steele, 2000). Because there is specific mention of cancer in these studies, they are described here in chronological order.

From September 1995 through May 1996, the Iowa Persian Gulf Study Group (1997) performed a cross-sectional telephone survey to solicit self-reported illness in Iowan military personnel active during the Gulf War (n = 4886). Members of the National Guard who had been deployed (n = 911) were more likely to report any cancer than nondeployed National Guards members (n = 831) (prevalence difference [PD] 1.3, 95% CI 0.6-2.0), but the prevalence was similar compared with the deployed (n = 985) and nondeployed regular military (n = 968) (PD 0.3, 95% CI −0.6-1.2). Specific reports of skin cancer followed a similar pattern.

The Canadian Department of National Defense commissioned Goss Gilroy, Inc., to assess the prevalence of health outcomes in Canadian forces deployed to the Gulf War (Goss Gilroy, 1998). In 1997, a questionnaire was administered to 3113 Gulf War deployed veterans and 3439 active but nondeployed Canadian veterans. Among the respondents 20-44 years of age, 0.8% of the deployed veterans and 0.5% of the nondeployed reported any cancer, and among the 45-65 year olds, the prevalence of any cancer was 4.2% in the deployed veterans and 2.5% in the nondeployed veterans.

Ishoy et al. (1999a) conducted a cross-sectional clinical examination study during 1997. Participants included Danish servicemembers deployed to the Gulf (n = 686) and eligible but nondeployed Danish servicemembers (n = 231). Skin cancer was assessed; however, results were not presented since the p-value comparing the two groups was greater than 0.05.

Kang et al. (2000) conducted a health survey comparing self-reported health outcomes for a population based sample of 15,000 deployed and 15,000 nondeployed US Gulf War veterans. Based on the responses from 11,441 deployed and 9476 nondeployed veterans, they estimated the population prevalence rates of various medical conditions. The estimated population prevalence for skin cancer was 1.5% for the deployed and 1.4% for the nondeployed veterans, with a significant difference (rate difference 0.15, 95% CI 0.11-0.19).

A population based survey of Kansas veterans deployed to the gulf (n = 1548) and nondeployed (n = 482) examined the health outcomes of deployment through automated telephone interviews to define and establish prevalence of "Gulf War illness" symptom complex (Steele, 2000). The incidence of disease diagnosed or treated by a physician was tracked through 1998. The OR for cancers, not including skin cancer (n = 18) was 1.21 (95% CI 0.40-3.69), and the OR for skin cancer (n = 23) was 1.17 (95% CI 0.47-2.90), adjusting for sex, age, income, and level of education.

In 1999, McCauley et al. (2002) conducted a telephone survey of 2918 active or reserve Army or National Guard veterans resident in Oregon, Washington, California, Georgia, or North Carolina. Among the 1263 deployed subjects, 21 incident cancers were reported, compared to 3 among the 516 nondeployed comparison group (OR 3.0, 95% CI 1.0-13.1). Details on year of diagnosis and type of cancer were obtained for 20 of the 24 cases. When all skin cancers (n = 7) and cases that were not confirmed at the time of telephone follow-up (n = 4) were excluded, the OR was 4.94 (95% CI 0.6-38.1) and there was no apparent trend for any specific type of cancer. Among the Gulf War veterans, there was no indication of an association of cancer risk with exposure to nerve agents at Khamisiyah, defined as being within a 50-km radius of Khamisiyah between March 4, 1991, and March 13, 1991 (OR for exposed vs unexposed 0.4, 95% CI 0.1-1.4).

A cohort study of Australian service personnel who had (n = 1456) or had not (n = 1588) been deployed to the gulf was designed to investigate the association of symptoms and medical conditions with immunizations and other Gulf War exposures (Kelsall et al., 2004a). This study was included in *Volume 4* as a major cohort study and specifically in the reviews of diseases of the circulatory system, diseases of the respiratory system, and symptoms in general. However, skin cancer, other than malignant melanoma, was also one of the 15 most frequently doctor-diagnosed medical conditions reported by the participants. After medical record review, 92 deployed veterans and 110 nondeployed veterans had a possible or probable diagnosis of the malignancy. The OR, adjusted for service type, rank, age, education, and marital status was 1.0 (95% CI 0.7-1.3).

Simmons et al. (2004) conducted a retrospective cohort study of male UK Gulf War deployed veterans (n = 23,358) and a comparable cohort of nondeployed veterans (n = 17,730) for self-reported health outcomes. Among the deployed veterans, 127 cancer cases, including malignant neoplasms and brain tumors were reported, compared to 88 among the nondeployed veterans (OR 1.1, 95% CI 0.9-1.5).

Finally, the Update committee identified two new secondary studies with information on cancer outcomes. From 1994 to 1996, Proctor et al. (2001a) evaluated health-related quality of life among 141 Gulf War deployed veterans and 46 veterans deployed to Germany, selected from active-duty, reserve and National Guard troops deployed through Fort Devens, Massachusetts. Among the Gulf War deployed veterans and the Germany deployed participants, 2.1% and 4.4% respectively, reported cancer, excluding skin cancer. In 2005, Kang and colleagues published a follow-up survey of the sample (15,000 deployed and 15,000 nondeployed US Gulf War veterans) described in the earlier study (Kang et al., 2000, 2009). Among the 6111 deployed and 3859 era veterans who responded, 1160 reported skin cancer diagnoses and 990 reported "other cancer." The risk ratios, adjusted for age, sex, race, body mass index, current cigarette smoking, rank, branch of service, and unit component, for skin cancer and other cancer were 1.09 (95% CI 0.97-1.22) and 1.09 (95% CI 0.96-1.24), respectively.

Summary and Conclusions

There is no consistent evidence of a higher overall incidence of cancer in veterans who were deployed to the Gulf War than in nondeployed veterans. An association of brain-cancer mortality with possible nerve-agent exposure (based on the 2000 DoD exposure model) was observed in one study discussed in *Volume 4* (Bullman et al., 2005), and the association holds up with an additional 4 years of follow-up in the same cohort (Barth et al., 2009). The association with exposure to smoke from oil-well fires became stronger with further follow-up. However, the numbers of cases of brain cancer who had possibly been exposed to nerve agents as a result of the Khamisiyah explosion was small, and there is little previous evidence of an association of sarin or organophosphate pesticides with brain cancer. Therefore, the committee concluded that there was insufficient/inadequate evidence of an association between Gulf War exposures and brain cancer. Mixed results for testicular cancer were reported by the Volume 4 committee; however, the Update committee did not identify any new studies of this cancer site. In general, many veterans are still too young for cancer diagnoses, and for most cancers the follow-up period after the Gulf War is probably too short to expect the onset of cancer. Therefore, the committee believes that further follow-up is necessary to be able to make a conclusion about whether there is an association between deployment during the Gulf War and cancer outcomes.

The committee concludes that there is insufficient/inadequate evidence of an association between deployment to the Gulf War and any cancer.

Recommendation: Due to the long latency period for cancer, there needs to be continued follow-up of Gulf War veterans and an appropriate comparison group to adequately determine any association.

TABLE 4-1 Cancer

Study	Design	Population	Outcomes	Results	Adjustments	Comments
Brain cancer						
Bullman et al., 2005 (Vol. 4)	Cohort mortality study (population from same source as Kang and Bullman, 1996, 2001)	100,487 US Army GWVs exposed to chemical warfare agents at Khamisiyah; 224,980 nonexposed Army GWVs; exposure determined from the DoD plume model	Brain cancer mortality through December 2000 ascertained from BIRLS and NDI	Exposed (25 cases) vs unexposed (27 cases) RR 1.94 (95% CI 1.12-3.34); Exposed 1 day: RR 1.72 (95% CI 0.95-3.10) Exposed 2+ days: RR 3.26 (95% CI 1.33-7.96)	Age at entry, race, sex, unit component, and rank	9-year follow-up likely too short to examine brain cancer risk (increases with time since exposure); multiple comparisons; death certificate diagnosis
Barth et al., 2009 (Update)	Mortality cohort study, follow-up through 2004 of same cohort as Kang and Bullman (2001)	621,902 US GWVs and 746,248 nondeployed era veterans; 98,406 GWVs exposed to Khamisiyah nerve agents; 123,478 GWVs exposed to oil-well fire smoke	Brain cancer mortality	GWVs (144 cases) compared to era veterans (228 cases) MRR 0.90 (95% CI 0.73-1.11) Khamisiyah exposed: MRR 2.71 (95% CI 1.25-5.87) Oil-well fire smoke exposed: MRR 1.81 (95% CI 1.00-3.27)	Race, service branch, type of unit, age, marital status, and sex	Similar results after 19 misclassified cancers were removed from analysis
Testicular cancer						
Knoke et al., 1998 (Vol. 4)	Cohort study (follow-up of Gray et al., 1996)	US, all regular, active-duty male servicemembers GWVs (n = 517,223) NDVs (n = 1,291,323)	First diagnosis of testicular cancer at US military hospitals worldwide (7/31/1991-3/31/1996)	GWVs (134 cases) vs NDVs (371 cases) RR 1.05 (95% CI 0.86-1.29)	Race or ethnicity, age, occupation	Short follow-up time, but right age range; no specific exposures evaluated; military hospitals only
Levine et al., 2005 (Vol. 4)	Population-based survey—pilot study	US, all personnel (including reserves) deployed to Gulf War (GWVs) and random sample of NDVs; GWVs (n = 621,902) NDVs (n = 746,248)	Testicular cancers diagnosed 1991-1999 and registered by DC or NJ Cancer Registries	GWVs (cases = 17) vs NDVs (cases = 11) (358 males with cancer) PIR 2.33 (95% CI 0.95-5.70)	Age, state of residence, deployment status, race	

Study	Design	Population	Outcomes	Results	Adjustments	Comments
Gray et al., 1996 (Vol. 4)	Hospitalizations from August 1991 through September 1993	547,076 active-duty GWVs, 618,335 non-GWVs	Hospital-discharge diagnoses of testicular cancer (ICD-9-CM Code 186)	GWVs vs nondeployed Last 5 months of 1991: 29 cases vs 14 cases, SRR 2.12 (95% CI 1.11-4.02) 1992: SRR 1.39 (95% CI 0.91-2.11) 1993: SRR 0.89 (95% CI 0.54-1.44)	Prewar hospitalization, sex, age, race, service branch, marital status, rank, length of service, salary, occupation	Limitations: restricted to persons remaining on active duty after the war, and thus does not include veterans who may have left the service due to poor health; no adjustment for other potential confounders
All cancers						
Kang and Bullman, 2001 (Vol. 4)	Cohort mortality study; follow-up from 1991 through 1997	Deployed GWVs (n = 621,902) compared to random sample of nondeployed era veterans (n = 746,248)	Overall cancer mortality ascertained from BIRLS, death certificates, and NDI	Males: GWVs (cases = 477) vs controls (cases = 860): RR 0.90 (95% CI 0.81-1.01) Females: GWVs (cases = 49) vs controls (cases = 103): RR 1.11 (95% CI 0.78-1.57)	Age, race, branch of service, unit component, marital status	Short latency; low age range; death certificates
Macfarlane et al., 2003 (Vol. 4)	Cohort (follow-up of Macfarlane et al., 2000)	51,721 UK GWVs, 50,755 NDVs; random samples Subgroup of 28,518 GWVs and 20,829 era veterans with records of smoking and alcohol use	Cancers identified from National Health Service Central Register; first diagnosis 4/1/1991-7/31/2002	GWVs (cases = 270) vs NDVs (cases = 269) Main study: RR 0.99 (95% CI 0.83-1.17) Subgroup: RR 1.12 (95% CI 0.86-1.45)	Main analysis: sex, age group, service branch, rank Subgroup: smoking, alcohol use	Follow-up period shorter than expected latency for most cancers; low age; grouped all cancer sites due to low numbers of occurrences
Gray et al., 2000 (Update)	Retrospective cohort, hospitalizations from August 1991 through December 1994	652,979 GWVs, 652,922 randomly selected NDVs 182,164 DoD hospitalizations; 16,030 VA hospitalizations; 5,185 COSHPD hospitalizations	Hospital-discharge diagnoses of neoplasms in DoD, VA, and COSHPD hospital systems	DoD PMR 0.98 (95% CI 0.94-1.01) VA PMR 0.88 (95% CI 0.78-0.98) COSHPD PMR 0.86 (95% CI 0.61-1.1)	Age, sex, race	Able to assess only illnesses that resulted in hospitalization; possible undetected confounders

Study	Design	Population	Outcomes	Results	Adjustments	Comments
Smith et al., 2006 (Update)	Hospitalizations cohort study (cohort data from DMDC)	Active-duty personnel with a single deployment to: Gulf War theatre (n = 455,465); Southwest Asia peacekeeping mission, 1991-1998 (n = 249,047); Bosnia, 1995-1998 (n = 44,341)	Postdeployment hospitalization events (1991-2000) for an ICD-9-CM diagnosis of malignant neoplasm (140-208), and for testicular cancer specifically	Veterans of Bosnia and veterans of SW Asia compared to GW veterans Any neoplasm: Bosnia HR 0.61 (95% CI 0.50-0.76) SW Asia HR 1.03 (95% CI 0.93-1.15) Testicular cancer: Bosnia HR 0.80 (95% CI 0.27-2.39) SW Asia HR 0.64 (95% CI 0.32-1.28)	Sex, age, marital status, pay grade, race/ethnicity, service branch, occupation, and predeployment hospitalization; time-dependent covariate to account for changing hospitalization methods, diagnostic criteria, and procedures	Active-duty personnel only; hospitalizations at DoD facilities only
DASA, 2009 (Update)	Summary statistics of causes of death from April 1, 1991 to December 31, 2007	UK GWVs (n = 53,409) vs era veterans (n = 53,143)	Mortality due to malignant neoplasms	GWVs (209 cases) compared to era veterans (228 cases) MMR 0.97 (95% CI 0.81-1.18) No significant difference in mortality rate was found for any of the specific classes of malignant neoplasm included in the study	Single years of age structure of the Gulf cohort at January 1, 1991	
Statistics Canada, 2005 (Update)	Retrospective cohort study (based on Goss Gilroy, 1998) Approximately 2200 members of the deployed cohort were in the gulf region during combat period	5117 Canadian GWVs; 6093 Canadian era veterans, frequency matched for age, sex, and military duty status	Mortality and cancer incidences determined from the CMD and CCD through 1999	Cancer mortality, HR 0.85 (95% CI 0.38-1.09) Incidence of any cancer (HR 0.86, 95% CI 0.54-1.39); cancer of the digestive system (HR 2.00, 95% CI 0.62-6.12); testicular cancer (HR 0.76, 95% CI 0.18-3.24); cancer of the lymph nodes (HR 0.65, 95% CI 0.16-2.62)	Age, rank	Limitations: Small sample size with low statistical power; young age of cohort; short follow-up period; no information on confounding factors

Study	Design	Population	Outcomes	Results	Adjustments	Comments
Macfarlane et al., 2005 (Update)	Mortality cohort; 13-year follow-up	51,753 UK GW deployed veterans and 50,808 era veterans, randomly selected, matched by age, sex, service branch, rank; also fitness for active service in the army and Royal Air Force	Mortality due to malignant neoplasms	GWVs (123 deaths) compared to era veterans (130 deaths): MRR 1.01 (95% CI 0.79-1.30)		Complete and long-term follow-up; cohort of moderate size; potentially other uncontrolled confounders such as smoking

NOTE: BIRLS = Beneficiary Identification Records Locator System; CCD = Canadian Cancer Database; CMD = Canadian Mortality Database; DMDC = Defense Manpower Data Center; GW = Gulf War; GWV = Gulf War veteran; HR = adjusted hazard ratio; MMR = mortality rate ratio; NDI = National Death Index; NDV = nondeployed veteran; NHSCR = National Health Service Central Register; PHQ = Patient Health Questionnaire; PIR = proportional incidence ratio; RR = adjusted risk ratio; SEER = Surveillance Epidemiology and End Results; SF-12 = 12-item short form health survey; SIR = standardized incidence ratio; SMR = standardized mortality ratio; SRR = standardized rate ratio.

DISEASES OF THE BLOOD AND BLOOD-FORMING ORGANS

Diseases of the blood and blood forming organs include conditions affecting blood cells (erythrocytes, leukocytes, platelets) as well as the organs where these cells are produced (bone marrow, lymph nodes, spleen). The etiology of these disorders is varied, including genetic conditions, exposure to toxins and medications, infections or nutritional deficiencies. Diseases of the blood were not considered separately from other conditions in *Volume 4*, thus, this section does not include a summary of that volume. Primary studies are summarized in Table 4-2.

Updated and Supplemental Literature

Primary Studies

A number of studies have compared hospitalizations for diseases of the blood in veterans deployed and nondeployed to the Gulf War. For the purpose of this review, those studies have been considered primary. In addition to hospitalization studies, three published reports have examined hematologic parameters using laboratory tests in deployed and nondeployed Gulf War veterans.

Gray et al. (1996) used a retrospective cohort approach comparing hospitalizations among 547,076 Gulf War deployed and 618,335 nondeployed active-duty personnel at DoD medical facilities. Hospitalizations for 14 ICD-9-CM diagnostic categories, which included "diseases of the blood," were assessed across three time periods following the war: August 1, 1991, to December 31, 1991; January 1, 1992, to December 31, 1992; and January 1, 1993, to September 30, 1993. Hospitalizations for diseases of the blood, primarily anemia, were increased among the Gulf War deployed personnel (vs nondeployed) during 1992 only. Differences, however, were not consistent over time and could be accounted for by deferred diagnoses during deployment. Limitations of this study include the relatively short follow-up, the lack of outpatient data, restriction to DoD hospitals, restriction to hospitalizations of those who remained on active duty after the war, and limited adjustment for potential confounders.

A later publication expanded the previous study to include hospitalizations for reservists and separated military personnel over the same three time periods as Gray et al. (1996). In addition to examining hospitalization data from DoD hospitals, this study also included hospital stays from the VA system and the California Office of Statewide Health Planning and Development for the years 1991-1994 (Gray et al., 2000). Denominator data for this analysis (the total number of veterans in each group) were not available, which led the researchers to use proportional morbidity ratios. The results did not provide evidence that blood diseases were more frequent among deployed than nondeployed veterans. Age and sex-adjusted proportional morbidity ratios for blood diseases in deployed versus nondeployed were 1.1 (95% CI 1.0-1.2) in DoD hospitals, 0.8 (95% CI 0.5-1.0) in VA hospitals, and 1.1 (0.2-2.0) in California hospitals. This analysis is limited since outpatient diagnoses were not included. Hospitalization rates were not estimated, and the analysis did allow for adjustment for confounding.

Hospitalizations for blood disorders were examined in an additional study comparing hospitalization rates in DoD hospitals through 2000 in three cohorts of veterans: Gulf War veterans, veterans deployed to Southwest Asia after the Gulf War, and veterans deployed to Bosnia (Smith et al., 2006). After adjustment for sex, age, marital status, pay grade, race/ethnicity, service branch, occupation, and predeployment hospitalizations, the rate of hospitalizations for blood diseases (identified according to ICD-9-CM discharge codes) was similar in the three cohorts (Southwest Asia vs Gulf War veterans: HR 0.93, 95% CI 0.80-1.07; Bosnia vs Gulf War veterans: HR 0.93, 95% CI 0.75-1.15).

An earlier analysis by Smith et al. (2002) compared postwar hospitalizations among 405,142 active-duty Gulf War veterans who left the region after the war. Data for DoD hospitals were compared through July 1999 according to levels of exposure to oil-well fires in 1991 ranging from unexposed to an average daily exposure of greater than 260 $\mu g/m^3$ for more than 50 days. The duration and length of exposure to particulate matter from the smoke were based on meteorological data, diffusion modeling and troop location data. This study did not observe a clear association between oil-well fire exposure and hospitalizations for blood disorders. The adjusted risk ratios for blood disorder hospitalization in those with the highest exposure to oil-well fires (> 260 $\mu g/m^3$ for > 50 days) was 0.9 compared to those with no exposure. As with other studies of hospitalizations in DoD hospitals, the main limitations of this study include the lack of information on outpatient diagnosis as well as hospitalizations among those who left the service.

Smith et al. (2003) also examined hospitalizations for blood disorders according to potential exposure to nerve agents from the Khamisiyah demolition. Exposure to nerve agents was modeled following the 2000 Khamisiyah gaseous hazard area modeling done by the DoD. Rate of hospitalizations in DoD hospitals for these disorders were equivalent in those potentially exposed and nonexposed (risk ratio 0.96, 95% CI 0.89-1.03).

Two studies measured hematologic parameters in deployed and nondeployed veterans. A study conducted in 1997 among 686 Danish Gulf War veterans and 231 Danish nondeployed controls measured hemoglobin and blood cell counts in both groups (Ishoy et al., 1999b). In bivariate analyses, no differences were observed between deployed and nondeployed in blood hemoglobin (9.3 mmol/L in both groups), erythrocyte count (4.8 million/L in both groups), hematocrit (0.44 in both groups), mean corpuscular volume (91 10^{-15} L per cell in both groups), and leukocyte count (5.8 10^9/L in deployed and 5.9 10^9/L in nondeployed). Leukocyte fractions were also comparable. Platelet counts were slightly lower in deployed compared to nondeployed (205 10^9/L vs 211 10^9/L, $p < 0.05$). Differences in response rate (84% in deployed and 58% in nondeployed) and lack of adjustment for potential confounders reduces the usefulness of these results.

The Australian Gulf War Veterans' Health Study (Sim et al., 2003) measured hemoglobin and other hematologic parameters in 1355 male and 30 female Gulf War veterans and in 1361 male and 32 female nondeployed veterans. In the males, hemoglobin (153.1 g/L vs 153.4 g/L), mean corpuscular volume (91.6 femtoliters $[fl]^2$ vs 91.5 fl^2), mean corpuscular hemoglobin (30.4 picograms$[pg]^3$ vs 30.5 pg)^3, platelets (227.8 10^9/L vs 231.3 10^9/L), and leukocytes (6.3 10^9/L vs 6.2 10^9/L) were similar in deployed and nondeployed veterans. No differences were observed for leukocyte fractions. In female veterans, deployed and nondeployed also presented similar hematologic parameters (hemoglobin: 131.8 g/L vs 134.3 g/L; mean corpuscular volume: 92.8 vs 93.4 fl; mean corpuscular hemoglobin: 29.8 pg vs 30.3 pg; platelets: 263.6 10^9/L vs 269.6 10^9/L; and lymphocytes: 2.0 10^9/L vs 2.1 10^9/L).

Secondary Studies

The committee did not identify any secondary studies of diseases of the blood or blood-forming organs in Gulf War veterans.

Summary and Conclusions

A number of studies have examined hospitalization rates for blood disorders in deployed and nondeployed veterans. Overall, these studies do not provide evidence that the incidence of blood disorders was different in deployed veterans compared with nondeployed veterans. However, limitations of these studies preclude drawing firm conclusions: hospitalizations were mostly restricted to DoD hospitals, studies did not include information on outpatient visits where patients with mild disorders are most likely to be seen, most studies lacked information on potential confounders, and none of these studies differentiated between potential hematologic disorders. Two additional studies measured hematologic parameters in deployed and nondeployed veterans. Taken together, these two reports did not show any major difference according to deployment status. They were limited, however, by differential participation rate and lack of adjustment for confounding variables. Additionally, some blood disorders typically have a long latency, and hospitalization and mortality studies have limited validity to detect their prevalence and incidence.

The committee concludes that there is inadequate/insufficient evidence to determine whether an association exists between deployment to the Gulf War and disorders of the blood and blood-forming organs.

TABLE 4-2 Diseases of the Blood and Blood-Forming Organs

Study	Design	Population	Outcomes	Results	Adjustments	Comments
Gray et al., 1996 (Update)	Retrospective cohort, hospitalizations from August 1991 through September 1993	547,076 active-duty GWVs, 618,335 NDVs	Hospital-discharge diagnoses of blood disease in DoD hospital system	Exact values not given 1991: OR about 0.9 (95% CI 0.8-1.05); 1992: OR about 1.1 (95% CI 1.0-1.2) 1993, OR about 1.05 (95% CI 0.9-1.15)	Prewar hospitalization, sex, age, race, service branch, marital status, rank, length of service, salary, occupation	Short follow-up period; no outpatient data; restriction to DoD hospitals and thus to persons remaining on active duty after the war; no adjustment for other potential confounders
Gray et al., 2000 (Update)	Retrospective cohort, hospitalizations from August 1991 through December 1994	652,979 GWVs, 652,922 randomly selected NDVs 182,164 DoD hospitalizations; 16,030 VA hospitalizations; 5185 COSHPD hospitalizations	Hospital-discharge diagnoses of blood disease in DoD, VA, and COSHPD hospital systems	DoD PMR 1.08 (95% CI 0.97-1.19) VA PMR 0.77 (95% CI 0.54-1.01) COSHPD PMR 1.09 (95% CI 0.22-1.96)	Age, sex, race (only for DoD PMR)	Able to assess only illnesses that resulted in hospitalization; possible undetected confounders; PMR has lower sensitivity than a comparison of hospitalization rates would have
Smith et al., 2006 (Update)	Retrospective cohort study (cohort data from DMDC)	Active-duty personnel with a single deployment to: Gulf War theatre (n = 455,465); Southwest Asia peacekeeping mission, 1991-1998 (n = 249,047); Bosnia, 1995-1998 (n = 44,341)	Postdeployment hospitalization events (1991-2000) for an ICD-9-CM diagnosis of a disease of the blood (280-289)	Compared to GW veterans, veterans of Bosnia showed similar risk (HR 0.93, 95% CI 0.80-1.07), as did veterans of Southwest Asia (HR 0.93, 95% CI 0.75-1.15)	Sex, age, marital status, pay grade, race/ethnicity, service branch, occupation, and predeployment hospitalization; time-dependent covariate to account for changing hospitalization methods, diagnostic criteria, and procedures	Limitations: active-duty personnel only; hospitalizations at DoD facilities only

Study	Design	Population	Outcomes	Results	Adjustments	Comments
Smith et al., 2002 (Update)	DoD hospitalizations 1991-1999; exposure modeling for oil-well fire smoke	405,142 active-duty GWVs who were in theater during the time of Kuwaiti oil-well fires	Hospitalization for diseases of the blood (ICD-9-CM codes 280-289)	No clear association between exposure and blood disease across all exposure levels	Adjusted for "influential covariates," defined as demographic or deployment variables with p values less than 0.15	Objective measure of disease not subject to recall bias; no issues with self-selection; however, only DoD hospitals, only active duty, no adjustment for potential confounders such as smoking
Smith et al., 2003 (Update)	DoD hospitalization study (1991-2000); analysis of health outcomes and exposure to nerve agents (follow-up of Gray et al., 1999b)	99,614 active-duty military considered exposed vs 318,458 nonexposed, according to revised DoD exposure model	First hospitalization for any blood disorder (ICD-9-CM codes 280-289)	Exposed vs unexposed: RR 0.96 (95% CI 0.89-1.03)		Restricted to DoD hospitals; restricted to hospitalizations for only Gulf War veterans who remained on active duty after the war; no adjustment for confounding exposures
Ishoy et al., 1999b (Update)	Cross-sectional	686 Danish peacekeepers deployed to gulf in 1990-1997 vs 231 age- and sex-matched armed forces nondeployed controls	Blood hemoglobin, erythrocyte count, hematocrit, mean corpuscular volume, leukocyte count, and platelet count	Hemoglobin (mmol/L): 9.3 (sd = 0.5) vs 9.3 (sd = 0.6); erythrocytes (million/L): 4.8 (sd = 0.3) vs 4.8 (sd = 0.3); hematocrit 0.44 (sd = 0.25) vs 0.44 (sd = 0.26); corp. vol. (10^{-15} L): 91 (sd = 3.6) vs 91 ((sd = 3.8); leukocytes (10^9/L): 5.8 (1.7) vs 5.9 (sd = 1.8); platelets (10^9/L): 205 (sd = 45) vs 211 (sd = 43), $p < 0.05$		Participation rate 83.6% deployed, 57.8% nondeployed; no adjustment for possible confounding factors
Sim et al., 2003 (Update)	Cross-sectional, mailed questionnaire and clinical	1355 male and 30 female Australian GWVs; 1361 male and 32 female	Hemoglobin, MCV, MCH, lymphocyte count, platelet count	Hemoglobin (g/L), men: 153.4 (sd = 9.5) vs 153.1 (sd = 9.1); women: 131.8 vs 134.3	Service type, rank, age, education, marital status	High participation in deployed veterans (male 81%, female 79%), but low participation in

Study	Design	Population	Outcomes	Results	Adjustments	Comments
	examination	nondeployed veterans		MCV (fl), men: 91.6 (sd = 4.7) vs 91.5 (sd = 4.5); women: 92.8 vs 93.4 MCH (pg), men: 30.4 (sd = 1.4) vs 30.5 (sd = 1.3); women: 29.8 vs 30.3 Lymphocyte count (10^9/L), men: 1.9 (sd = 0.5) vs 1.9 (sd = 0.6); women: 2.0 vs 2.1 Platelets (10^9/L), men: 227.8 (sd = 44.4) vs 231.3 (sd = 48.5); women: 263.6 vs 269.6		control group (male 57%, female 44%) possibly leading to participation bias

NOTE: CI = confidence interval; COSHPD = California Office of Statewide Health Planning and Development; DMDC = Defense Manpower Data Center; DoD = Department of Defense; fl = femtoliter; GW = Gulf War; HR = adjusted hazard ratio; MCH = mean corpuscular hemoglobin; MCV = mean corpuscular volume; MRR = mortality rate ratio; OR = adjusted odds ratio; pg = pictogram; PHQ = Patient Health Questionnaire; PMR = patient medical record; RR = adjusted risk ratio; sd = standard deviation; VA = Department of Veterans Affairs.

ENDOCRINE, NUTRITIONAL, AND METABOLIC DISEASES

Among the general US population, the most frequent disorders in this group of diseases are diabetes, thyroid disease, and obesity. In *Volume 4* of this series, diabetes was grouped together with cardiovascular diseases. Other specific endocrine, nutritional, or metabolic outcomes were not considered. In this chapter, we will present, separately, studies reporting hospitalizations for endocrine and metabolic disorders, mortality studies and studies reporting associations of deployment with specific diseases (diabetes, thyroid disorders, and obesity). See Table 4-3 for a summary of the primary papers reviewed for endocrine, nutritional, and metabolic disorders.

Diabetes

Diabetes is an endocrine disorder characterized by abnormally elevated levels of blood glucose. The two major types of diabetes are type 1 diabetes, caused by destruction of the pancreatic cells that produce insulin, and type 2 diabetes, caused by peripheral resistance to insulin action and impaired insulin secretion, with increased blood glucose levels. Type 1 usually affects young people, while type 2 is more prevalent in adults and is strongly associated with obesity.

Summary of *Volume 4*

Primary Studies

Volume 4 included one primary study examining the association of deployment with 12 primary health outcomes, including diabetes, ascertained from a medical examination (Eisen et al., 2005). The study evaluated 1061 Gulf War deployed and 1128 nondeployed veterans who had been randomly selected from 11,441 Gulf War deployed and 9476 nondeployed veterans who previously participated in the National Health Survey of Gulf War Era Veterans and Their Families. Based on physical examinations conducted 10 years after the Gulf War, the prevalence of diabetes in deployed and nondeployed veterans was 4.2% and 3.5% (OR 1.52, 95% CI 0.81-2.85). Results for self-reported conditions were similar. A major limitation was the low participation rate, with only 53% of Gulf War veterans and 39% of nondeployed Gulf War veterans participating.

Secondary Studies

Studies relying on self-reported diabetes diagnoses, without additional confirmation, were considered secondary.

In a study of Kansas Gulf War veterans, prevalence of self-reported diabetes was similar in 1545 deployed veterans and 435 nondeployed (about 1% in both groups; OR 1.2, 95% CI 0.45-3.3) (Steele, 2000). Kang and colleagues (2000) found a very similar prevalence of self-reported diabetes in 11,441 deployed and 9476 nondeployed veterans (0.1% in both groups) in the National Health Survey of Gulf War Era Veterans and Their Families conducted in 1995. Among Seabee commands, no differences in prevalence of self-reported diabetes between Gulf War deployed Seabees (1.0%), those deployed elsewhere (0.9%), and nondeployed Seabees (1.6%) (OR 1.1, 95% CI 0.7-1.7 and OR 0.8, 95% CI 0.5-1.2, respectively) (Gray et al., 2002). Finally, in a multistate study of Gulf War deployed veterans (McCauley et al., 2002), being deployed near the Khamisiyah demolition site was not related to the prevalence of self-reported diabetes (OR 1.0, 95% CI 0.4-2.9). In this same report, being deployed (versus nondeployed) was not associated with the prevalence of diabetes (OR 1.0, 95% CI 0.5-2.4).

Updated and Supplemental Literature

Primary Studies

A study conducted in 1997 on 686 Danish Gulf War veterans and 231 nondeployed veterans found that mean insulin levels, which are predictive of diabetes risk, were similar in deployed (48 pmol/L) and nondeployed (52 pmol/L) (Ishoy et al., 1999b). It should be noted that Danish veterans served mostly as peacekeepers after the end of the conflict.

Finally, the Australian Gulf War veterans study (Sim et al., 2003) obtained random glucose levels in a sample of 1365 male and 30 female deployed veterans and 1365 male and 32 female controls. Levels of blood glucose were comparable in both groups: among deployed and nondeployed men, median plasma glucose was 4.7 mmol/L in both groups, while among deployed and nondeployed women, the average plasma glucose was 5.0 mmol/L and 4.5 mmol/L, respectively. In this study, response rates were higher among deployed (81% in men, 79% in women) than nondeployed veterans (57% in men, 44% in women), which could lead to selection bias. Also, blood glucose levels were not obtained from fasting blood, which limits their value to diagnose diabetes.

McDiarmid and colleagues measured levels of blood glucose in a cohort of deployed veterans exposed to depleted uranium (DU) from friendly-fire followed up with biennial exams. Though these veterans have been observed many times since 1991, levels of blood glucose have been only reported in publications corresponding to the 2005 and 2007 assessments (McDiarmid et al., 2007a, 2009). The authors did not observe any important difference in blood glucose levels between those exposed to low and high levels of DU, though these results are limited due to the small sample size of the cohort (n = 34 in the 2007 publication, corresponding to the 2005 exam; n = 35 in the 2009 publication, corresponding to the 2007 exam), and the lack of adjustment for potential confounders.

Secondary Studies

A number of large-scale epidemiologic studies included self-reported endocrine and metabolic disorders, including diabetes, with onset after the Gulf War. These studies were regarded as secondary studies for the purpose of this review.

Simmons et al. (2004) surveyed all 51,581 male UK veterans who served in the Gulf War and a demographically similar comparison cohort of 51,688 UK male veterans who were not deployed to the gulf. Among the 23,358 deployed men who responded, 0.2% reported having diabetes with onset after 1990, as did 0.4% of 17,730 nondeployed men who responded, for an OR of 0.7 (95% CI 0.5-1.0) adjusted for age at the time of the survey, service and rank at the time of the Gulf War, serving status at the time of the survey, alcohol consumption, and smoking.

A follow-up survey to the 1995 National Health Survey of Gulf War Era Veterans and Their Families conducted in 2004-2005 compared self-reported health status of deployed Gulf War veterans and nondeployed Gulf War veterans (Kang et al., 2009). This survey included 6111 deployed and 3859 nondeployed veterans, out of 15,000 in each group (response rates of 41% in deployed and 26% in nondeployed veterans). The prevalence of a self-reported diagnosis of diabetes was similar in deployed and nondeployed veterans (prevalence ratio 1.11, 95% CI 0.99-1.25), after adjustment for sociodemographic and lifestyle variables. The prevalence of "other endocrine (nondiabetes) disorders," however, was slightly higher among the deployed (prevalence ratio 1.24, 95% CI 1.11-1.39), but these disorders were not specified.

Also in the context of the National Health Survey of Gulf War Veterans Study, the frequency of self-reported diabetes was compared among Gulf War veterans according to their potential exposure to the Khamisiyah demolition (Page et al., 2005). Prevalence of diabetes (OR 0.92, 95% CI 0.57-1.48) or other endocrine disorders (OR 0.92, 95% CI 0.65-1.30) was similar in those potentially exposed and unexposed.

In a mailed survey conducted in 1997, Canadian male Gulf War veterans (n = 2924) reported a prevalence of diabetes similar to that for nondeployed male veterans (n = 3241) (0.6% vs 0.4% in those aged 20-44 years and 2.0% vs 3.8% in those aged 45-64 years) (Goss Gilroy, 1998). Another study conducted in New England between 1994 and 1996 included 141 Gulf War veterans and 46 veterans deployed to Germany. The prevalence of self-reported diabetes was comparable in the two groups (2% in Gulf War veterans vs 0% in Germany-deployed veterans) (Proctor et al., 2001a).

Smith et al. (2006) compared hospitalizations in Gulf War deployed veterans with veterans deployed in the Persian Gulf after the war (Southwest Asia veterans) and in Bosnia (details on this study are provided in the section on hospitalizations for endocrine disorders). This study is considered secondary for diabetes, since diabetes discharge codes have low sensitivity and specificity for the diagnosis of diabetes (see, for example, Kieszak et al., 1999). The incidence of diabetes was similar among Gulf War veterans and Southwest Asia veterans (rate ratio 0.95, 95% CI 0.69-1.30, comparing Southwest Asia veterans to Gulf War veterans), but lower among veterans in Bosnia (rate ratio 0.54, 95% CI 0.29-1.00). This study was limited by including only hospitalizations occurring in DoD hospitals among active-duty personnel.

Thyroid Disease

The most frequent disorders of the thyroid gland are hypothyroidism and hyperthyroidism, characterized respectively by low or high levels of thyroid hormones. Many different causes can lead to these disorders, including autoimmune diseases, infections, malnutrition, exposure to some drugs or toxins, or neoplasias. Thyroid disease was not specifically studied in *Volume 4*.

Updated and Supplemental Literature

Primary Studies

Thyroid disease was included as an outcome in the study by Eisen and colleagues (2005). The study has been mentioned above under diabetes. Briefly, it evaluated 1061 Gulf War deployed and 1128 nondeployed veterans from those participating in the National Health Survey of Gulf War Era Veterans and Their Families. Based on physical examinations, the prevalence of hypothyroidism (defined as having an untreated thyroid-stimulating hormone level of 10.0 mU/mL or greater, or taking medication for hypothyroidism) and hyperthyroidism (defined as having an untreated thyroid-stimulating hormone level less than 0.1 mU/mL, or taking medication for hyperthyroidism) in deployed veterans were 1.6% and 0.3%, respectively. The corresponding prevalences in nondeployed were 1.2% and 0.1% (OR of hypothyroidism: 1.70, 95% CI 0.75-3.87; OR of hyperthyroidism 4.86, 95% CI 0.68-34.58). This study had a low participation rate, which limits the reliability of its results.

A small cohort of Gulf War veterans exposed to DU as a result of friendly-fire accidents has been followed biennially for 16 years to identify uranium-related changes in health, including serum concentrations of free thyroxine and thyroid-stimulating hormone (TSH) as measures of thyroid function (McDiarmid et al., 2000, 2001, 2004, 2006, 2007a,b, 2009). Overall, consistent differences in mean concentrations of free thyroxine and TSH have not been observed when comparing those with high to those with low urinary uranium concentrations. One exception occurred when mean free thyroxine concentrations were found to be lower in the high uranium-exposed group at the 2001 evaluation, but no differences were observed in subsequent evaluations occurring in 2003, 2005, or 2007 (McDiarmid et al., 2007a, 2009; Squibb and McDiarmid, 2006). Although up to 77 DU-exposed Gulf War veterans have been evaluated in this cohort over time, at any single time point only a small subset of individuals were assessed. For example, 35 members underwent clinical evaluation during the most recent 2007 follow-up (McDiarmid et al., 2009). Thus, comparisons are based on small numbers. Additionally, the authors did not adjust for potential confounders between the two groups.

Secondary Studies

Three secondary studies assessed thyroid function in Gulf War veterans on the basis of self-reports. In 1997, a mail survey of the entire Canadian military contingent of 2924 male veterans who served in the Gulf War and 3241 Canadian veterans who were in the military but had not been posted to the gulf region were asked about the presence of goiter (a form of thyroid disease) or thyroid trouble. Positive responses were reported by 0.9% of the Gulf War veterans and 0.7% of the nondeployed veterans 20-44 years old and by 2.0% of deployed and 1.3% of nondeployed veterans 45-64 years old; the median age of the deployed was 36 years, and that of the nondeployed was 37 years (Goss Gilroy, 1998).

In a study conducted among Kansas veterans, deployed veterans were more likely than their nondeployed counterparts to report thyroid conditions (OR 2.32, 95% CI 0.81-6.67), but numbers were small and therefore estimates of association imprecise (Steele, 2000). Gray et al. (2002), examining Seabee commands, observed an increase in thyroid conditions among the Gulf War deployed Seabees when compared to Seabees deployed elsewhere (OR 1.87, 95% CI 1.16-3.03) but not when compared to the nondeployed members of this cohort (OR 1.49, 95% CI 0.89-2.50).

Obesity

Obesity is a state of excess adipose tissue mass. The most widely used method to measure obesity is through the body mass index (BMI), defined as the weight in kilograms divided by the square of the height (in meters). Overweight is usually defined as a BMI ≥ 25 kg/m^2, while the cutoff point for obesity is a BMI ≥ 30 kg/m^2. In the year 2000, the prevalence of obesity in the United States was approximately 30%, while more than 60% of adults older than 20 were overweight. Genetic factors, sedentary lifestyles, and diet are the major determinants of obesity. Obesity was not studied separately in *Volume 4*.

Updated and Supplemental Literature

Primary Studies

A study of 686 Danish Gulf War veterans and 231 nondeployed veterans included measurements of weight and height (Ishoy et al., 1999b). The exams were conducted in 1997.

Average weight and waist circumference were slightly higher in deployed (84.2 kg and 90.2 cm, respectively) than in nondeployed veterans (81.9 kg and 88.3 cm).

In the study of Australian Gulf War veterans (Sim et al., 2003), researchers obtained direct measures of BMI and waist circumference in a sample of 1384 male and 30 female deployed veterans and 1379 male and 32 female nondeployed controls examined in 2002. BMI was comparable in deployed and nondeployed groups. Comparisons were adjusted for service type, rank, age, education, and marital status. In deployed men, the mean (standard deviation) of BMI was 28.1 kg/m^2 (sd = 4.1) while in nondeployed men it was 28.3 kg/m^2 (sd = 4.1) (adjusted difference: −0.3, 95% CI −0.6-0.02). Their corresponding mean waist circumference was 97.7 cm (sd = 10.7) and 98.2 cm (sd = 10.7) (adjusted difference: −0.6, 95% CI −1.4-0.2). Among female veterans, both deployed and nondeployed had an average body mass index of 26 kg/m^2, and similar waist circumferences (86.3 cm in deployed and 83.4 cm in nondeployed). Given the small sample size in this group, the authors did not conduct statistical comparisons among women.

Secondary Studies

A small study of 111 deployed and 133 nondeployed UK veterans compared different clinical parameters, objectively measured, in the two groups (Ismail et al., 2008). These parameters included BMI, glycemia, and blood levels of thyroxine-stimulating hormone. No differences were observed between the groups. These veterans were selected from a group of approximately 12,000 UK veterans who were contacted by mail and reported physical disability according to the Short Form 36 (SF-36) Physical Functioning Scale. Being a selected subgroup of deployed and nondeployed veterans, it is unclear how these results apply to the entire veteran population.

Hospitalization Studies

Summary of *Volume 4*

A DoD study examined hospitalizations in relation to possible exposure to sarin and cyclosarin as a result of demolishing weapons at Khamisiyah, Iraq, in March 1991 (Smith et al., 2003). As an update to a previous report (Gray et al., 1999b), the investigators analyzed hospitalizations from 1991 to 2000 among 431,762 active-duty military deployed to the Gulf War theater during the time of the Khamisiyah demolition. Investigators studied discharge diagnoses from 15 ICD-10 categories, including "endocrine, nutritional, and metabolic diseases." The incidence of hospitalizations for endocrine and metabolic diseases was the same in veterans exposed and nonexposed to the Khamisiyah plume (risk ratio 1.00, 95% CI 0.94-1.06). Limitations of this study include: diagnoses not severe enough to require hospitalization would not be captured in these data, lack of outpatient data, restriction to DoD hospitals in those on active duty, and limited adjustment for potential confounding exposures.

Updated and Supplemental Literature

Since the publication of *Volume 4*, four additional primary studies reporting hospitalizations for endocrine and metabolic disorders have been identified (Gray et al., 1996, 2000; Smith et al., 2002, 2006). Like Smith et al. (2003), however, these studies evaluated hospitalizations for major diagnostic categories, and thus were limited to assessing events serious enough to warrant hospitalization.

Gray et al. (1996) compared DoD hospitalizations among Gulf War deployed and nondeployed active-duty personnel. Discharge diagnoses for 14 ICD-9-CM categories, which included "endocrine, nutritional, and metabolic diseases," were assessed across three time periods following the war: August 1, 1991, to December 31, 1991 (included 1,165,411 subjects on active duty on the first day of this time period); January 1, 1992, to December 31, 1992 (1,075,430 subjects); and January 1, 1993, to September 30, 1993 (839,389 subjects). Hospitalizations for endocrine and metabolic diseases were not increased among the Gulf War deployed personnel (vs nondeployed) during any of the three time periods. Limitations of this study include the relatively short follow-up, the lack of outpatient data, restriction to DoD hospitals, restriction to hospitalizations of those who remained on active duty after the war, and limited adjustment for potential confounding exposures.

The authors later expanded the study above to include reserve and former military personnel hospitalized in non-DoD hospitals (Gray et al., 2000). Hospitalization for the 14 major discharge diagnoses during the period of August 1, 1991, and December 31, 1994, were compared for Gulf War veterans and nondeployed veterans in three hospital systems (DoD, VA, and the California Office of Statewide Health Planning and Development). Because the population eligible for hospitalization in the VA and California systems could not be identified to calculate hospitalization rates, the investigators estimated proportional morbidity ratios (PMRs) within each hospital system. Gulf War veterans did not experience an increased probability of hospitalizations for endocrine, nutritional, and metabolic diseases compared to nondeployed veterans during the 4 years after the war. This finding was consistent among hospitalizations within the DoD (n = 182,164), VA (n = 16,030), and California (n = 5185) hospital systems. The authors acknowledge the proportional morbidity approach is likely to be less sensitive for detecting differences in hospitalizations than a comparison of hospitalization rates. However, the results within the DoD system were consistent with the finding reported in Gray et al. (1996), which observed no differences in the odds of hospitalization for endocrine and metabolic disorders over the 2-year observation period.

Postwar hospitalizations in US military personnel were also examined in relation to exposure to smoke from oil-well fires (Smith et al., 2002). Hospitalizations within DoD treatment facilities were identified for 405,142 active-duty personnel who were in the Gulf War theater of operations during the Kuwaiti oil-well fires (February 2, 1991, to October 31, 1991) and did not remain in the region after the war. Hospitalizations for "endocrine, nutritional and metabolic diseases" and other major ICD-9-CM categories were evaluated over an 8-year follow-up period. Exposure to oil-well fire smoke was estimated by combining smoke-plume modeling data and troop unit location. Exposure was categorized into seven levels based on combinations of average daily dose (none, 1-260 $\mu g/m^3$, > 260 $\mu g/m^3$) and duration of exposure (1-25 days, 26-50 days, > 50 days). When compared to those with no exposure to smoke from oil-well fires, there was no increase in the incidence of hospitalization for endocrine and metabolic diseases at any level of exposure (adjusted risk ratio comparing those with the highest exposure to those with no exposure, 0.84). The limitations of this study are the same as those described above for Gray et al. (1996) and Smith et al. (2003).

More recently, the hospitalization experience of the Gulf War veterans (n = 455,465) was compared with that of veterans deployed to Southwest Asia after the Gulf War (n = 249,047) and veterans deployed to Bosnia (n = 44,341) (Smith et al., 2006). Only hospitalizations occurring in DoD hospitals through the end of 2000 while the veteran was on active duty were considered. Compared to veterans deployed to the Gulf War, the rate ratio of hospitalizations for endocrine and metabolic disorders was 1.02 (95% CI 0.92-1.13) in those deployed to Southwest Asia after the conflict and 0.69 (95% CI 0.57-0.84) in those deployed to Bosnia. As with other studies of hospitalizations in DoD hospitals, a major limitation of this analysis is the exclusion of hospitalizations in other hospitals and the restriction to active-duty personnel.

Mortality Studies

Updated and Supplemental Literature

For the purpose of this review, mortality studies of endocrine, nutritional, and metabolic diseases were considered secondary, given the expected low sensitivity of death certificates for the accurate identification of these disorders.

Only one report of mortality for endocrine, nutritional, or metabolic diseases was identified (Macfarlane et al., 2005). This study examined mortality from 1991 through June 30, 2004, of 51,753 UK Gulf War veterans and 50,808 nondeployed veterans in service on January 1, 1991. Nondeployed veterans were matched with deployed by age, sex, service branch, rank, and fitness for active service. Vital status and cause of death, if applicable, was obtained from linkage with the National Health Service central register. Only three deaths (one in Gulf War veterans, two in nondeployed veterans) were attributed to endocrine, nutritional, or metabolic disorders (mortality rate ratio 0.5, 95% CI 0.1-5.8).

Summary and Conclusions

Primary studies found no clinically relevant differences in prevalence of different endocrine and metabolic disorders, including diabetes, thyroid disease, and obesity, between deployed and nondeployed veterans. Because five of the eight primary studies were limited to hospital discharge data, conditions not requiring hospitalization have not been sufficiently evaluated. Furthermore, the grouping of all endocrine, nutritional, and metabolic disorders into a single outcome, as presented in all hospitalization studies, may obscure potential associations with specific conditions. Results from secondary studies were similarly inconclusive, with deployment status unrelated to the prevalence of self-reported diabetes but with less consistent findings observed for "other endocrine disorders." Overall, existing evidence does not support an increased risk of endocrine, nutritional, or metabolic disorders among Gulf War veterans compared to other veterans. However, the Gulf War veteran population is still relatively young, and an increased risk of type 2 diabetes in deployed veterans might not be evident yet. The committee recommends that future assessments of Gulf War veterans include obtaining hemoglobin A1c samples as a more reliable indicator of type 2 diabetes.

The committee concludes that there is inadequate/insufficient evidence to determine whether an association exists between deployment to the Gulf War and endocrine, nutritional, and metabolic diseases.

TABLE 4-3 Endocrine, Nutritional, and Metabolic Diseases

Study	Design	Population	Outcomes	Results	Adjustments	Comments
Eisen et al., 2005 (Vol. 4)	Cross-sectional, prevalence, population-based (Derived from Kang et al. 2000)	1061 GWVs and 1128 NDVs	Diabetes, hypothyroidism, hyperthyroidism	Diabetes (OR 1.52, 95% CI 0.81-2.85); hypothyroidism (OR 1.70, 95% CI 0.75-3.87); hyperthyroidism (OR 4.86, 95% CI 0.68-34.58); no outcomes tested were significant	Age, sex, race, smoking, duty type, service branch, education, rank (hyperthyroidism not adjusted for service branch or rank)	Low participation rates, deployed (53%), nondeployed (39%)
Smith et al., 2003 (Vol. 4)	DoD hospitalization study (1991-2000) of those potentially exposed to nerve agent	99,614 active-duty military considered exposed vs 318,458 nonexposed, according to revised DoD exposure model	Hospitalization due to endocrine, nutritional, and metabolic diseases (ICD-9 classification)	RR 1.00 (95% CI 0.94-1.06)	One or more hospitalizations in a specific diagnostic category	Diagnoses not requiring hospitalization not captured; no outpatient data; DoD hospitals and active duty only; not possible to adjust for confounding exposures
Ishoy et al., 1999b (Update)	Cross-sectional	686 Danish peacekeepers deployed to gulf in 1990-1997 vs 231 age- and sex-matched armed forces nondeployed controls	Plasma insulin levels Avg. weight and waist circumference	No significant difference in insulin levels between deployed (48 pmol/L) and nondeployed (52 pmol/L) Weight and waistline were higher ($p < 0.05$) for deployed (84.2 kg, 90.2 cm) than for nondeployed (81.9 kg, 88.3 cm)		Participation rate 83.6% deployed, 57.8% nondeployed
Sim et al., 2003 (Update)	Cross-sectional, mailed questionnaire and clinical examination	1384 male and 30 female Australian GWVs; 1379 male and 32 female NDVs (Only 1365 GWVs and 1365 for plasma glucose analysis)	Plasma glucose; BMI; waist circumference	Plasma glucose, men: 85 mg/dL in both groups; women: 90 mg/dL vs 81 mg/dL BMI, men: 28.1 kg/m^2 (sd = 4.1) vs 28.3 kg/m^2 (sd = 4.1), OR -0.3 (95% CI -0.6, 0.02); women: 26 kg/m^2 in both groups Waist circumference, men:	Service type, rank, age (< 20, 20-24, 25-34, ≥ 35 years), education and marital status	High participation in deployed veterans (male 81%, female 79%), but low participation in control group (male 57%, female 44%) possibly leading to participation bias

Study	Design	Population	Outcomes	Results	Adjustments	Comments
				97.7 cm (sd = 10.7) vs 98.2 cm (sd = 10.7), OR −0.6 (95% CI −1.4, 0.2) ; women: 86.3 cm vs 83.4 cm		
McDiarmid et al., 2007a, 2009 (Update)	Case series	Population for 2005 exam (2007a study): n = 34 Population for 2007 exam (2009 study): n = 35	Blood glucose	Low-uranium compared to high-uranium group: 107 mg/dL vs 109 mg/dL in 2005 exam (p = 0.67), 111 mg/dL vs 90 mg/dL in 2007 exam (p = 0.07)	None	Very small sample size, no adjustment for potential confounders
Smith et al., 2003 (Vol. 4)	DoD hospitalization study (1991-2000); analysis of health outcomes and exposure to nerve agents (follow-up of Gray et al. 1999b)	99,614 active-duty military considered exposed vs 318,458 nonexposed, according to revised DoD exposure model	First hospitalization for any endocrine, nutritional, and metabolic diseases (ICD-9-CM codes 240-279)	Exposed vs unexposed: RR 1.00 (95% CI 0.94, 1.06)		Restricted to DoD hospitals; restricted to hospitalizations for only Gulf War veterans who remained on active duty after the war; no adjustment for confounding exposures; diagnoses not severe enough to require hospitalizations are not captured
Gray et al., 1996 (Update)	Retrospective cohort, hospitalizations from August 1991 through September 1993	547,076 active-duty GWVs, 618,335 NDVs	Hospital-discharge diagnoses of endocrine, metabolic, or nutritional system diseases in the DoD hospital system (ICD-9 classification)	OR about 0.85-0.90 (95% CI 0.80-0.95) across all three years, 1991-1993. Exact values not given	Prewar hospitalization, sex, age, race, branch of service, marital status, rank, length of service, salary, occupation	Very short follow-up period; no outpatient data; restriction to DoD hospitals, and thus to persons remaining on active duty after the war; no adjustment for potential confounders
Gray et al., 2000 (Update)	Retrospective cohort, hospitalizations from August	652,979 GWVs, 652,922 randomly selected NDVs 182,164 DoD	Hospital-discharge diagnoses for endocrine, nutritional, and metabolic disease in	DoD PMR 0.99 (95% CI 0.93-1.06) VA PMR 1.08 (95% CI 0.92-1.24)	Age, sex, race (only for DoD PMR)	Able to assess only illnesses that resulted in hospitalization; possible undetected confounders

Study	Design	Population	Outcomes	Results	Adjustments	Comments
	1991 through December 1994	hospitalizations; 16,030 VA hospitalizations; 5185 COSHPD hospitalizations	three hospital systems: DoD, VA, COSHPD	COSHPD PMR 0.81 (95% CI 0.48-1.14)		PMR has lower sensitivity than a comparison of hospitalization rates would have
Smith et al., 2002 (Update)	DoD hospitalizations 1991-1999; exposure modeling for oil-well fire smoke	405,142 active-duty GWVs who were in theater during the time of Kuwaiti oil-well fires	Association of exposure level with hospitalizations for endocrine, nutritional, and metabolic disease	No significant difference between RR for exposure at any level vs nonexposed	Adjusted for "influential covariates," defined as demographic or deployment variables with p values less than 0.15	Objective measure of disease not subject to recall bias; no issues with self-selection; however, only DoD hospitals, only active duty, no adjustment for potential confounders such as smoking
Smith et al., 2006 (Update)	Retrospective cohort study; cohort data from DMD	Active-duty personnel with a single deployment to: Gulf War theater (n = 455,465); Southwest Asia peacekeeping mission, 1991-1998 (n = 249,047); Bosnia, 1995-1998 (n = 44,341)	Postdeployment hospitalization events (1991-2000) for an ICD-9-CM diagnosis of an endocrine disease (240-279)	Veterans of Bosnia, HR 0.69 (95% CI 0.57-0.84) Veterans of SW Asia, HR 1.02 (95% CI 0.92-1.13)	Sex, age, marital status, pay grade, race/ethnicity, service branch, occupation, and predeployment hospitalization; time-dependent covariate to account for changing hospitalization methods, diagnostic criteria, and procedures	Limitations: active-duty personnel only; hospitalizations at DoD facilities only

NOTES: BMI = body mass index; CI = confidence interval; COSHPD = California Office of Statewide Health Planning and Development; DMDC = Defense Manpower Data Center; DoD = Department of Defense; GWV = Gulf War veterans; NDV = nondeployed veterans; OR = adjusted odds ratio; PHQ = Patient Health Questionnaire; PMR = patient medical records; RR = risk ratio; sd = standard deviation; VA = Department of Veterans Affairs.

MENTAL AND BEHAVIORAL DISORDERS

War is a known risk factor for psychiatric conditions (Pizarro et al., 2006; Wessely, 2005). The description of the extent and type of psychiatric affliction and its course has depended on the development of modern psychiatric diagnostic systems and epidemiologic methods. The development of a structured diagnostic system and diagnostic instruments has facilitated the diagnosis of behavioral disorders. Moreover, the prevalence of psychiatric disorders in epidemiologic samples drawn from the general population has become available (Kessler et al., 2005a,b) and provides baseline data with which to compare data from specific inquiries. Thus, after the Persian Gulf War, many methodological and scientific details were in place to support an assessment of the psychological consequences of war. The Persian Gulf War was highly unusual in that the air war lasted 40 days and the ground war concluded in 5 days, so there was a limited theater and set of conditions amenable in many respects to scientific study. In fact, each of the large cohort studies of Gulf War veterans, described in Chapter 3, included items pertaining to mental health. Nested within them was analysis of mental health characteristics based on direct interview techniques or validated symptom scales.

Types of psychiatric ill health that could be associated with the Gulf War, particularly posttraumatic stress disorder (PTSD), were predicted on the basis of their descriptions from previous wars (O'Toole et al., 1996; Roy-Byrne et al., 2004). Psychiatric disorders in the general population are not uncommon, and are often disabling and chronic (Kessler et al., 2005a,b). Diagnosable psychiatric disorders are found in about one-third of the US adult population at any given time, but their prevalence in military populations is lower, which may be largely as a result of the healthy-warrior effect. Psychiatric disorders can be grouped into several classes, such as mood disorders (that is, depression and bipolar disorder); anxiety disorders (that is, generalized anxiety disorder, obsessive-compulsive disorder, panic disorder, PTSD, and social phobia); disorders involving perceptions of physical symptoms and health, which are called somatoform disorders (for example, hypochondriasis and somatization disorder); and substance use disorders (for example, abuse of and dependence on drugs and alcohol). Specific criteria for diagnosing those mental health disorders are given in the *Diagnostic and Statistical Manual of Mental Disorders-IV* (*DSM-IV*) (American Psychiatric Association, 2000) or the ICD-10 *Classification of Mental and Behavioural Disorders: Diagnostic Criteria for Research*.

The specification of characteristics of mental diagnoses has made research on their incidence and prevalence possible, so that there are guidelines differentiating them from transient experiences of distress or sadness that do not signify the presence of mental disease. Major depression, a type of mood disorder, is characterized by lifelong vulnerability to episodes of depressed mood and loss of interest and pleasure in daily activities accompanied by other symptoms such as sleeping too little or too much, reduced appetite and weight loss or increased appetite and weight gain, restlessness, irritability, difficulty concentrating, feeling guilty, hopeless or worthless, and thoughts of suicide or death. A major depressive episode is categorized as major depressive disorder (MDD) or, when it accompanies mania, as bipolar disorder. PTSD is a subtype of anxiety disorder.

PTSD is diagnosed on the basis of exposure to a traumatic event. After this exposure, the person experiences a specific constellation of symptoms such as severe distress on recollection of the event, avoidance of reminders of the situation, numbing of general responsiveness, and such signs of hyperarousal as irritability, sleep disturbance, or exaggerated startle reflexes. The presence of a few PTSD symptoms after a trauma is common and does not signify the presence of disease, but the presence of the full syndrome itself is much less common and is associated with significant disability.

Substance abuse is defined as a maladaptive pattern of substance use (there are many types of abused substances, but alcohol abuse is the most common) that results in a failure to fulfill major social roles (such as work or family-care performance), that involves use of the substance despite physical hazards and in association with legal consequences, and that involves use despite deleterious social and interpersonal consequences.

Substance use disorders include substance abuse and substance dependence. Substance abuse is defined as a maladaptive pattern of substance use that results in a failure to fulfill major social roles (such as work or family-care performance), that involves use of the substance despite physical hazards and in association with legal consequences, and that involves use despite deleterious social and interpersonal consequences. Substance dependence involves persistent and sustained maladaptive desire for and/or preoccupation with the substance, manifesting physiologically as symptoms of *withdrawal* when the substance is not taken, or as *tolerance*—a need to imbibe markedly increased amounts of the substance in order to continue to feel the desired outcome. Psychological manifestations of substance use disorders dependence include taking the substance over longer periods than intended, making unsuccessful efforts to cut down, and/or continuing to use the substance despite knowledge of having a significant physical or psychological problem resulting from its use. There are many types of substances for which abuse and dependence can be diagnosed; in most societies nicotine dependence is the most common and hazardous substance use disorder, currently responsible for half a billion deaths a year worldwide (Ezzati and Lopez, 2003). The studies of Gulf War veterans were generally limited, however, to assessment of the use of alcohol and illegal drugs, and therefore, the committee restricts its comments to these substances.

The prevalence of those disorders among young and middle-aged adults in the general population has now been addressed in several large studies, including the National Survey of Drug Use and Health, the National Epidemiologic Survey on Alcohol and Related Conditions, and the US National Comorbidity Survey Replication, a nationally representative face-to-face household survey conducted from February 2001 to April 2003 (Kessler et al., 2005a,b). The most recent data show that the prevalence estimates for all anxiety disorders were 28.8% (lifetime) and 18.1% (in the last 12 months); for all mood disorders, 20.8% (lifetime) and 9.5% (in the last 12 months); and for all substance use disorders, 14.6% (lifetime) and 3.8% (in the last 12 months). It should be noted that there is substantial variation by gender, and also by age group, even within the limited age range covered. It is also well established that because of difficulties associated with recall, lifetime prevalences tend to provide underestimates of the likelihood that an individual has had a particular condition, and recall about whether the condition has occurred in the last 12 months is more accurate (Susser and Shrout, 2009).

The prevalence estimates for the general population are generally higher than those in deployed veterans exposed to combat and much higher than in the control nondeployed veteran populations. As noted above, this is partly explained by a healthy warrior outcome. Thus, both military screening and self-selection are likely to ensure that individuals enter the military with better mental and physical health than the general population.

Primary studies provided the basis of the committee's findings on the relationship between deployment to the Gulf War and psychiatric outcomes (see Table 4-4). Primary studies were those in which veterans were categorized as deployed, not deployed, or deployed to a nonwar zone (for example, Germany). To diagnose psychiatric disorders, primary studies also included an in-person standardized diagnostic interview. Some studies used clinician interviews such as the Structured Clinical Interview for DSM-III-R (SCID); the Schedule for Clinical Assessment and Diagnosis (SCAN); or for PTSD, the Clinician Administered PTSD Scale (CAPS). Others used interviews administered by trained lay interviewers, such as the Composite International Diagnostic Interview (CIDI), a comprehensive and standardized diagnostic interview that is very widely used. The CIDI has been adapted to many forms that limit the diagnoses covered and the length of interview, and these alternative forms often produce less precise diagnoses. Studies of Gulf War veterans often used versions of the CIDI that were abbreviated from the full standard CIDI. Secondary studies typically failed to use diagnostic interviews to diagnose mental health disorders and often screened for mental health disorders using symptom checklists such as the PTSD Checklist developed by the VA.

Summary of *Volume 4*

Primary Studies

Many of the large epidemiologic studies of Gulf War veterans' health included items pertaining to mental health. Moreover, there was often a nested case-control study of mental health characteristics in the primary epidemiologic cohort studies that used direct-interview techniques. In *Volume 4*, eight primary studies were reviewed that used direct-interviews of the large Gulf War cohorts described in Chapter 3. These studies often used validated instruments, such as the CIDI, SCID, and CAPS, to complement the interview. Black et al. (2004b) reanalyzed the population-based, telephone interviews from the Iowa cohort of 4886 randomly selected veterans (military and reserve), deployed and nondeployed (Iowa Persian Gulf Study Group, 1997). The initial cohort study had uncovered higher than anticipated levels of anxiety; therefore, this analysis of the interview data looked more carefully into the features of anxiety in that population. The original cohort was interviewed by telephone using the Primary Care Evaluation of Mental Disorders (PRIME-MD), the Post Traumatic Stress Disorder Checklist-Military (PCL-M), and the CAGE[2] to estimate alcoholism. Additional structured questions identified medical conditions and military preparedness. Compared with nondeployed veterans, deployed veterans had a twofold increase in the prevalence of generalized anxiety disorder, panic disorder, PTSD, and any anxiety disorder (OR 2.3, 95% CI 1.5-3.5). Participation in combat increased the likelihood of the development of anxiety disorders, particularly PTSD (OR 2.1, 95% CI 1.7-4.2). Anxious Gulf War veterans were more likely to have had a pre-existing psychiatric condition, to have taken psychotropic medications, or to have had a psychiatric hospitalization prior to deployment. Anxiety conditions were comorbid with several psychiatric and medical conditions, particularly symptoms of cognitive dysfunction, any depression, major depression, and symptoms of fibromyalgia.

Barrett et al. (2002) analyzed the same data as Black et al. (2004b) to assess PTSD. A score of 50 or more on the PCL-M defined PTSD. PTSD-positive veterans had a mean score of 58.7, whereas those without PTSD had a mean score of 19.7; the prevalence of PTSD was 1.09%. The PTSD score was significantly associated with decreased functioning and quality of life, as well as increased reporting of symptoms and medical conditions.

---

[2]The CAGE is a four-item scale to assess cutting down (C), feeling annoyed by people criticizing your drinking (A), feeling guilty about drinking (G), and using alcohol as an eye-opener in the morning (E).

In a nested case-comparison study, Black et al. (2004a) conducted face-to-face interviews with 602 veterans in 1999-2002. They used the SCID with a random group of veterans drawn from strata of the PRIME-MD-interviewed group who reported one or more of the following symptom-based conditions during their previous interview: depression (major or minor depression), widespread chronic pain (established criteria for generalized, severe, and chronic pain), and cognitive dysfunction (amnesia or cognitive impairment of a moderate and prolonged intensity). Veterans were stratified by each symptom combination (one, two, or all) and by deployed or nondeployed status. Controls had not met screening criteria for any of these conditions and might have been deployed or not deployed. The veterans were selected randomly for interview from each stratum to optimize the match between cases and controls.

Personality disorders were screened for with the Schedule for Nonadaptive and Adaptive Personality (SNAP). Level of functioning was assessed using the SF-36. The Whiteley Index was used to determine hypochondriasis. The study found that 32% of the veterans met the criteria for a lifetime depression diagnosis (all types), and that rate was the same in deployed and nondeployed veterans (36.6% vs 30.3%, not significant). There were few diagnostic differences between the depressed deployed and the depressed nondeployed veterans, except for lifetime and current PTSD (OR 4.50, 95% CI 1.80-11.27 and OR 7.13, 95% CI 2.10-24.20, respectively), any lifetime and current anxiety disorders (OR 2.89, 95% CI 1.52-5.47 and OR 3.19, 95% CI 1.62-6.27, respectively), and any current psychiatric disorder (OR 2.00, 95% CI 1.0-3.74). The deployed depressed veterans were also more likely to have a diagnosis of any lifetime, but not current, substance-use disorder (OR 2.15, 95% CI 1.15-4.03), particularly lifetime alcohol-use disorder (OR 2.0, 95% CI 1.07-3.74). What was most surprising about the direct interview analysis was that there was little difference between the deployed and the nondeployed veterans in aspects of depression; the largest difference was found in the prevalence of any anxiety disorder (51.5% for deployed vs 25.0% for nondeployed).

Kang et al. (2003) conducted a population-based stratified random sample of 15,000 US Gulf War troops compared to a similar sample of nondeployed troops. Phase 1 was a mail survey and phase 2 was a telephone-based survey of PTSD symptoms using the PCL-M and chronic fatigue symptoms. In the interview cohort, 12.1% of Gulf War veterans and 4.3% of other veterans had symptoms of PTSD, with an adjusted OR of 3.1 (95% CI 2.7-3.4) for PTSD in the Gulf War group; 5.6% of the Gulf War veterans, and 1.2% of the other veterans (OR 4.8, 95% CI 3.9-5.9) had chronic fatigue symptoms. It was interesting to note that PTSD symptoms showed a dose-response relationship to intensity of war stress, whereas the chronic fatigue symptoms did not show any relationship to war stress. Estimates of PTSD as determined by a cutoff score of 50 or above tracked rates of stressors closely. Deployment, but not war stress, was associated with chronic fatigue symptoms.

Wolfe et al. (1999a,b) and Proctor et al. (1998) examined cohorts of veterans randomly sampled and stratified from the Fort Devens, Massachusetts, and New Orleans Gulf War veterans, as well as a cohort deployed to Germany. The Gulf War deployed veterans from Fort Devens were followed longitudinally from the day of their arrival home from the gulf (time 1) to about 2 years later (time 2) with a 78% participation rate. The Fort Devens cohort was mainly male, caucasian, and National Guard; rates of PTSD measured at time 1 were 3%. From those cohorts, stratified random samples were selected for closer study with direct interview (220 of the Fort Devens cohort, 73 of the New Orleans cohort, and 48 of the Germany deployed). The researchers used questionnaires (the 52-item expanded Health Symptoms Checklist [HSC] and the Expanded Combat Exposure Scale), a neuropsychologic test battery, an environmental interview, and psychiatric diagnostic instruments (the Clinician-Administered PTSD Scale [CAPS] or the Mississippi Scale for Combat-Related PTSD) (Proctor et al., 1998). Current PTSD (time 2) was diagnosed in 8.1% of the Fort Devens group, 7.6% of the New Orleans group, and none of the Germany group based on the CAPS. Health status and function were lower in the Gulf War deployed cohorts than the Germany deployed cohort (19.7-20.7% of deployed cohorts reported fair or poor health vs 6.4% of Germany deployed cohort). The three most prevalent symptoms in the Fort Devens group were "forgetfulness," "fatigue," and "unsatisfactory sleep" (Proctor et al., 1998).

Wolfe et al. (1999b) also recruited cases from the Fort Devens, New Orleans, and Germany cohorts with a stratified random-sampling strategy (148 from the Fort Devens group, 56 from the New Orleans group, and 56 from the Germany group). They used the Laufer Combat Scale to assess exposure to combat situations and the Mississippi Scale for Combat-Related PTSD to assess PTSD. The deployed Fort Devens group had significantly ($p < 0.05$) higher levels of current and lifetime PTSD (5.4% and 6.5%, respectively) and current and lifetime MDD (6.6% and 22.5%, respectively) than the Germany group (0% for both). Deployed personnel from New Orleans also had higher levels of current and lifetime PTSD (7.2% and 8.2%, respectively) and current and lifetime MDD (4.5% and 10.2%, respectively) than the Fort Devens or Germany deployed groups, although the difference was not significant. The prevalence of the other eight psychiatric disorders was similar between the three groups. Compared with the PTSD prevalence in the general population (7.8%) (Kessler et al., 1995), the Germany group (controls) had much lower rates of PTSD (0%). However, the low prevalence estimates in the controls increases from zero to 5-8% when the veterans are deployed to active war situations. A strength of this study is that it is characterized by direct interview.

In another analysis of these data (Wolfe et al., 1999a) looked at the course and predictors of PTSD and found that there was a higher rate of PTSD at time 2 (8%) than at time 1 (3%) (OR 3.2), indicating the development of new cases. Responders at time 2 were more likely to be younger, belong to racial minorities, and be deployed; however, the absence of differences in PTSD rates due to those characteristics indicates a lack of selection bias at time 2. Women were significantly more likely to have PTSD than men at either time (OR 3.2 at time 1, 95% CI 1.9-5.5; OR 2.3 at time 2, 95% CI 1.5-3.5), although their numbers were very low at each assessment. For men, 1% exceeded the cutpoint for PTSD at time 1 and time 2, 1% exceeded it at time 1 only, and 6% exceeded it at time 2 only.

Brailey et al. (1998) studied Gulf War veterans on their return from service (an average of 9 months after their return) with a face-to-face debriefing and psychological assessment with self-administered questionnaires, comparing Gulf War deployed ($n = 876$) with nondeployed veterans ($n = 396$ mobilized but not deployed), including National Guard and reserve troops. A subset of 349 received a followup assessment an average of 16 months later. Investigators used standard psychiatric rating scales for their assessments including: the Beck Depression Inventory (BDI), the State Anger, the State Anxiety, the Brief Symptom Inventory (BSI) Depression, BSI Anxiety, BSI Hostility, and the HSC. The deployed veterans had higher scores than the nondeployed on the BDI, the State Anger, the BSI Anxiety, and the HSC. When the Gulf War deployed veterans were reassessed on average of 16 months later, they showed increases on all scales, including the BDI, the State Anger, the BSI Anxiety, the BSI Hostility, HSC, and on both PTSD scales (the 17-item DSM-III R PTSD Checklist and the Mississippi Scale for Desert Storm War Zone Personnel). They showed increased rates of depression (6.9% to 13.8%), PTSD (2.3% to 10.6%), and hostility (4.9% to 13.8%). The authors correlated war stress with those symptoms and found that the higher the war-zone stress, the more severe the depressive and anxiety symptoms. Compared with nondeployed troops, troops who were assigned to high-risk activities, such as grave registration, showed a high prevalence of PTSD (0% vs 48%).

Ikin et al. (2004) conducted a comprehensive health assessment of 1424 male Gulf War veterans (86.5% Navy) and 1548 male Australian Defence Force members who were not deployed to the Gulf War, including an interview-administered psychological health assessment with the Composite International Diagnostic Interview (CIDI), a structured interview of demonstrated reliability and validity. The CIDI data allowed them to make an estimate of pre-Gulf War disorder, post-Gulf War disorder, and current (last 12 months) disorder. Those interview data were used with postal questionnaire data to form a complete workup of 1381 Gulf War veterans, and 1377 comparison veterans. Both the veterans and the controls completed the health assessment and the postal questionnaire. The two groups were demographically similar, although the Gulf War veterans were significantly younger, more likely to have been in the Navy, and less highly ranked than the comparison veterans. The two veteran groups were similar in prevalence of prewar psychiatric disorders. However, the Gulf War veterans were more likely than the comparison group to have developed any disorder after the war (31% vs 21%). The greatest risks were for the anxiety disorders, for example, PTSD (OR 3.9, 95% CI 2.3-6.5), major depression (OR 1.6, 95% CI 1.3-2.0), and alcohol dependence/abuse (OR 1.5, 95% CI 1.2-2.0). The rates of somatoform disorders (referred to as "any somatic disorders" by the study authors) were low in both groups (OR 1.9, 95% CI 0.8-4.5). In addition, the Gulf War group was significantly more likely to have any anxiety disorder (OR 2.2, 95% CI 1.6-3.2), PTSD (OR 4.1, 95% 2.4-7.2), obsessive-compulsive disorder (OCD) (OR 5.2, 95% CI 1.6-16.7), social phobia (OR 3.4, 955 CI 1.7-6.6), or panic disorder (OR 2.6, 95% CI 1.0-6.3), than the comparison group in the preceding 12 months. On average, the Gulf War veterans had twice as many current psychiatric disorders as the comparison veterans. The strengths of this study were the large sample, the comparable control group, the use of well-validated psychological interviews, and the analyzed participation bias, which was estimated to be low.

A study of DoD postwar hospitalizations for mental disorders (June 1, 1991, to September 30, 1993) using 10 categories from the International Classification of Diseases, 9th revision, Clinical Modification, 6th edition (ICD-9-CM) was conducted by Dlugosz and colleagues (1999). It compared all active-duty personnel during the Gulf War era (n = 1,984,996) with those who did not serve. It also sought to identify risk factors for hospitalization. Nearly half the postwar hospitalizations were for alcohol-related disorders. Gulf War veterans were at greater risk for hospitalizations than nondeployed veterans due to drug-related disorders (RR 1.29, 95% CI 1.10-1.52) and acute reactions to stress (RR 1.45, 95% CI 1.08-1.94). Adjustments were made for age, sex, and military service branch. Although the database of ICD-9 codes does not allow determination of whether stress reactions expressly included PTSD, the authors noted that if posttraumatic stress was diagnosed, it would probably have been coded as an unspecified acute reaction to stress (ICD-9 code 308.9). Alcohol-related diagnoses were not increased. Exposure to the ground war in Iraq was associated with a greater risk of alcohol-related hospitalizations in men (RR 1.13, 95% CI 1.04-1.23). Serving as support for the ground war without being in direct combat was associated with a greater risk of drug-related hospitalizations in men (RR 1.42, 95% CI 1.03-1.96) and women (RR 3.61, 95% CI 1.70-7.66). The limitation of this study is that it examined only hospitalizations and thus was not representative of most psychiatric disorders that require outpatient treatment rather than hospitalization. It also did not include veterans who left the military after the Gulf War.

Secondary Studies

Findings on many other major cohorts of Gulf War veterans support what has been found in primary studies (Gray et al., 2002; McCauley et al., 2002). The most important limitation was their reliance on self-reports of "physician-diagnosed disorders" rather than measurement of symptoms with validated questionnaires or face-to-face interviews. In the UK cohort studied by Unwin et al. (1999), investigators asked some questions taken from the Mississippi Scale for Combat-Related PTSD but did not administer the entire questionnaire. They found that some symptoms were about 2-3 times more likely in deployed than in two nondeployed groups. The magnitude of the increase is consistent with that seen in the primary studies. Several other secondary studies have found an association between serving in the Gulf War and psychiatric disorders (Holmes et al., 1998; Magruder et al., 2005; Simmons et al., 2004; Steele, 2000; Stretch et al., 1996a,b; Sutker et al., 1995).

Goss Gilroy (1998) assessed all 3113 Canadian Gulf War veterans deployed to the war zone and a comparison group of nondeployed veterans with a mail questionnaire. Using the PCL-M, the investigators found that symptoms of PTSD were 2.5 times more prevalent in the deployed than in the nondeployed veterans (OR 2.69, 95% CI 1.7-4.2). Using the PRIME-MD, the investigators found that the deployed had higher prevalences of major depression (OR 3.67, 95% CI 3.0-4.4), chronic dysphoria, and anxiety. Anxiety and depression were more severe in lower-income veterans.

The studies of psychological outcomes in Australian Gulf War veterans were distinguished by inclusion of the entire deployed population (unclear what is meant by "direct assessment"). The instruments described below are self-administered screening questionnaires. McKenzie et al. (2004) used the SF-12, the PCL-M, and the GHQ-12 (12-item version of the General Health Questionnaire) to assess 1424 male Gulf War veterans (86.5% Navy) and 1548 male Australian Defence Force members who were not deployed to the Gulf War. On those self-rating instruments, the Gulf War-deployed had overall poorer psychological health (OR 1.4, 95% CI 1.2-1.6) and more PTSD-like symptoms (OR 2.0, 95% CI 1.5-2.9) than control veterans. The psychological distress increased with age in the comparison group but decreased with age in the Gulf War veterans (that is, the youngest Gulf War veterans had the worst psychological ill health). Moreover, the perceived level of exposure to war stress was associated with both psychological ill health and PTSD-like symptoms, although very few experienced direct combat.

Updated and Supplemental Literature

The Update committee identified four new primary studies (Fiedler et al., 2006; Ismail et al., 2002; Kang et al., 2009; Toomey et al., 2007) and five new secondary studies (Al-Turkait and Ohaeri, 2008; Axelrod et al., 2005; Black et al., 2006; Kang et al., 2005; Rona et al., 2007).

Primary Studies

Using a standardized clinician interview, Ismail and colleagues (2002) assessed mental health of random samples of UK Gulf War veterans who reported disability (n = 111) and those who did not (n = 98) and compared them to random samples of era veterans and Bosnia veterans reporting disability (n = 54 and 79, respectively). Individuals who had a known disease or serious medical condition were excluded from the study. One-month prevalences of DSM-IV disorders were assessed using the WHO schedule of clinical assessment in neuropsychiatry, a clinician-administered interview on which they achieved good inter-rater reliability. This is the only study that used a clinician-administered interview and reported kappa values for inter-rater reliability. It was also unique in that it compared rates of unexplained physical disability between veterans who served in the Gulf and veterans who served in other wars. The main result was that a great majority of disabled Gulf War veterans (76%) did not have a formal psychiatric disorder. Indeed, the prevalence of mental disorders was similar for veterans disabled after the Gulf War and veterans disabled after other Gulf War-era deployments (prevalence of any psychiatric disorder 24% vs 19%); 12% of nondisabled Gulf War veterans had any psychiatric disorder. Compared with disabled veterans from Bosnia or era veterans, disabled Gulf War veterans were no more likely to have an alcohol-related disorder (OR 1.9, 95% CI 0.4-9.1), mood disorder (OR 1.0, 95% CI 0.3-3.2), anxiety disorder (OR 1.4, 95% CI 0.4-4.3), PTSD (OR 1.1, 95% CI 0.1-9.1), sleep disorder (OR 1.1, 95% CI 0.4-3.2), or any psychiatric disorder (OR 1.3, 95% CI 0.5-3.4); only the presence of somatoform disorder approached significance (OR 3.1, 95% CI 1.0-9.6). When compared to nondisabled Gulf War veterans, disabled Gulf War veterans were at increased risk only for anxiety disorders (OR 6.8, 95% 1.4-33.4). The authors inferred that psychiatric disorders do not explain the elevation in self-reported ill health in Gulf War veterans.

This study also compared disabled with nondisabled Gulf War veterans. There was a more than twofold increase (16% for disabled vs 7% for nondisabled) in undifferentated somatoform disorder (OR 3.3, 95% CI 0.8-13.8), which represents the presence of one or more unexplained medical symptoms. Also, the overall prevalence of psychiatric disorders was twofold higher (24% in disabled Gulf War veterans vs 12% in nondisabled Gulf War veterans; OR 2.4, 95% CI 0.8-7.2). It should be noted, however, that the prevalences of some specific disorders—notably PTSD and alcohol-related disorders—were not significantly different between the disabled and nondisabled veterans.

Ten years after the war, Fiedler and colleagues (2006) conducted telephone interviews using the CIDI Short Form. In a random sample drawn from all US troops deployed and not deployed to the Gulf War from August 1990 to July 1991, the response rates were 59% for deployed and 51% for nondeployed veterans. This study used the largest random sample of US Gulf War deployed and era veterans in which a layperson-administered structured interview was used to assess 12-month prevalences of psychiatric disorders. When compared with era veterans, those deployed to the Gulf War had significantly higher prevalences of psychiatric disorders. Thus, there were increases in the prevalence of MDD (14.2% in deployed vs 7.2% nondeployed male veterans and 25.3% vs 11.8% for deployed vs nondeployed female veterans); PTSD (3.4% vs 0.7% for male veterans and 4.0% vs 2.2% for female veterans); and of substance dependence (5.3% vs 3.3% male veterans and 2.7% vs 2.2% in female veterans). Comparing all deployed veterans with nondeployed veterans, the OR for anxiety disorder was 1.81 (95% CI 1.34-2.45) and the OR for MDD was 2.07 (95% CI 1.50-2.85). Lower rank, female gender, and divorced or single marital status were significant independent predictors of psychiatric disorders other than substance use disorders. For substance use disorders, being male, having lower rank, divorced or single marital status, and deployment other than to the Persian Gulf were significant independent predictors.

These results are consistent with those found by Ikin et al. (2004) who used the CIDI to assess 1381 deployed Australian Gulf War veterans and 1377 nondeployed veterans. They also reported elevated rates of any depressive disorder (OR 1.7, 95% CI 1.3-2.1) and any anxiety disorders (OR 2.9, 95% CI 2.0-4.2), specifically MDD (OR 1.6, 95% CI 1.3-2.0), PTSD (OR 3.9, 95% CI 2.3-6.5), OCD (OR 5.6, 95% CI 1.7-24.2), or social phobia (OR 3.1, 95% 1.6-6.0), but no cases of somatization disorder. It is important to note that somatization disorder is not a measure of the presence or absence of physical (somatic) symptoms because it does not include medically explained symptoms, only medically unexplained symptoms. Unfortunately, prevalences of somatic symptoms were not measured in these studies, and the rate of somatization disorder does not provide a basis for estimating prevalences of somatic symptoms.

Approximately 10 years after the Gulf War, Toomey et al. (2007) used clinical interviews to estimate the current prevalence of mental disorders that had onset during the Gulf War. They studied a subset of deployed (n = 1061, participation rate = 53%) vs nondeployed (n = 1128, participation rate = 39%) veterans who had been interviewed in the National Health Survey of Gulf War Veterans and their Families (Kang et al., 2000). The interviews were carried out between 1998 and 2001. Gulf War-onset mental disorders were more prevalent in deployed (18.1%) versus nondeployed veterans (8.9%). with increased rates of PTSD as measured by the CAPS in Gulf War veterans (6.2% vs 1.1%; OR 5.78, 95% CI 2.62-12.74). Elevations in anxiety disorders, other than PTSD, as measured by the CIDI were elevated almost fourfold (OR 3.79, 95% CI 1.8-7.99) as was MDD (7.1% vs 4.1%; OR 1.81, 95% CI 1.03-3.19). Approximately 10 years after the war, era-onset major depression continued to be more prevalent among deployed (3.2%) versus nondeployed veterans (0.8%), as were rates of PTSD (1.8% vs 0.6%), although both decreased over time and for PTSD, the difference was no longer significant at 10 years. Somatoform disorders were rare in both groups (1.0% in deployed vs 0.3% in nondeployed), and the difference was not significant in this category overall. There was a significant difference in pain disorder (0.9% vs 0.01%) that represents the presence of one unexplained pain symptom. There was no significant difference in rates of somatization disorder between deployed and nondeployed veterans. Independent predictors of war-era onset mental disorders included female gender, higher levels of combat exposure, and the presence of prewar mental disorders.

Six years after the Gulf War, Al-Turkait and Ohaeri (2008) conducted a cross-sectional study in a stratified random sample of 200 Kuwaiti military men who had served in the Gulf War, using both self-administered questionnaires and a validated interview, the CAPS. Subjects were divided into four groups of 50 men each: retired from the military before the war, active duty but not in combat, active duty and in combat, and prisoners of war (POWs). The overall prevalence of PTSD as determined by the CAPS was 31.7%. The rate was highest for the most highly exposed group, POWs (48%), 22% for those with frontline combat exposure, 32% for those who were active-duty but had not been exposed to combat, and 24% for the retired control group. Higher rates of PTSD were associated with higher rates of depression and anxiety and lower self-esteem. Although this study included comparison groups and diagnostic interviews, the timeframe for prevalence is not reported, which limits its usefulness.

Secondary Studies

The committee identified five secondary studies (Axelrod et al., 2005; Black et al., 2006; Kang et al., 2005, 2009; Rona et al., 2007). Two of these studies focused on women veterans (Kang et al., 2005; Rona et al., 2007) and are discussed in the section on female veterans at the end of this chapter. Secondary studies also focused on borderline personality traits and the possibility that there may be an interaction between these traits and PTSD after deployment.

Axelrod et al. (2005) assessed 94 Operation Desert Storm veterans from the Connecticut National Guard study at several points following their return from the gulf for PTSD symptoms, combat exposure, and personality traits. The study asked retrospectively about pre- and postwar traits associated with borderline personality disorder, a chronic condition characterized by mood instability and difficulty with relationships. They reported that the presence of prewar borderline personality traits was associated with the development of some features of PTSD after combat exposure, and that PTSD symptoms at 1 month were associated with increases in endorsement of borderline personality traits at 6 months postwar.

In 2005, a third survey of the National Health Survey of Gulf War Era Veterans and Their Families population was conducted by Kang and colleagues (2009). This survey used self-administered questionnaires, rather than validated diagnostic interviews on a much larger sample of deployed (n = 6111) versus era veterans (n = 3859), although the overall response rate was low (34%). The study reported elevations in all mental disorders among those deployed to the Persian Gulf when compared to era veterans. In contrast to the previous report, which found no persistent significant differences in rates of PTSD, this study reported persistent two to threefold elevations in the rates of PTSD (in the past 4 weeks) in deployed versus nondeployed veterans based on the PCL-C (15.2% vs 4.6%; OR 2.98, 95% CI 2.54-3.50) as well as persistent elevations in major depression (in the past 4 weeks) (14.9% vs 5.8%; OR 2.34, 95% CI 2.03-2.70). Rates of functional impairment and reports of physical symptoms were also elevated about twofold in those deployed to the Gulf War when compared with the nondeployed. The authors did not report on whether PTSD or the presence of mental disorders was associated with the presence or magnitude of physical symptoms or disability.

Summary and Conclusion

The Committee draws four main conclusions on the relationship between deployment to the Gulf War and mental disorders.

First, combat exposure in the Gulf War was causally related to PTSD. Although the available evidence from Gulf War studies is somewhat limited, it is, however, sufficient to support the conclusion that the causal relationship of combat exposure to PTSD shown for other wars also pertains to combat exposure and the development PTSD in the Gulf War. In addition, the Gulf War studies suggest that future research should evaluate whether, in some instances, deployment to a war zone, without combat experience, could be a cause of PTSD.

Second, there is sufficient evidence of an association between deployment to the Gulf War and several other psychiatric disorders. These include generalized anxiety disorder, depression, and substance abuse, particularly alcohol abuse. For these disorders, the available evidence is not sufficient to establish whether or not the association is due to a causal relationship between the deployment and the psychiatric outcome.

Third, the associations between Gulf War deployment and psychiatric disorders were still evident 10 years after deployment (Fiedler et al., 2006; Kang et al., 2009; Toomey et al., 2007). For many of the psychiatric disorders that were measured in long-term follow-up studies, their prevalence even 10 years after the war was more than twofold higher in veterans who had been deployed compared with nondeployed veterans.

Fourth, from several lines of evidence, it can be inferred that the high prevalence of medically unexplained disability in Gulf War veterans cannot be reliably ascribed to any known psychiatric causes or disorders. It is not possible to attribute the high prevalence of medically unexplained disability in Gulf War veterans to somatoform disorder, based on available evidence. For example, a comparison of disabled Gulf War veterans with disabled veterans from other wars did not support such an attribution (Ismail et al., 2002), although veterans with known diseases or serious medical conditions were excluded from the disabled groups in this study. The majority of disabled Gulf War veterans did not have a diagnosable psychiatric disorder. Moreover, the prevalence of psychiatric disorder among disabled Gulf War veterans was similar to the prevalence among disabled veterans of other wars. Reports on somatization disorder in Gulf War veterans also do not support such an attribution. Somatization disorder, which is rare, requires eight symptoms that are not caused by a medical illness. Fiedler et al. (2006) and Toomey et al. (2007) found almost no cases of somatization disorder among Gulf War veterans, nor was there a significant elevation in somatization disorder among deployed versus nondeployed veterans. Therefore, somatization disorder cannot account for the high prevalence of medically unexplained disability in Gulf War veterans.

Finally, studies of somatoform disorder in Gulf War veterans also do not support the hypothesis that their medically explained symptoms results from this disorder. Somatoform disorder includes many specific diagnoses, of which the most relevant for this report is undifferentiated somatoform disorder. This disorder requires only one symptom without known medical causes, and is therefore a relatively common and nonspecific diagnosis. In the study by Ismail et al. (2002), somatoform disorder was more common in deployed versus nondeployed Gulf War veterans (16% vs 6%) and also more common in disabled Gulf War veterans than in disabled veterans from other wars (16% vs 7%). It was, however, present in only a small minority of disabled Gulf War veterans (after exclusion of those with known diseases, see above). Furthermore, the medical investigations in this study were not sufficiently comprehensive to rule out medical explanations for the symptoms in those who did have somatoform disorder.

Therefore, the committee concludes there is sufficient evidence of a causal relationship between traumatic war exposures experienced during deployment to the Gulf War and PTSD. The committee also concludes that there is sufficient evidence of an association between deployment to the Gulf War and other psychiatric disorders, including generalized anxiety disorder and substance abuse, particularly alcohol abuse. Furthermore, these disorders persist for at least 10 years after deployment. Finally, the excess of unexplained medical symptoms reported by deployed Gulf war veterans cannot be reliably ascribed to any known psychiatric disorder.

TABLE 4-4 Mental and Behavioral Disorders

Study	Design	Population	Outcomes	Results	Adjustments	Comments
Black et al., 2004b (Vol. 4)	Population-based interview study, by telephone; stratified random sample with proportional allocation (Iowa Persian Gulf Study Group, 1997)	1896 deployed vs 1799 nondeployed veterans listing Iowa as home state at time of enlistment	PRIME-MD (major depression, panic disorder, GAD) PCL-M, combat exposure assessed in basic demographic questionnaire. CAGE questionnaire (alcohol abuse)	Panic disorder (OR 2.2, 95% CI 1.2-3.8); GAD (OR 2.5, 95% CI 1.5-4.1); PTSD (OR 2.5, 95% CI 1.2-5.0); any anxiety disorder (OR 2.3, 95% CI 1.5-3.5)	Age, sex, race, branch of military, rank, military status, prior mental-health condition	Large, population-based sample
Barrett et al., 2002 (Vol. 4)	Population-based survey; completed telephone survey about their health status	3682 GWVs and control subjects	PCL-M, SF-36	Persons screened positive for PTSD more likely to have been deployed to Gulf War (OR 2.02, 95% CI 0.97-4.23) PTSD associated with: Current smoking status (OR 3.83, 95% CI 1.40-10.46) Number of self-reported symptoms (19.83 symptoms with PTSD vs 3.64 with no PTSD, $p < 0.0001$) Number of medical conditions (1.73 conditions with PTSD vs with no PTSD 10.18) Lower SF-36 scores for physical functioning (93 vs 66, $p < 0.0001$) and general health (80 vs 33, $p < 0.0001$)	Deployment status, age, sex, race, rank, branch, military status, and smoking status	Brief PTSD screen used; used 50 as the cutoff score with the PCL-M; low number of subjects who screened positive for PTSD; the sample from Iowa might not be representative of all US military personnel
Black et al., 2004a (Vol. 4)	Nested case-comparison; face-to-face interviews	602 veterans and controls	SCID (face-to-face interviews); SNAP; SF-36; Whitely Index	PTSD (27% vs 5% in deployed vs controls, OR 7.1, 95% CI 2.1-24.2); anxiety disorders (52% vs 25%, OR 3.2, 95% CI 1.6-6.3); any disorder (68% vs 52%, OR 2.0, 95% CI 1.0-3.7)	Validated PTSD checklist against SCID (70.4% sensitivity and 86.2% specificity of questionnaire	

Study	Design	Population	Outcomes	Results	Adjustments	Comments
					for the 192/602 subjects who met the criteria for depression)	
Kang et al., 2003 (Vol. 4)	Cross-sectional; population-based stratified random sample of GWV deployed compared with those deployed elsewhere	11,441 deployed vs 9476 nondeployed	Mail survey and telephone-based survey of PTSD symptoms	GWV (12.1%) compared to era veterans (4.3%); OR 3.1 (95% CI 2.7-3.4)	Sex, age, marital status, rank, and unit component	Nationally representative sample, questionnaire only
Wolfe et al., 1999a,b; Proctor et al., 1998 (Vol. 4)	Cross-sectional survey and interviews from larger cohorts followed longitudinally	220 Fort Devens vs 73 New Orleans vs 48 Germany; New Orleans and Germany cohorts only studied at time 2	Health Symptom Checklist, Mississippi PTSD Scale (times 1 and 2), SCID, CAPS (clinician diagnostic interviews, time 2 only)	Risk factors for PTSD were being female (time 1 OR 3.2, 95% CI 1.9-5.5; time 2 OR 2.3, 95% CI 1.5-3.5) and having high combat exposure (time 1 OR 1.22, time 2 OR 1.12, $p < 0.05$ for both); PTSD also highly correlated with current major depression ($r = 0.35$, $p < 0.001$) Lifetime occurrence of PTSD more prevalent in Fort Devens (8.1%) and New Orleans (7.6%) vs Germany (0%), no p-value reported Prevalence of PTSD increased from time 1 (3%) to time 2 (8%) in Fort Devens, 2% of the study group had PTSD at both time 1 and time 2, 1% had PTSD at time 1 but not time 2, and 6% had PTSD at time 2 but not time 1	Sex, reported health symptoms	Small sample deployed to Germany, 78% participation rate; Wolfe et al., 1999b, used direct interviews
Brailey et al., 1998 (Vol. 4)	Longitudinal; psychological interviews 9 months after war,	876 deployed (349 at time 2, 16 months later) vs 396	BDI-II, State Anger; State Anxiety; the BSI Depression; BSI Anxiety; BSI	Prevalence of depression increased over time in deployed veterans from time 1 (6.9%) to time 2 (13.8%), as did prevalence of PTSD (2.3% to	Age, education	Large attrition by time 2 (39.8% response rate at follow-up)

Study	Design	Population	Outcomes	Results	Adjustments	Comments
	and subgroup follow-up at 16 months; Louisiana National Guard and Reserve troops (Marine, Army, Air Force, Navy)	nondeployed	Hostility, the HSC, PTSD Checklist, and the Mississippi Scale	10.6%) and hostility (4.9% to 13.8%); no p-values reported		
Ikin et al., 2004 (Vol. 4)	Cross sectional survey of all Australian deployed veterans	1381 GWVs vs 1377 comparison veterans	CIDI	Prevalence of any disorder: 31% in GWVs vs 21% in comparison group; PTSD: OR 3.9 (95% CI 2.3-6.5); major depression: OR 1.6 (95% CI 1.3-2.0); alcohol abuse: OR 1.5 (95% CI 1.2-2.0)	Service type, rank, age, education, marital status	GWVs younger, more likely in the Navy, and lower ranked than comparison group Large sample, well-validated psychological interview tool; low participation bias
Dlugosz et al., 1999 (Vol. 4)	Post-war hospitalizations June 1991-September 1993	Active-duty men (1,775,236) and women (209,760) June 1991-September 1993; GWVs vs NDV	ICD-9 CM categories for 10 mental disorders	GWVs had increased risk of hospitalizations due to: acute reactions to stress (RR 1.45, 95% CI 1.08-1.94); drug-related disorders (RR 1.29, 95% CI 1.10-1.52) No general increase in alcohol-related diagnoses, but serving in ground war in Iraq associated with alcohol-related hospitalizations in men (RR 1.13, 95% CI 1.04-1.23)	Age, sex, service-branch adjusted rates	Active duty only; no assessment of outpatient treatment

Study	Design	Population	Outcomes	Results	Adjustments	Comments
Ismail et al., 2002 (Update)	Two-phase cohort study	Random sample of UK GWVs with reported disability (n = 111) and no disability (n = 98) and era and Bosnia veterans with disability (n = 54) and no disability (n = 79); Disability defined as score < 72.2 on SF-36	DSM-IV disorders assessed during clinician-administered interview	Disabled GWVs compared to disabled controls: No increase in prevalence of any mental disorder except undifferentiated somatoform disorder (OR 3.1, 95% CI 1.0-9.6)		Response rate good in GWV (67% disabled and 62% non-disabled), but low in controls (55% and 43%) Strength: clinician administered interview
Fiedler et al., 2006 (Update)	Cross-sectional, random sampling of all US troops deployed vs nondeployed (era veterans); assessment by computer-assisted telephone interview	967 deployed vs 784 nondeployed veterans	CIDI	Deployed veterans had significantly higher 12-month prevalence of any psychiatric disorder compared to nondeployed, (26.1% vs 16.1%, $p < 0.05$) Increase in major depressive disorder (14.2% vs 7.2% for males and 25.3% vs 11.8% for females) and PTSD (3.4% vs 0.7% for males and 4.0% vs 2.2% for females), no p-value reported All deployed vs all controls: Any anxiety disorder (OR 1.81, 95% CI 1.34-2.45); depression (OR 2.07, 95% CI 1.50-2.85) Males: alcohol dependence (4.8% vs 3.3%, NS); drug dependence (1.2% vs 0.0% $p < 0.05$)		Response rate 59% for deployed, 51% for era veterans Female gender, divorced, and lower rank were significant independent risk factors

Study	Design	Population	Outcomes	Results	Adjustments	Comments
Toomey et al., 2007 (Update)	Cross-sectional survey; stratified random sample of deployed vs nondeployed veterans; structured interview, self-report of symptoms	1061 deployed vs 1128 nondeployed US veterans (same cohort as Eisen et al., 2005)	CAPS; CIDI; PTSD Checklist; BDI-II; BAI; SF-36; QoLI; CES	Gulf War era onset: PTSD (6.2% deployed vs 1.1%, nondeployed), (OR 5.78, 95% CI 2.6-12.7); non-PTSD anxiety disorders (4.3% deployed vs 1.4% nondeployed), (OR 3.79, 95% CI 1.8-8.0); major depression (7.1 % deployed vs 4.1% nondeployed), (OR 1.81, 95% CI 1.0-3.2) 10 years post-Gulf War era: PTSD (1.8% vs 0.06% deployed vs nondeployed, p = 0.12); non-PTSD anxiety disorders (2.8% vs 1.2% deployed vs nondeployed, p = 0.01); major depression (3.2% deployed vs 0.8% nondeployed, p = 0.01) Symptom self report: deployed reported more severe symptoms of PTSD, depression, anxiety; lower level quality of life; SF-36 scores significantly lower	Age, sex, ethnicity, years of education, duty type (active vs reserve/guard), service branch, rank	Response rate: 53% for deployed; 39% for nondeployed Prevalence of non-PTSD anxiety disorders significantly higher in deployed (12.5%) vs nondeployed (9.2%), p = 0.02
Al-Turkait and Ohaeri, 2008 (Update)	Retrospective Cohort; stratified random sampling of four groups of veterans: retired from military prior to war; active duty with no combat; active duty with combat; POW	200 Kuwaiti Gulf War veterans, 50 from each group	PTSD, determined by CAPS	POWs: 48.4% Combat: 32% No combat: 22% Retired: 24% Higher rates of anxiety, depression, and low self-esteem in those with PTSD compared to those without PTSD (p = 0.0001)		Potential bias resulting from application of questionnaire to a foreign population

NOTES: BAI = Beck Anxiety Inventory; BDI-II = Beck Depression Inventory; BSI = Bried Symptom Inventory; CAPS = Clinician Administered PTSD scale; CES = Combat Exposure Scale; CIDI = Composite International Diagnostic Interview; GAD = generalized anxiety disorder; GWV = Gulf War veteran; HSC = Health Symptoms Checklist; NS = not significant; PCL-M = PTSD Checklist-Military Version; POW = prisoner of war; PRIME-MD = Primary Care Evaluation of Mental Disorders; PTSD = posttraumatic stress disorder; QoLI = Quality of Life Inventory; SCID = Structured Clinical Interview for DSM Disorders; SF-36 = 36-Item Short Form Health Survey; SNAP = Special Needs Assessment Profile.

NEUROCOGNITIVE AND NEUROBEHAVIORAL OUTCOMES

This section contains an overview and update on neurocognitive and neurobehavioral performance in Gulf War veterans compared with nondeployed veterans. In *Gulf War and Health, Volume 4: Health Effects of Serving in the War* the committee defined primary studies as "high-quality studies that used neurobehavioral tests that had previously been used to detect adverse effects in population-based research on occupational groups." Furthermore the committee presented findings separately for those studies that (a) compared neurobehavioral performance in deployed veterans and nondeployed veterans, and (b) compared neurobehavioral performance in deployed veterans reporting symptoms that met various definitions of Gulf War syndrome with neurobehavioral performance in deployed veterans who did not report symptoms.

The major issues that distinguished secondary studies from primary studies were lack of adjustment for potential confounding effects of age, sex, education, native intellectual ability (as measured by the Wechsler Adult Intelligence Scale, National Adults Reading Test [NART], Armed Forces Qualifying Test [AFQT]), and lack of blinding of testers to deployment and/or symptom status. Studies in which neurocognitive and neurobehavioral performance was measured only based on self-report were not included. Table 4-5 summarizes the primary studies for neurocognitive and neurobehavioral outcomes.

Summary of *Volume 4*

Studies in Nonsymptomatic Veterans

In consideration of the comparison of neurobehavioral performance in Gulf War deployed veterans compared with nondeployed veterans there were two primary studies (David et al., 2002; Proctor et al., 2003) and three secondary studies (Axelrod and Milner, 1997; Vasterling et al., 2003; White et al., 2001).

David et al. (2002) compared 209 UK veterans deployed to the Persian Gulf with 54 UK Bosnian peacekeepers and 78 nondeployed veterans. In this analysis no differences were found in neurobehavioral performance taking into account age, education, the National Adults Reading Test, and a depression score (Beck Depression Inventory). In the study of Proctor et al. (2003) the findings were verified with no differences found between 143 Danish Gulf War veterans and 72 non deployed veterans of the Danish military.

Of the secondary studies, only one (Axelrod and Milner, 1997) found differences between deployed and nondeployed veterans on the Stroop test of directed attention, following adjustment for age and education. White et al. (2001) combined two quite different samples (a cohort from Fort Devens and a second cohort from New Orleans) and compared this group to a small group of Germany-deployed veterans.

Studies in Symptomatic Veterans

In considering the neurobehavioral performance of symptomatic versus nonsymptomatic Gulf War veterans, two primary studies (David et al., 2002; Storzbach et al., 2001) and six secondary studies (Axelrod and Milner, 1997; Bunegin et al., 2001; Goldstein et al., 1996; Hom et al., 1997; Lange et al., 2001; Sillanpaa et al., 1997) were identified in *Volume 4*. Overall the definition of symptomatic was variable ranging from "any one of memory loss, confusion, mood swings, etc." to categorization based on SF-36 scores. The committee identified the core symptoms as cognitive in all of the studies except Lange et al. (2001), in which the only symptom was fatigue.

One of the primary studies, David et al. (2002), categorized Gulf War veterans as ill (n = 151) and well (n = 188) based on SF-36 physical function scores. Subjects were also classified as symptom reporting (n = 65) or symptom not reporting (n = 33) based on the Centers for Disease Control and Prevention (CDC) working definition of Gulf War-related symptoms (Fukuda et al., 1998). Following adjustment for age, education, the National Adults Reading Test, and depression, and correction for multiple testing, there were no identified differences in neurobehavioral performance.

Storzbach et al. (2001) compared 239 Gulf War veterans who reported at least one symptom associated with Gulf War syndrome with 112 nonsymptomatic Gulf War veterans. This analysis found poorer performance among the symptomatic group on the Oregon Dual Task Procedure errors and latency, Digit Span Backward, and the Simple Reaction Time. Results were adjusted for age, education, AFQT, and for multiple testing.

There were six secondary studies that compared symptomatic to nonsymptomatic Gulf War veterans. These studies varied in design including the definition of *symptomatic* although in general the same performance tests were used. All but one found performance differences between symptomatic and nonsymptomatic Gulf War veterans. However, only two studies included an adjustment for age and education, and only one took multiple comparisons into account.

Updated and Supplemental Literature

The Update committee identified two additional studies both of which were classified as secondary (Proctor et al., 2006; Toomey et al., 2009).

Proctor et al. (2006) was considered secondary (rather than primary) because the comparison was not between deployed Gulf War veterans and nondeployed veterans but across deployed Gulf War veterans classified within putative sarin exposure categories. In this study, a subset of the Fort Devens cohort neurobehavioral/neurocognitive performance was assessed in 1994-1995 and examined in relation to putative sarin exposure during the Gulf War. Sarin exposure was based on the 2000 Khamisiyah plume analyses, which produced four modeled hazard areas—one for each day between March 10 and March 13, 1991, when it was believed that sarin and cyclosarin were released following the detonations. Individuals in the study were classified in an exposure category based on the estimated dosages assigned to the 11 Fort Devens cohort study units. Study participants who served in units with exposure levels of greater than 0.072 mg-min/m^3 were classified as having high exposure (n = 23); those in units with exposure levels greater than the general population limit of 0.01296 mg-min/m^3 but no more than > 0.072 mg-min/m^3 were defined as moderately exposed (n = 47). Those participants in areas where no exposure level was estimated because they were not in an area within the plume areas were classified as low-to-no exposure (n = 70).

The outcomes of interest were based on neuropsychological tests of five cognitive domains: attention, executive function, psychomotor function, visuospatial abilities, and short-term memory. The selected tests were chosen from those known to be sensitive to the effects of neurotoxicants that were believed to have been present in the Gulf War. The authors reported that sarin and cyclosarin exposure were associated with a reduced proficiency on functional domains of psychomotor function (Purdue pegboard) and visuospatial abilities (WAIS block designs. The high-exposure group and the moderate-exposure group had significantly poorer performance in these tests than the low-to-no exposure group. The analysis adjusted for age, sex, unit group, rank, PTSD scores, handedness, and history of head injury. The authors interpreted these reductions in proficiency on the Purdue pegboard test for an individual with an estimated exposure of 0.1 mg-min/m^3 as being approximately one point lower than individuals in the low-to-no exposure group. This difference is equivalent to a performance of someone approximately 20 years older on the task. For the block designs for the same hypothetical individual the estimated difference would be approximately 4 points or the equivalent of being 15 years older.

A particular strength of this study was that the neurobehavioral and neurocognitive testing was performed in the vast majority of subjects (95%) prior to the 1996 public announcement that the munitions at Khamisiyah contained sarin. Limitations of this study include the fact that, like others studies, there was no predeployment testing available for comparison, and there may have been misclassification of individuals across the three exposure categories.

In 2009, Toomey et al. published a study that examined the neuropsychological functioning of Gulf War veterans 10 years after deployment. This study was classified as a secondary (rather than primary) study for several reasons. First, the study was conducted 10 years after the Gulf War, thus the findings were interpreted under the assumption that any observed differences in neuropsychological functioning in a subgroup of deployed versus nondeployed veterans is attributable to deployment and there was no account taken of events that took place in the years since the Gulf War. While this may be the case, one would also wish to consider life events and comorbidities that may have occurred in the 10-year period between the Gulf War and the time of assessment. This is particularly problematic given that there are no predeployment baseline neuropsychological measures with which to compare the measures at 10 years. In addition, the participation rates for both deployed and nondeployed are low (53% in the deployed and 39% in the nondeployed) and quite different, possibly resulting in selection bias (Toomey et al., 2009). While in an earlier study the same group of authors report on an assessment of the differences between participants and nonparticipants in both the deployed and nondeployed groups (Eisen et al., 2005), in the discussion Toomey et al. (2009) concede that the low study participation may have "biased results."

The source of participants for this study was the National Health Survey of Gulf War Era Veterans and Their Families Study (Eisen et al., 2005). Based on the 11,441 deployed and 9476 nondeployed participants in the 1995 study, 1996 and 2003 veterans, respectively, were solicited to participate. In the deployed group, 1061 (53%) agreed to participate, and only 39% (1128/2883) of the nondeployed agreed to participate. Measures of neuropsychological functioning were based on those that had been suggestive of differences in the deployed and nondeployed cohorts previously and included measures of general intelligence, attention/executive functioning, motor ability, visuospatial processing, and verbal and visual memory. Factor analysis was used to derive eight neuropsychological test variables (verbal memory, attention/working memory, visual memory, executive functioning, perceptual motor speed, visual organization, motor speed, and sustained attention) from 27 individual variables. Deployed and nondeployed veterans were compared on mean factors scores as well as on the mean scores of the 27 individual variables included in the factor analysis.

In comparing the factor scores, the results of this study indicated that participants in the deployed group did worse on two of the eight factors, motor speed ($p = 0.03$) and sustained attention ($p = 0.04$), while nondeployed participants did worse on visual organization. Concerned about an education effect the authors conducted a sensitivity analysis excluding those participants with postgraduate education and the worse performance on motor speed and sustained attention remained. In the comparison between the two participant groups across the 27 individual variables and controlling for multiple testing using a Bonferroni adjustment, the deployed veterans performed worse only on the Trails B–Trails A time ($p = 0.002$, which was equal to the Bonferroni correct p value). The authors themselves concluded from this study that "Gulf War deployment is associated with subtle declines in motor speed and sustained attention, despite overall intact neuropsychological functioning."

Summary and Conclusions

The Volume 4 committee concluded that the primary studies reviewed in that volume showed nonsignificant trends of poorer neurobehavioral performance when Gulf War veterans were compared with nondeployed veterans or those deployed to Germany. However, when PTSD (White et al., 2001) or depressed mood (David et al., 2002) was treated as a confounder in the statistical analyses those trends disappeared. The results were adjusted for depression because it is often found to coexist with PTSD. That adjustment could have made it impossible to detect cognitive differences.

One study concluded that Gulf War veterans who report symptoms associated with the Gulf conflict performed more poorly on neurobehavioral tests than veterans who did not report symptoms (Storzbach et al., 2001). Another study found substantial neurobehavioral deficits in deployed veterans but had intentionally recruited veterans who experienced a high prevalence of post-Gulf War illness (Hom et al., 1997). That study, however, failed to adjust for key confounders and for the large number of statistical comparisons in their study, raising doubt about the validity of their findings.

In this update, two studies were added to those presented in *Volume 4*. While each of these studies presents some results indicating an effect of either deployment (Toomey et al., 2009) or putative sarin exposure amongst deployed soldiers (Proctor et al., 2006), the differences between and the limitations within these studies suggests that they may only be considered as secondary studies.

In conclusion, primary studies of deployed Gulf War veterans versus veterans not deployed to the Gulf do not demonstrate differences in cognitive and motor measures as determined through neurobehavioral testing. However, returning Gulf War veterans who had at least one symptom commonly reported by Gulf War veterans (fatigue, memory loss, confusion, inability to concentrate, mood swings, somnolence, gastrointestinal distress, muscle or joint pain, or skin or mucous membrane complaints) demonstrated poorer performance on cognitive tests than returning veterans who did not report such symptoms.

Therefore, the committee concludes that there is inadequate/insufficient evidence to determine whether an association exists between deployment to the Gulf War and neurocognitive and neurobehavioral performance.

TABLE 4-5 Neurobehavioral and Neurocognitive Outcomes

Reference	Study Design	Population	Outcomes	Results	Adjustments	Comments
David et al., 2002 (Vol. 4)	Case-control, clinical evaluations	200 male UK GWVs, 54 Bosnia-deployed, 78 era nondeployed soldiers randomly selected from larger cohort of UK veterans who participated in earlier postal survey (see Unwin et al., 1999)	WAIS-R scaled scores: Vocabulary Digit span Arithmetic Similarities Picture arrangement Block design Object assembly Digit symbol PASAT Sustained attention to response task Stroop Trail-making test, A & B WMS: Logical memory (Immediate and delayed recall) Verbal paired associates (Immediate and delayed recall) Camden recognition memory test Purdue pegboard Individually administered tests, blinded examiners	GWVs had significantly lower scores on 5 cognitive tests after demographic confounder and LSD corrections: Digit symbol Trail-making Stroop PASAT Verbal associates After final Bonferroni adjustments for multiple comparisons and BDI, only the results of the Purdue pegboard remained significantly different	ANCOVA adjusted for education, age, NART, BDI; multiple comparison adjustment for least significant difference procedure and Bonferroni adjustments	Careful treatment of potential confounders, such as depression, mood, IQ, education
Proctor et al., 2003 (Vol. 4)	Cross-sectional	143 male Danish GWVs, 72 male nondeployed troops randomly selected from 84% and 58% of total Danish armed forces deployed and nondeployed, respectively, at time of Gulf War	WAIS-R Information subscale, continuous performance test, trail making, WCST, Purdue pegboard, WAIS-R block design, CVLT, WMS visual reproductions, TOMM; individually administered tests except in computer-based NES; blinded examiners	No overall differences in neuropsychologic domains, significant test differences in domains ($p \leq 0.05$) for CVLT and WCST	MANCOVA by neuropsychologic domain, adjusted for age	Response rate 75%

Reference	Study Design	Population	Outcomes	Results	Adjustments	Comments
Storzbach et al., 2001 (Vol. 4)	Case-control	239 randomly selected male and female GWVs with symptoms vs 112 deployed with no symptoms; case = one of memory loss, confusion, inability to concentrate, mood swings, somnolence, gastrointestinal distress, fatigue, muscle and joint pain, skin or mucous membrane lesions lasting 1 month or longer, starting during or after service in gulf, and present during 3 months before questionnaire received	Symbol digit Serial digit learning ODTP Selective attention test Digit span Simple reaction time BARS computer-based testing system Blinded examiners	Cases significantly worse than controls on: Digit span backward Simple reaction time ODTP Errors Latency (including a slow group of 13% of sample with scores > 2 sd slower than control mean latency) PCA showed the slow ODTP (slow case in 1999) were responsible for group differences in neurobehavioral performance; 2 of 354 excluded for possible poor motivation because of excess errors in ODTP	ANCOVA, adjusted for age, sex, and AFQT, but effect was small so t-tests were used; Bonferroni correction for multiple comparisons	

NOTE: AFQT = Armed Forces Qualifying Test; ANCOVA = analysis of covariance; BARS = Behavioral Assessment and Research System; BDI = Beck Depression Inventory; CVLT = California Verbal Learning Test; GWV = Gulf War veteran; IQ = intelligence quotient; MANOVA = multivariate analysis of variance; NART = National Adult Reading Test; ODTP = Oregon Dual Task Procedure; PASAT = Paced Auditory Serial Addition Test; PCA = principal-components analysis; TOMM = Test of Memory Malingering; WAIS = Wechsler Adult Intelligence Scale; WCST = Wisconsin Card Sorting Test; WMS = Wechsler Memory Scale.

DISEASES OF THE NERVOUS SYSTEM

Neurologic diseases are common afflictions, with risk for specific disorders dependant on such factors as age, family history, and environmental exposures. The battlefield environment might be associated with an increase in risk for a variety of neurologic problems. These range from the known consequences of traumatic brain and nerve injury, which can include epilepsy, cognitive disturbances, headache, and nerve or bodily pains, to the likely relationship between battlefield deployment and an increase in risk for amyotrophic lateral sclerosis (ALS or Lou Gehrig's disease). Multiple sclerosis (MS) is another neurologic disorder of interest in this context, as risk for MS has been associated with exposure to highly stressful experiences including war. Immune-mediated neuropathies, including Guillain Barré syndrome, are also known to follow a variety of infectious illnesses or vaccinations to which servicemembers may have been exposed. The special circumstances of the Gulf War theater, with exposures to extreme heat, poor sanitation in some circumstances, exposure to unfamiliar biological agents, as well as known and unknown exposures to drugs such as pyridostigmine bromide (PB), pesticides, fumes, and other environmental toxins might contribute to the development of a variety of neurologic disorders. As examples, peripheral neuropathy or myopathy are known to occur with exposures to a number of different toxins and drugs, and Parkinson's disease is associated with pesticide exposure. For these reasons, a broad analysis was undertaken to review the literature on a wide range of neurologic outcomes identified to date in servicemembers who participated in the Gulf War mission. The review is organized by specific neurologic afflictions including peripheral neuropathy and myopathy, MS, ALS, and other neurologic disorders. Some common neurologic disorders such as Parkinson's and Alzheimer's diseases rarely ever occur until later in life (after age 60), and it is highly unlikely that Gulf War veterans would have developed these disorders to date, even though a very long latency period of decades for such health outcomes is a possibility. Thus current studies have insufficient follow-up time to allow drawing any conclusions on increases of risk for these disorders among Gulf War veterans. Other disorders of unknown but possible neurologic etiology, including chronic fatigue syndrome, fibromyalgia, and multisystem illness, are discussed in other sections.

Peripheral Neuropathy and Myopathy

This section reviews studies of peripheral neuropathy, polyneuropathy, or neuromuscular symptoms, as identified by the investigators' conducting the studies. Peripheral neuropathy, broadly defined, is a disease of the peripheral nerve tissues (that is, nerve fibers ensheathed by Schwann cells, including nerve roots), which transmit information from the brain and spinal cord to other parts of the body.

Numerous types of peripheral neuropathy have been characterized, each with its own set of symptoms, patterns of development, and prognosis. Peripheral neuropathy can be classified by a variety of factors, such as the population of nerve fibers affected (for example, motor, sensory, or autonomic). Additionally, neuropathy can be classified by the time course (acute, subacute and chronic, remitting, or relapsing) and by pathology (axonal, demyelinating, or other). Peripheral neuropathy might be inherited (for example, resulting from inborn errors in the genetic code or mutations) or acquired (for example, from physical injury, tumors, toxins, autoimmune responses, nutritional deficiencies, alcoholism, vascular and metabolic disorders, or infections from conditions such as leprosy, human immunodeficiency virus, herpes simplex and zoster, or hepatitis associated) (National Institute of Neurological Disorders and Stroke, 2006, 2009). Polyneuropathy is a neurologic disorder characterized by progressive weakness and impaired sensory function in arms and legs. The committee notes that an objective inquiry of peripheral neuropathy depends on clinical recognition of absent ankle reflexes, distal symmetric leg and foot weakness and atrophy, sensation loss in toes and feet, and abnormalities in nerve conduction. The committee also regards studies with objective and quantitative measures, such as those with nerve-conduction tests, to be optimal. The importance of obtaining neurophysiologic studies is especially helpful in determining the presence of neuropathy whenever the clinical evaluations alone are inconclusive or the type of neuropathy is uncertain (for example, does the disorder primarily affect the myelin sheath or the axon of the nerve cell?). For disorders that affect small nerve fibers (resulting in pain, temperature, and autonomic symptoms only) more sophisticated neurophysiologic tests and in some cases nerve biopsies may be required to reveal the underlying pathology.

Summary of *Volume 4*

The best population-based questionnaire study for assessment of peripheral neuropathy is that of Cherry and colleagues (Cherry et al., 2001a,b), who studied UK troops deployed to the Gulf War. Almost 35% of Gulf War veterans who reported handling pesticides for more than a month indicated numbness or tingling on mannequin diagrams compared with 13.6% of veterans who did not report handling pesticides. The handling of pesticides and side effects of handling nerve agent prophylaxis were associated with self-reports of peripheral neuropathy (OR 1.26; $p < 0.001$). However, although the study was well designed and suggested a dose-response relationship, it was limited by recall bias, lack of clinical evaluations, and the absence of nerve-conduction studies. Self-reporting of peripheral neuropathy symptoms has poor diagnostic accuracy (Franse et al., 2000). Because of those limitations, the committee defined primary studies as requiring, at a minimum, medical evaluations.

Primary Studies

In the medical evaluation component of the large, population-based cohort assembled by the VA, Davis and colleagues (2004) reported on the presence of distal symmetric polyneuropathy in deployed and nondeployed veterans. That condition was evaluated through history, physical examination, and standardized electrophysiological assessment of motor and sensory nerves in 1047 deployed veterans and 1121 nondeployed veterans. Spouses of deployed and nondeployed veterans were also studied, as was a population of 240 Khamisiyah-exposed veterans. Exposure to potential nerve agents was assessed with one of the first DoD models of atmospheric dispersion (Winkenwerder, 2002). Blood studies were performed to rule out metabolic causes of neuropathy. Although the study provided results on distal symmetric polyneuropathy as distal sensory or motor neuropathy identified on the basis of the neurologic examination, nerve conduction study, or both, the committee favored distal symmetric polyneuropathy identified with a nerve conduction study as the best, most reliable measure of peripheral neuropathy. No significant differences between adjusted population prevalence of distal symmetric polyneuropathy in deployed and nondeployed veterans were found (OR 0.65, 95% CI 0.33-1.28). There also were no differences on physical examination or self-reported peripheral neuropathy, although at the time of examination, deployed veterans reported more numbness and tingling than did nondeployed veterans. The veterans exposed to the Khamisiyah ammunition depot explosion did not differ significantly from nonexposed deployed veterans (OR

1.04, 95% CI 0.25-4.37). The prevalence of distal symmetric polyneuropathy in the spouses of deployed and nondeployed veterans also did not differ; however, the measure of distal symmetric polyneuropathy was obtained through self-reports as opposed to medical evaluation or nerve conduction study. One limitation of the study is potential participation bias: only 53% of deployed veterans and 39% of nondeployed veterans invited to participate were actually examined.

Neuromuscular symptoms of UK veterans were evaluated with objective testing of peripheral nerves, skeletal muscles, or neuromuscular junctions in a case-control study (Rose et al., 2004; Sharief et al., 2002). Ill veterans (with more than four neuromuscular symptoms and lower functioning according to the SF-36) were compared with healthy deployed veterans, 13 symptomatic Bosnian veterans, and 22 symptomatic Gulf War-era controls. All groups had been randomly selected from 8195 male military personnel. In the first publication, veterans underwent nerve-conduction studies, quantitative sensory and autonomic testing, and concentric needle and single-fiber electromyography. In the second, they underwent quantitative myometry through the ischemic forearm exercise test, the subanaerobic bicycle exercise test, and a muscle biopsy. The studies revealed no significant differences between deployed and nondeployed veterans who had symptoms of Gulf War illness. The sole exception was the greater effort required for the bicycle exercise test with increased lactate production; this finding could reflect mitochondrial damage or inactivity resulting from ill health. See Table 4-6 for a summary of the peripheral neuropathy findings.

Secondary Studies

Other studies supporting the absence of findings include those of Amato et al. (1997), Eisen et al. (2005), Pasquina et al. (2004), and Rivera-Zayas et al. (2001). Eisen et al. (2005) appear to have reported in less detail on the peripheral neuropathy findings in the same cohort as previously reported by Davis and colleagues (2004), but the precise relationship between the two publications is not clear. The Pasquina et al. study (2004), a retrospective review of electrophysiologic testing of 56 Gulf War veterans and 120 nondeployed veterans, showed no objective evidence of a higher incidence of neuromuscular disease in deployed veterans than in nondeployed veterans. In the Rivera-Zayas et al. (2001) study, 12 of 162 Gulf War veterans tested electrophysiologically with positive questionnaires for neuropathy had normal results except for two subjects who had carpal tunnel syndrome. Amato et al. (1997) showed that in 20 Gulf War veterans who had severe muscle fatigue, weakness, and myalgias, nerve conduction studies, repetitive nerve stimulation, quantitative and single-fiber electromyography, and muscle biopsies were inconclusive.

Updated and Supplemental Literature

Kelsall et al. (2005) performed a cross-sectional analysis of the entire cohort of 1871 Australian Gulf War veterans and a comparison group of 2924 nondeployed veterans, matched by age, sex, and service type. Postal and telephone questionnaires were administered followed by evaluations at 10 clinics across the country. Increased reporting of lower-extremity symptoms possibly indicative of neuropathy was present in the deployed Gulf War group (OR 1.6; 95% CI 1.0-2.7), Increased reporting of lower-extremity symptoms possibly indicative of neuropathy was present in the deployed Gulf War group (OR 1.6; 95% CI 1.0-2.7), but results of neurologic examinations were similar in both groups. There was no clinical evidence of an increased risk of myopathy or muscle weakness. An increase in the reporting of neurological symptoms was associated with self-reports of immunizations and exposure to various chemical agents including

PB and pesticides. Symptoms possibly indicative of neuropathy were not associated with self-reports of immunizations or chemical exposures however (conclusion stated in paper but data not presented). Electrophysiologic studies were not performed.

Summary and Conclusions

Several well-designed studies from the United States, United Kingdom, and Australia found no evidence of excess peripheral neuropathy in Gulf War veterans. Several other secondary studies supported a conclusion of no excess risk. Some studies, such as that of Cherry et al. (2001a), did report higher rates of peripheral neuropathy, but they used self-reports, which the committee did not accept as a reliable measure of peripheral neuropathy. Furthermore, because researchers use different case definitions of peripheral neuropathies, there are problems of ascertainment, which makes comparisons among groups difficult.

The committee finds no increase in the prevalence of peripheral neuropathy in deployed versus nondeployed veterans, as defined by history, physical examination, and electrophysiologic studies. Detailed quantitative analyses to investigate small-fiber polyneuropathy have not, as yet, been reported in Gulf War veterans.

Therefore the committee concludes that there is limited/suggestive evidence of no association between deployment to the Gulf War and peripheral neuropathy.

Multiple Sclerosis

MS is a chronic inflammatory disease of the brain and spinal cord. It is caused by an immune-mediated attack on the myelin membrane that surrounds and insulates nerve fibers (axons) that are responsible for normal transmission of electrical and chemical information in the nervous system. Strong circumstantial evidence indicates that MS is an autoimmune disease in which normal myelin, and perhaps also nerve cells themselves, are misread as “foreign” by the immune system. Numerous immune cell types—T cells, B cells, and microglia—as well as a variety of immune molecules including antibodies, cytokines, and chemokines are all believed to contribute to destruction of myelin and scarring (gliosis) that are the hallmarks of MS. MS can vary from a relatively benign illness to a rapidly evolving and incapacitating disease. Symptoms of MS—such as weakness of the limbs, numbness, visual loss or blurring, pain, imbalance, fatigue, slowed thinking, and bladder/bowel/sexual dysfunction—reflect the loss of neural connections required for normal function. Treatments are available for many people with relapsing forms of MS; however, no useful therapies exist for progressive symptoms.

MS is a common disease in most parts of the developed world; it affects about 350,000 people in the United States and 2.5 million people worldwide. In Western societies, MS is second only to trauma as a cause of neurologic disability beginning in early to mid adulthood.

MS is approximately three times more common in women than men. The age of onset is typically between 18 and 40 years of age, but the disease can present across the lifespan. MS also appears to be increasing in frequency, especially in women. The environmental factors that lead to MS are not known; however, evidence implicates a lack of sun exposure associated with vitamin D deficiency, and exposure to Epstein Barr virus resulting in a strong antibody response to the virus, as possible contributors.

Several aspects of the Gulf War theater could, in theory, heighten the risk of MS. The first relates to exposure to the hot desert environment. Symptoms of MS may first appear, or can transiently worsen, upon exposure to heat; this is due to the “short-circuiting” of impulses carried across demyelinated nerves when the core body temperature is raised. Second, a variety of infections can increase the risk of MS attacks, and it is well established that soldiers in both the Gulf War and in the conflicts in Iraq and Afghanistan experienced numerous infectious illnesses (see IOM, 2007). A third potential deployment-related risk is that of multiple vaccinations; however, there is no convincing evidence that any vaccinations are risk factors for MS (reviewed in Compston, 2006). Finally, it is possible that psychological and physical stress associated with war might increase MS risk, as has been recently reported from Israel (Golan et al., 2008).

Updated and Supplemental Literature

Primary Study

There was no information related to MS at the time of the last IOM review in 2006. Barth et al. (2009) reviewed mortality from MS as well as from ALS, Parkinson's disease, and brain cancer from 621,902 veterans who served in the Gulf War between August 1, 1990, and March 1, 1991, and compared these with 746,248 veterans who served concurrently but were not deployed to the gulf. Follow-up was terminated on December 31, 2004. Records from the VA database Beneficiary Identification and Records Locator Subsystem (BIRLS), a file consisting of all veterans eligible for VA benefits, and the SSA Death Masterfile were examined. Death certificates and medical records were reviewed by experts who were blinded to deployment status and classified using the McDonald criteria (McDonald et al., 2001). A total of 19 deaths due to MS were identified; 6 in the deployed group and 13 nondeployed. The adjusted relative risk estimates for MS mortality did not suggest an increased risk of mortality from MS (RR 0.67, 95% CI 0.24-1.85; Cox proportionate hazard model).

Secondary Studies

Kelsall et al. (2005) performed a cross-sectional analysis of the entire cohort of 1871 Australian Gulf War veterans, and a comparison group of 2924 nondeployed veterans, matched by age, sex and service type. Postal and telephone questionnaires were administered followed by evaluations at 10 clinics across country. MS was self-identified in one Gulf War veteran and in three in the comparison group (OR 0.3, 95% CI 0.00-3.5). Because of the small size and limitations of this study, and the fact that MS was determined by self-report, no conclusions can be drawn about the prevalence of MS in this cohort; therefore, this study is considered to be secondary for this health outcome.

Summary and Conclusions

No excess in MS mortality was identified in Gulf War veterans in a single well-executed primary study. However, for several reasons the design of the study is likely to be insensitive to the detection of any MS risk associated with deployment. First, the study could detect deaths from MS within 13 years or less from the time of deployment, yet epidemiologic data suggest that the interval between a critical environmental exposure and the clinical onset of MS may be a decade or longer. Second, any excess mortality due to MS is likely to be only minimal during the first 15 years of the illness. Thus a mortality endpoint with a short duration study is unlikely to have power to detect an increase in the occurrence of clinical MS among those deployed in the 1990-1991 conflict.

Therefore, the committee concludes that there is inadequate/insufficient evidence to determine whether an association exists between deployment to the Gulf War and multiple sclerosis.

Recommendation: Well-designed, adequately powered studies of MS incidence following deployment are needed.

Amyotrophic Lateral Sclerosis

ALS is a neuromuscular disorder; it is often referred to as Lou Gehrig's disease and might also be called motor neuron disease or Charcot's disease. It affects approximately 20,000 to 30,000 people in the United States (ALS Association, 2008; National Institute of Neurological Disorders and Stroke, 2006, 2009). ALS affects all races and ethnic backgrounds, and the risk is higher in men than women of the same age (Annegers et al., 1991). The disease is often relentlessly progressive and almost always fatal. The rate of progression is quite variable from patient to patient.

ALS causes degeneration of the motor neurons in the cerebral motor cortex (called upper motor neurons) and the brain stem and spinal cord (called lower motor neurons) (Rowland, 2000). The motor neurons are nerve cells that provide communication between the highest levels of the nervous system and the voluntary muscles of the body (National Institute of Neurological Disorders and Stroke, 2006). When the upper motor neurons degenerate, their connections to the lower motor neurons and spinal interneurons are disrupted. That disruption leads to weakness of muscles in a characteristic distribution and the development of spasticity. Lower motor neuron degeneration disrupts nerve contact to the muscles resulting in muscle atrophy. Spontaneous muscle activity, called fasciculation, occurs. Eventually, affected people are unable to move their arms and legs and cannot speak or swallow. When the connection is disrupted between the neurons and the muscles responsible for breathing, patients either die from respiratory failure or require mechanical ventilation to continue to breathe. The majority of persons with ALS die from respiratory failure within 5 years from the onset of symptoms. To be diagnosed with ALS, patients must have signs and symptoms of both upper and lower motor neuron damage that cannot be attributed to other causes (such as progressive muscular atrophies and varieties of peroneal muscular atrophy, Kennedy's syndrome, or multifocal motor mononeuropathy).

Five to ten percent of ALS cases are familial (inherited), and the remainder are sporadic (Rowland, 2000; Siddique et al., 1999). Only one parent needs to carry the mutant gene for ALS to occur in about half of the children in cases of familial ALS. The specific gene mutations causing the majority of familial ALS cases are unknown. However, about 20% of familial cases are believed to be caused by a mutation in a gene that encodes the enzyme superoxide dismutase 1 (National Institute of Neurological Disorders and Stroke, 2006).

The cause of sporadic ALS is unknown. Despite a number of epidemiologic studies examining occupations (for example, farmers and electricians), occupational toxins (such as lead or pesticides), physical trauma, transmissible agents (such as viruses or other microorganisms) strenuous physical activity (for example, Italian professional soccer players), lifestyle factors (for example, diet, body mass index, cigarette use, and alcohol consumption), race/ethnicity, socioeconomic status, and possibly latitude (such as a north-south gradient of risk), to date there are no accepted nongenetic risk factors for ALS (Armon, 2003, 2004; Armon et al., 1991; Cermelli et al., 2003; Chio et al., 2005; Kamel et al., 2002; McGuire et al., 1996, 1997; Nicolson et al., 2002; Rowland, 2000; Valenti et al., 2005).

Summary of *Volume 4*

Primary Studies

Horner and colleagues (2003) conducted a nationwide, epidemiologic case-ascertainment study to determine if Gulf War veterans have elevated rates of ALS relying on both active and passive methods of case ascertainment. Active methods included screening of inpatient, outpatient, and pharmacy medical databases of VA or DoD. Passive methods included establishment of a toll-free telephone number, solicitations through relevant Internet sites, and mass mailings of study brochures to practicing neurologists in the VA and to members of the American Academy of Neurology. The ALS diagnosis in study participants was verified by medical record review.

Among nearly 2.5 million eligible military personnel active during the Gulf War period, nearly 700,000 had been deployed to the Gulf War between August 1990 and July 1991. Mostly based on active ascertainment methods, this study identified 107 eligible cases of ALS (40 in the Gulf War deployed and 67 in the nondeployed troops), for an overall occurrence of 0.43 per 100,000 persons per year between August 1990 to December 1999. The ALS risk was estimated to be about twofold for all deployed compared to the nondeployed military personnel (RR 1.92, 95% CI 1.29-2.84) with an attributable risk (that is, the risk difference or excess risk) due to deployment estimated as 18% (95% CI 4.9-29.4). The foremost limitation of the study was potential underascertainment of cases, particularly among nondeployed veterans, because nondeployed veterans had less incentive to participate. Because of the rarity of ALS, underascertainment of a few cases, particularly if it is greater among the nondeployed, can substantially exaggerate the risk among the deployed by comparison. The finding that the incidence of ALS in deployed veterans was actually lower than that of an age-matched sample from Washington state (McGuire et al., 1996) contributed to this concern; however, such a difference between military personnel and the general population might also reflect a healthy warrior bias. Another but less important study limitation raised in a letter by another ALS researcher was failure to consider smoking as a possible confounding factor in the study design under the assumption that smoking is a risk factor for the development of ALS (Armon et al., 2004; Nelson et al., 2000). In response, the authors of the original study pointed out that there is little reason to believe that smoking rates are different among deployed and nondeployed veterans reducing the likelihood for confounding bias.

More importantly, however, the same authors undertook a secondary analysis to address concerns about differential case ascertainment among deployed versus nondeployed veterans. In this secondary analysis (Coffman et al., 2005) they assessed case ascertainment bias by estimating the occurrence of ALS employing three capture–recapture analysis methods: log-linear models, sample coverage, and ecologic models. The investigators concluded that there might have been some modest underascertainment of cases in nondeployed military personnel but little underascertainment in the deployed. After correcting the rates for underascertainment, the investigators still found a higher age-adjusted risk of ALS among the deployed than among the nondeployed (RR 1.77, lower bound 1.21, with log-linear model). These analyses confirmed the original findings of an increase in ALS among deployed veterans assuming that the modeling assumptions they had to make for this exercise are correct. See Table 4-6 for a summary of the primary ALS studies discussed above.

Secondary Studies

Haley (2003) found an excess incidence of ALS among deployed veterans in comparison with the expected incidence based on US vital statistics. Similar to the first Horner et al. study (2003), this analysis spanned a short war or postwar period from 1991 to 1998 only. In the first half of that period an increased incidence was not apparent; from 1995 to 1998, the incidence more than doubled (standardized mortality ratio [SMR] 2.27, 95% CI 1.27-3.88). Although the study used passive and active means of case ascertainment similar to those of Horner et al., it differed in several key aspects: it restricted cases to those below the age of 45 years (instead of all ages); it used 8 years of follow-up (instead of 10 years), and it used for comparison the age-adjusted rates from US mortality statistics (instead of the age-adjusted rates in nondeployed veterans). Use of mortality statistics for the general population to estimate an "expected" incidence is a major limitation (Armon et al., 2004), since this assumes that the case ascertainment methods for the comparison population are similar to those for the deployed military population when deriving SMRs. The case ascertainment methods used by Haley (2003) are not comparable to those in the general population and may have overascertained cases among veterans.

Several US and UK mortality studies have not found an excess risk of ALS, but they did not have sufficiently long follow-up or sufficiently detailed methods (DASA, 2005; Kang and Bullman, 1996; Macfarlane et al., 2000). Recently, the original Kang and Bullman (1996) mortality study has been updated (Barth et al., 2009) and included data through December 2004. This study did not find any increase in ALS mortality in Gulf War veterans compared to nondeployed veterans (adjusted RR 0.96; 95% 0.56-1.62), but these results were based on less than half the number of ALS cases identified in the primary study by Horner et al. (2003) (23 cases in deployed and 38 in nondeployed veterans). A hospitalization study (Smith et al., 2000) also found no difference in relative risk of ALS (RR 1.66, 95% CI 0.62-4.44), but the authors acknowledge that they had too few cases to make valid comparisons between deployed and nondeployed veterans. The study was also limited by inclusion of only active-duty military personnel and only 6 years of follow-up. Nicolson and colleagues, studying eight Gulf War veterans with ALS and two other comparison populations, found that ill Gulf War veterans had the highest frequency of systemic mycoplasm infections (Nicolson et al., 2002). Although the authors suggest that mycoplasma might be involved in the pathogenesis or progression of ALS, insufficient information was given regarding the selection of cases and controls to evaluate bias in ascertainment.

Updated and Supplemental Literature

Horner et al. (2008) extended their follow-up for 1 year to December 2001 and investigated temporal patterns of ALS occurrence. Among all 2.5 million military personnel on active duty during the 1991 Gulf War a total of 124 ALS cases were confirmed; 48 of these cases occurred among those deployed, while 76 cases were found among the nondeployed; the percentage of young onset cases (< 45 years of age) was similar in both groups (69% vs 64%). The main increase in ALS cases in this study occurred within the decade following the war, that is, prior to 1999. The authors proposed that Gulf War-specific neurotoxins may have caused the short-period increase in ALS rates after the war among deployed military personnel. The results for nondeployed troops—found as in the original study to have experienced lower rates of ALS than the western Washington State population—contrast with another high-quality study that reported increased rates among men who had served in the military or had been deployed to a war zone between 1910 and 1982 (Weisskopf et al., 2005). On the basis of this study a previous IOM committee (2006) termed the evidence for ALS and military deployment as limited and suggestive. Horner et al. (2008), however, also emphasized that their follow-up period was still too short to draw any conclusions about ALS in nondeployed military personnel when compared to a general population. However, due to small numbers of cases overall, it remains unclear whether the observed pattern represents random fluctuations in ALS rates among the deployed or an episodic post war increase as suggested by the authors.

Summary and Conclusions

One primary study with extended follow-up and one secondary study found that deployed veterans appear to be at increased risk for ALS. The primary study by Horner et al. (2003, 2008) possibly underascertained cases in the nondeployed population. However, they investigated ascertainment bias analytically and concluded that it was unlikely to explain their results (in Coffman et al., 2005); they also extended follow-up through 2001 and described a short-term increase in ALS risk in the deployed during the decade after the war. These analyses together support an estimate of a nearly doubling in risk among deployed veterans compared with nondeployed veterans. A secondary study by Haley (2003), using general population rates for comparison purposes, found a similar increase in relative risk. Other US and UK mortality studies and a hospitalization study have not found excess risk of ALS.

> **Therefore, the committee concludes that there is limited but suggestive evidence of an association between deployment to the Gulf War and ALS; however, further follow-up is warranted.**

Other Neurodegenerative Diseases

Alzheimer dementia is the most common neurodegenerative disorder in the elderly population and Parkinson's disease—primarily considered a movement disorder—is the second most common. Both have progressive courses and no known cure. The dopaminergic neurodegeneration in Parkinson's disease is thought to be caused by a combination of repeated, prolonged, or chronic exposures to toxicants, genetic factors, gene–toxicants interactions, and aging-related effects. Over the last decade and a half, evidence has accumulated that exposure to certain pesticides can produce the anatomical, neurochemical, behavioral, or neuropathological features of Parkinson's disease in animal models (Sherer et al., 2001), and recently some high-quality studies have confirmed the pesticide hypothesis for Parkinson's disease in humans (Elbaz et al., 2009; Kamel et al., 2007; Ritz et al., 2009).

Environmental factors are also suspected to contribute to Alzheimer disease to a lesser degree. High-quality human studies are not available except for lead exposures (Shih et al., 2007), for which data from both animal experiments and human epidemiologic studies suggest an influence of lead exposure on Alzheimer-like cognitive impairment. Of special importance for Gulf War veterans is that brain injuries are an established risk factor for Alzheimer dementia, especially among susceptible individuals (for example, carriers of the APOE 4 allele). Brain injury has been shown to result in widespread hippocampal damage in mice and may lead to Alzheimer disease in humans (reviewed in Van Den Heuvel et al., 2007).

The committee was unable to identify any studies of dementia or Alzheimer's disease in Gulf War veterans and only one study on Parkinson's disease. Barth et al. (2009) compared mortality from neurological disease in 621,902 deployed and 746,248 nondeployed veterans between May 1991 and December 2004. The adjusted mortality rate ratio for Parkinson's disease was 0.77 (95% CI 0.17-2.99); there were three cases among the deployed male veterans, eight cases among the nondeployed males, and no cases in either group of female veterans.

Summary and Conclusion

Parkinson's and Alzheimer's diseases generally present late in life (usually after age 60); thus, it is unlikely that Gulf War veterans would manifest symptoms or signs of these neurodegenerative disorders until they reach at least the sixth decade of life. The Update committee strongly believes that a very long latency period for these health outcomes is a possibility, and current studies have inadequate follow-up time to assess whether risk for these disorders is increased among Gulf War veterans.

> **Therefore, the committee concludes that there is inadequate/insufficient evidence of an association between deployment to the Gulf War and other neurodegenerative diseases. The committee recommends continued monitoring of Gulf War veterans (both deployed and nondeployed) for neurologic outcomes such as Parkinson's disease, Alzheimer's disease, and dementia.**

Other Neurological Outcomes

Haley and colleagues performed detailed neurologic assessments in several case-control studies of the original cohort of Seabee reservists. The cases were veterans who had met criteria for factor-derived syndromes. Under the hypothesis that those veterans were ill from neurotoxic exposures, especially to organophosphates, the assessments covered broad neurologic function (Haley and Kurt, 1997), autonomic function (Haley et al., 2004), vestibular function (Roland et al., 2000), basal ganglia injury (Haley et al., 2000a,b), normalized regional cerebral blood flow (Haley et al., 2009); and paraoxonase (PON) genotype and serum concentrations (Haley et al., 1999). Separate groups of investigators also studied PON genotype or activity (Hotopf et al., 2003; Mackness et al., 1997). A case-control study of neuropsychologic functioning (Hom et al., 1997) is discussed elsewhere in this chapter.

The committee regarded those case-control studies as secondary studies primarily because of their lack of generalizability and strong potential for selection bias. Although their study design was characterized as nested case-control, the studies of Haley et al. were not true nested case-control studies. Cases were, appropriately, selected from the original cohort, but controls were not. Ten of the 20 controls were from 150 newly discovered members of the battalion who had not been deployed. Those 10 were not from the original cohort, and there is no indication that they were tested to determine whether they should be treated as cases. The selection of those controls raises the possibility of selection bias. With regard to the other concern, lack of generalizability, the authors selected as cases the most severely affected veterans—that is, those who scored highest on factor analysis-derived syndromes—rather than a random sample of those who met a particular case definition.

Summary and Conclusion

Haley and colleagues found evidence of basal ganglia injury and other abnormalities with detailed neurologic assessments in several case-control studies. The committee regarded the studies as secondary because of their lack of generalizability and their strong potential for selection bias.

Therefore, the committee concludes that there is inadequate/insufficient evidence of an association between deployment to the Gulf War and other neurologic outcomes.

TABLE 4-6 Nervous System Diseases

Study	Design	Population	Outcomes	Results	Adjustments	Comments
Peripheral Neuropathy and Myopathy						
Davis et al., 2004 (Vol. 4)	Cross-sectional, prevalence, medical evaluation, exposure-specific component	1047 deployed veterans vs 1121 nondeployed veterans; 240 Khamisiyah-exposed deployed veterans vs 807 non-Khamisiyah-exposed deployed veterans	Distal symmetric polyneuropathy identified by nerve-conduction study[a]	Deployed vs nondeployed veterans: OR 0.65 (95% CI 0.33-1.28); Khamisiyah-exposed veterans vs non-Khamisiyah-exposed veterans: OR 1.04 (95% CI 0.25-4.37)	Excludes coexisting conditions[b]	Low participation rate: 53% in deployed veterans, 39% in nondeployed veterans
Rose et al., 2004; Sharief et al., 2002 (Vol. 4)	Case-control	49 symptomatic deployed UK veterans vs 26 healthy deployed UK veterans, 13 symptomatic Bosnia deployed veterans, 22 symptomatic Gulf War-era veterans	Nerve-conduction studies, quantitative sensory and autonomic testing, concentric needle and single-fiber, electromyography, ischemic forearm exercise test, subanaerobic bicycle exercise test, muscle biopsy	No significant differences between symptomatic deployed and nondeployed veterans, except deployed veterans had increased lactate production in bicycle exercise test		Positive finding from bicycle test could reflect mitochondrial damage or inactivity resulting from ill health
Kelsall et al., 2005 (Update)	Cross-sectional survey	1382 Australian male GWVs, 1376 nondeployed male era veterans frequency matched by age and service type (Same study population as Kelsall et al., 2004a,b)	Self-reported neurologic symptoms corroborated during neurological examination; SF-12; modified NIS	Lower limb neurological type symptoms and signs: OR 1.6 (95% CI 1.0-2.7) Neuropathy Score: GWV (2.0, sd = 4.3) vs controls (2.0, sd = 4.7) RoM 1.1 (95% CI 0.9-1.3) Association of neurological symptoms in self-reported nonexposed compared to exposed: PB (RoM 1.5, 95% CI 1.2-1.8) Antibiological warfare	Age, rank, service type, current marital status, highest level of education, alcohol consumption, and history of diabetes	Exposure data self-reported; response rate 80.5% for deployed, 56.8% for nondeployed

Study	Design	Population	Outcomes	Results	Adjustments	Comments
				tablets (RoM 1.8, 95% CI 1.3-2.5) Solvents (RoM 1.8, 95% CI 1.4-2.2) Pesticides (RoM 1.7, 95% CI 1.4-2.0) Insect repellents (RoM 1.3, 95% CI 1.1-1.5) No association with self-reports of immunizations or chemical exposure		
Multiple Sclerosis						
Barth et al., 2009 (Update)	Mortality cohort study, follow-up through 2004 of same cohort as Kang and Bullman (2001)	621,901 US male GWVs and 746,247 nondeployed male veterans	Mortality due to multiple sclerosis (McDonald criteria)	GWVs (6 cases) compared to era veterans (13 cases) MRR 0.67 (95% CI 0.24-1.85)	Race, service branch, type of unit, age, marital status	
Amyotrophic Lateral Sclerosis (ALS)						
Horner et al., 2003 (Vol. 4)	Retrospective cohort	All active, GWVs (1990-1991) compared with NDVs	ALS	All deployed forces, significant increased risk of ALS (RR = 1.92, 95% CL −1.29-2.84)	Age-adjusted average, annual 10-year incidence; attributable risk	Case ascertainment through screening of VA and DoD medical databases and benefit files (and TriCare) by ICD-9 code for ALS or riluzole use; toll-free telephone enrollment; Internet notices; mass mailings to neurologists, VA centers, and veteran service organizations

Study	Design	Population	Outcomes	Results	Adjustments	Comments
Coffman et al., 2005 (Vol. 4)	Capture–recapture reanalysis of Horner et al., cohort	See Horner et al., 2003	ALS	Found no underascertainment of ALS cases among deployed	Log-linear models; sample coverage; ecologic models	Possible slight undercounts not likely to substantively affect results
Horner et al., 2008 (Update)	Retrospective cohort, follow-up from 1991-2001 (follow-up of Horner et al., 2003)	All active, Gulf War-deployed military personnel (n = 696,118), compared with NDVs	ALS	Deployed (48 cases) vs nondeployed (76 cases), no significant difference in SIR during additional follow-up period Similar percentage of young onset between deployed (69%) and controls (64%)	Age-adjusted average, annual 10-year incidence; attributable risk	Small number of cases and short follow-up period limit the ability of the study to determine long-term trends

NOTES: CI = confidence interval; GWV = Gulf War veteran; MRR = mortality rate ratio; NDV = nondeployed veteran; NIS = Neuropathy Impairment Score (Mayo Clinic version); OR = odds ratio; PB = pyridostigmine bromide; RoM = ratio of means; sd = standard deviation; SF-12 = 12-item Short Form Health Survey; SIR = standardized incidence ratio.

[a]Although the study defined distal symmetric polyneuropathy as distal sensory or motor neuropathy identified on basis of neurologic examination, nerve conduction study, or both, the committee defined it by nerve-conduction study alone.
[b]Alcohol dependence, diabetes mellitus, renal insufficiency, hypothyroidism, AIDS/HIV, collagen vascular disease, and neurotoxic medications.

DISEASES OF THE CIRCULATORY SYSTEM

Cardiovascular disease is a broad term for any disorder of the heart or the blood vessels, such as artherosclerosis and hypertension. Cardiovascular disease, which includes coronary heart disease and stroke, is the leading cause of death of both women and men in the United States. In 2005, 864,480 people (53% of them women) died of cardiovascular disease, accounting for 34% of all US deaths. The age-adjusted death rate was 262.9 per 100,000 of population. Over 40% of deaths in those aged 65 or older is the result of cardiovascular disease (Lakatta, 2002). Major risk factors for cardiovascular disease include hypercholesterolemia, diabetes, smoking, obesity, and physical inactivity. Primary studies for circulatory system diseases are presented in Table 4-7.

Summary of *Volume 4*

Primary Studies

Volume 4 included two primary studies considering cardiovascular outcomes. The first study (Eisen et al., 2005) examined the prevalence of different health outcomes in a group of 1061 Gulf War deployed veterans and 1128 nondeployed veterans between 1999 and 2001; veterans were part of the larger National Health Survey of Gulf War Era Veterans and Their Families, who had completed mailed questionnaires about their health status in 1995 (Kang et al., 2000). Hypertension, defined as systolic blood pressure greater or equal than 140, diastolic blood pressure greater or equal than 90 mmHg, or use of antihypertensive medication, was equally prevalent in deployed and nondeployed veterans (adjusted OR 0.90, 95% CI 0.60-1.33). The major limitation of this study was the differential, low response rate (53% in Gulf War veterans and 39% in nondeployed).

The second study examined hospitalizations in DoD hospitals among Gulf War veterans according to their exposure to the demolition of the Khamisiyah weapons depot. An initial report of this analysis, published in 1999 (Gray et al., 1999b), was updated in a later publication (Smith et al., 2003). Among those potentially exposed to sarin and cyclosarin the risk ratio of being hospitalized with a cardiovascular condition was 1.07 (95% CI 1.01-1.13) compared to nonexposed. The increased risk was specific for cardiac dysrhythmias (risk ratio 1.23, 95% CI 1.04-1.44). This study could not ascertain outpatient diagnoses as well as hospitalizations in those who did not remain in active duty after the war.

Secondary Studies

Several large epidemiologic studies examined self-reported cardiovascular outcomes occurring in Gulf War veterans. The committee classified studies relying on self-report of cardiovascular disease as secondary. In an Australian study, prevalence of self-reported physician-diagnosed high blood pressure was similar in 1456 veterans deployed to the Gulf War and 1588 nondeployed (OR 1.2, 95% CI 0.9-1.6) (Kelsall et al., 2004a). Similarly, Kansas veterans were as likely as their nondeployed counterparts to report physician-diagnosed high blood pressure (OR 1.24, 95% CI 0.82-1.89) or heart disease (OR 1.56, 95% CI 0.69-3.56) (Steele, 2000). In a study including 11,441 Gulf War veterans and 9476 nondeployed veterans, Kang and colleagues (2000) found an increased prevalence of self-reported high blood pressure in deployed versus nondeployed veterans (prevalence difference 3.84%, 95% CI 3.75-3.93) and a similar prevalence of stroke (−0.01%, 95% −0.003-−0.01). Studying all Seabee commands, Gray and colleagues (2002) found a higher prevalence of self-reported hypertension in those deployed to the Gulf War versus those deployed elsewhere (OR 1.63, 95% CI 1.36-1.95). A study including 2918 Gulf War veterans from five US states (California, Georgia, North Carolina, Oregon, and Washington) did not find differences in self-reported conditions among deployed veterans potentially exposed to nerve agents from the Khamisiyah demolition compared to deployed but unexposed veterans. Compared with nondeployed veterans, however, deployed veterans (exposed and nonexposed combined) did have a higher prevalence of self-reported high blood pressure (OR 1.7, 95% CI 1.3-2.4) and heart disease (OR 2.5, 95% CI 1.1-6.6) (McCauley et al., 2002). Finally, one study of UK male Gulf War veterans found a higher prevalence of self-reported high blood pressure in 3284 deployed veterans compared to 1815 veterans deployed to Bosnia (OR 1.3, 95% CI 1.0-1.8) or 2408 nondeployed Gulf War era veterans (OR 1.2, 95% CI 1.0-1.6) (Unwin et al., 1999). The main limitation, shared by these secondary studies, is the use of self-reported information and, therefore, the potential for differential misclassification if deployed veterans were more likely to report cardiovascular conditions than their nondeployed counterparts.

Updated and Supplemental Literature

Primary Studies

Since the publication of *Volume 4*, a series of studies examining hospitalizations and mortality for cardiovascular diseases have been identified. The committee considered that cardiovascular disease hospitalizations and mortality had adequate validity and, therefore, studies considering these outcomes should be classified as primary studies.

Gray et al. (1996) compared DoD hospitalizations among Gulf War deployed and nondeployed active-duty personnel. Hospitalizations for 14 ICD-9-CM diagnostic categories, which included "circulatory system diseases," were assessed across three time periods following the war: August 1, 1991, to December 31, 1991 (included 1,165,411 subjects on active duty on the first day of this time period); January 1, 1992, to December 31, 1992 (1,075,430 subjects); and January 1, 1993, to September 30, 1993 (839,389 subjects). Hospitalizations for cardiovascular diseases were not increased among the Gulf War deployed personnel versus nondeployed during any of the three time periods. Limitations of this study include the relatively short follow-up, the lack of outpatient data, restriction to DoD hospitals, restriction to hospitalizations of those who remained on active duty after the war, and limited adjustment for potential confounding exposures.

A later publication complemented the above study adding reserve and former military personnel hospitalized in non-DoD hospitals (Gray et al., 2000). Hospitalizations for the 14 major discharge diagnoses during the period of August 1, 1991, and December 31, 1994, were compared for Gulf War veterans and nondeployed veterans in three hospital systems (DoD, VA, and the California Office of Statewide Health Planning and Development). Because the population eligible for hospitalization in the VA and California systems could not be identified to calculate hospitalization rates, the investigators estimated proportional morbidity ratios within each hospital system. Gulf War veterans did not experience an increased proportion of hospitalizations for "diseases of the circulatory system" compared to nondeployed veterans during the 4 years after the war. This finding was consistent among hospitalizations within the DoD (n = 182,164), VA (n = 16,030), and California (n = 5185) hospital systems (PMRs ranged between 0.85 and 0.94). The use of proportional morbidity ratios results in a lower sensitivity for detecting differences in hospitalizations than does a comparison of hospitalization rates.

Postwar hospitalizations in US military personnel were also examined in relation to exposure to smoke from oil-well fires (Smith et al., 2002). Hospitalizations within DoD treatment facilities were identified for 405,142 active-duty personnel who were in the Gulf War theater of operations during the Kuwaiti oil-well fires (February 2, 1991, to October 31, 1991) and did not remain in the region after the war. Hospitalizations for "diseases of the circulatory system" and other major ICD-9-CM categories were evaluated over an 8-year follow-up period. Exposure to oil-well fire smoke was estimated by combining smoke-plume modeling data and troop unit location. Exposure was categorized into seven levels based on combinations of average daily dose (none, 1-260 $\mu g/m^3$, > 260 $\mu g/m^3$) and duration of exposure (1-25 days, 26-50 days, > 50 days). When compared to those with no exposure to smoke from oil-well fires, there was no increase in the incidence of hospitalization for cardiovascular disorders at any level of exposure: risk ratios ranged between 0.9 and 1.2 for the different levels of exposure (all 95% CIs included 1.0), without a clear dose-response trend. Considering hospitalizations for ischemic heart disease as the outcome, veterans exposed to oil-well fires had a slightly lower risk than unexposed veterans (risk ratio 0.82, 95% CI 0.68-0.99). The limitations of this study are the same as those described for other hospitalization studies in the DoD system.

A more recent study compared hospitalizations in DoD hospitals among Gulf War veterans and other veterans and found no evidence of an increased risk of cardiovascular disease among the former group (Smith et al., 2006). Specifically, this study compared incidence of postdeployment hospitalizations among active-duty servicemembers deployed to the Gulf War (n = 455,465) to those deployed to Southwest Asia following the Gulf War (n = 249,047) or those deployed to Bosnia (n = 44,341). Electronic information on hospitalizations was collected from DoD hospitals through December 2000. The incidence of hospitalizations for diseases of the circulatory system was similar in Southwest Asia veterans and Gulf War veterans (HR 1.06, 95% CI 0.97-1.16). Incidence of hospitalizations for cardiovascular disease in Bosnia veterans was lower than in the Gulf War veterans (HR 0.70, 95% CI 0.59-0.83). All analyses were adjusted for potential confounding factors (sex, age, marital status, pay grade, race/ethnicity, service branch, occupation, and predeployment hospitalizations). Limitations of the study include the inclusion of active-duty personnel only and restricting the outcomes to those identified in DoD hospitals only.

Five published reports have examined mortality for cardiovascular diseases in Gulf War veterans. Kang and Bullman (2001) compared cardiovascular mortality from 1991 through the end of 1997 in 621,902 US Gulf War veterans and 746,248 nondeployed veterans, by sex, adjusting for age, race, marital status, branch of service, and type of unit. Adjusted mortality rate ratios for cardiovascular diseases in deployed versus nondeployed were 0.90 (95% CI 0.81-1.01) in men and 0.96 (95% CI 0.55-1.69) in women. Limitations of this study include the lack of adjustment for predeployment health status and for lifestyle variables, such as smoking or alcohol consumption.

Another study in US Gulf War veterans compared cardiovascular mortality through 2000 according to potential exposure to nerve agents from the Khamisiyah demolition (Bullman et al., 2005). Analyses were adjusted for age, sex, race, rank, and unit component. Among 100,487 potentially exposed veterans, 170 cardiovascular deaths were identified, while 407 were identified among 224,980 unexposed veterans (adjusted risk ratio 0.89, 95% CI 0.74-1.06).

Results were similar when exposed veterans were further classified as having 1 day of exposure or 2 or more days of exposure.

The Canadian Persian Gulf Cohort Study explored total and cause-specific mortality in 5117 Gulf War deployed and 6093 nondeployed Canadian veterans (Statistics Canada, 2005). Mortality and cause of death through the end of 1999 was ascertained from the Canadian Mortality Data Base. Analyses were adjusted for age, sex, rank, and marital status. During the 8-year follow-up, 17 cardiovascular deaths were identified. The adjusted mortality rate ratio (MRR) of cardiovascular mortality in deployed versus nondeployed veterans was 0.49 (95% CI 0.17-1.40). Limitations of this study include its limited sample size (and therefore low statistical power to detect associations if these exist), the relatively short follow-up (which would not allow the identification of long-term effects of deployment), and the lack of information on potential confounding factors, such as smoking and other lifestyle factors.

Two publications reported cardiovascular mortality among UK Gulf War veterans. Macfarlane et al. (2005) compared mortality from April 1991 to June 2004 among 51,753 UK Gulf War veterans and a cohort of 50,808 military personnel not deployed to the Persian Gulf, matched by age, sex, rank, service and level of fitness. Mortality was determined through linkage with the National Health Service central register. Cardiovascular mortality was similar in both cohorts (adjusted mortality rate ratio 0.87, 95% CI 0.66-1.14). A later publication, extending the follow-up of these cohorts through the end of 2007 found comparable results (adjusted rate ratio 0.87, 95% CI 0.70-1.07) (DASA, 2009).

A study conducted in Denmark measured blood pressure in a group of 686 Danish veterans deployed to the Gulf area between August 1990 and December 1997, and 231 nondeployed controls (Ishoy et al., 1999b). In bivariate analysis, systolic blood pressure was similar in deployed and nondeployed: means were 127 mmHg (sd = 12) and 126 mmHg (sd = 11), respectively. Differences were also absent for diastolic blood pressure (78 mmHg, sd = 9 and 76 mmHg, sd = 10, respectively).

In addition to obtaining self-reports of diagnoses of medical conditions, including high blood pressure (Kelsall et al., 2004a), the study of Australian Gulf War veterans included physical examinations of 1424 Gulf War male veterans and a sample of 1548 nondeployed male veterans conducted by April 2002 (Sim et al., 2003). Response rates were 81% among eligible deployed veterans and 57% among nondeployed. All analyses in this study were adjusted for age, service type, rank, education, and marital status. Levels of blood pressure were similar in deployed and nondeployed. In polytomous logistic regression, adjusted ORs of high-normal blood pressure and hypertension in deployed (n = 1371) versus nondeployed (n = 1368) were 1.1 (95% CI 0.9-1.3) and 1.1 (95% CI 0.9-1.4), respectively. Likewise, the prevalence of hypertension was the same (3%) among 30 female Australian Gulf War veterans compared to a control group of 32 nondeployed women (Sim et al., 2003). Response rates for female veterans were comparable to their male counterparts: 79% in deployed and 44% in nondeployed.

Secondary Studies

Seven studies provided self-reported prevalence of different cardiovascular disorders, including high blood pressure, palpitations, stroke, heart attacks, and unspecified heart problems by deployment status. Given the low validity of self-reported information to diagnose cardiovascular disease, these studies are considered to be secondary.

A mailed survey assessed health status of 4334 veterans in Pennsylvania and Hawaii, 1739 of them deployed as result of Operation Desert Shield/Storm (Stretch et al., 1995). Results of this survey conducted within 2 years of deployment were reported separately for active-duty and reserve personnel. Self-reported high blood pressure was more frequent in deployed versus nondeployed veterans (23% vs 10% in active-duty veterans, and 11% vs 4% in reserve veterans). Similarly, heart problems were more frequently reported in deployed than nondeployed veterans (7% vs 2% and 4% vs 1% in active-duty and reserve veterans, respectively). Limitations of this study included the low response rate (31%) and the lack of adjustment for potential confounders.

Proctor and colleagues (1998) studied 186 Gulf War deployed veterans from New England, 66 deployed veterans from New Orleans, and a group of 48 veterans deployed to Germany during the Gulf War. Information on cardiovascular conditions was collected using mailed questionnaires. Prevalence of palpitations (described as irregular heart beat or racing heart) was approximately twice as frequent among the deployed than nondeployed veterans in analyses adjusted for age, sex, and education (ORs ranged from 1.8-4.1). In a later publication comparing the same Gulf War deployed New England cohort with the Germany deployed cohort (Proctor et al., 2001a), self-reported prevalence of hypertension was higher among Gulf War veterans (14% vs 4%), but the prevalence of other heart problems was similar between the Gulf War deployed compared with those deployed to Germany (3% vs 4%).

A follow-up survey to the 1995 National Health Survey of Gulf War Era Veterans and Their Families (Kang et al., 2000) assessed the self-reported prevalence of different health outcomes in Gulf War veterans and a group of nondeployed veterans (Kang et al., 2009). Information on health status was collected through mailed questionnaires or phone calls. Of 30,000 eligible participants, 9970 participated (34% response rate; 40% among Gulf War veterans, 27% among nondeployed veterans). In a multivariable analysis, deployment to the Gulf War was associated with a higher prevalence of self-reported tachycardia (RR 1.42, 95% CI 1.26-1.60), stroke (RR 1.32, 95% CI 1.14-1.52), coronary heart disease (RR 1.22, 95% CI 1.08-1.39), and hypertension (RR 1.11, 95% CI 1.04-1.19). This study, however, has limited validity given the low participation rate and the lack of objective confirmation of the outcomes.

Self-reported cardiovascular disorders were assessed in 1995-1997 for 5555 Gulf War veterans included in the 1995 National Health Survey of Gulf War Veterans. Veterans were categorized as to whether they had potential exposure to nerve gas from the Khamisiyah demolition (n = 1898) or were unexposed (n = 3336) (Page et al., 2005). Information was obtained from mailed or telephone surveys. Analyses were adjusted for age, sex, race, rank, marital status, and unit component. Palpitations were reported with the same frequency for exposed (5.1%) and unexposed (5.7%) veterans (OR 0.88, 95% CI 0.69-1.11). Likewise, the prevalence of self-reported heart disease (OR 0.98, 95% CI 0.64-1.48), hypertension (OR 1.03, 95% CI 0.90-1.07), stroke (OR 0.89, 95% 0.42-1.88), and tachycardia (OR 0.92, 95% CI 0.79-1.07) were similar for the potentially exposed and unexposed groups.

In 1997, a mail survey of the Canadian military contingent of 2924 male veterans who served in the Gulf War and 3241 Canadian veterans who were in the military but had not been deployed to the gulf region asked about the presence of heart disease or circulatory problems. The prevalence of circulatory problems was higher in deployed than nondeployed veterans (5% vs 2%) and in those younger than 45 versus older veterans (6% vs 5%), while the prevalence of self-reported heart disease was similar in deployed and nondeployed (1% in younger veterans, and 4-5% in older ones) (Goss Gilroy, 1998).

Finally, a study was conducted among 23,358 male UK Gulf War veterans and 17,730 nondeployed veterans who answered a mailed questionnaire collecting information on a number of health conditions (Simmons et al., 2004). Self-reported prevalence of cardiovascular disorders with incidence after 1990 was higher in deployed than nondeployed veterans (OR 1.3, 95% 1.1-1.4) after adjustment for age, service, rank, serving status at time of survey, alcohol, and smoking. A low response rate (53% in deployed and 42% in nondeployed veterans) could introduce selection bias, limiting the results of this study.

Summary and Conclusions

Several studies have explored whether deployment to the Gulf War was associated with higher risk of cardiovascular disease. Available primary studies did not report an increased risk of cardiovascular hospitalizations or mortality in those deployed compared to nondeployed veterans during the 10-15 years after the Gulf War. The few studies measuring blood pressure in deployed and nondeployed veterans similarly did not find differences between the two groups. The only study that found an increase in cardiovascular disease was limited to hospitalizations in deployed veterans who were possibly exposed to the Khamisiyah plume and those who were not exposed. The increase was due entirely to a higher risk of cardiac dysrhythmia (Smith et al., 2003). No studies have confirmed this association in other populations. In the secondary studies, deployed veterans were generally more likely to self-report hypertension, palpitations, and other cardiovascular disease, but those reports were not confirmed in medical evaluations. Additionally, many of those studies could be affected by selection bias. Therefore, their validity is poor.

The committee concludes that there is limited/suggestive evidence of no association between deployment and mortality from cardiovascular disease in the first 10 years after the war, and that there is inadequate/insufficient evidence to determine whether an association exists between deployment to the Gulf War and cardiovascular disorders.

TABLE 4-7 Circulatory System Diseases

Study	Design	Population	Outcomes	Results	Adjustments	Comments
Eisen et al., 2005 (Vol. 4)	Population-based; cross-sectional; prevalence; medical evaluation; 1999-2001	1061 deployed, 1128 nondeployed	Hypertension = blood pressure > 140/90 mmHg or history of hypertension and use of antihypertensive medications	Hypertension: OR 0.90 (95% CI 0.60-1.33)	Age, sex, race, years of education, smoking, duty type, service branch, rank	Low response rates, especially in control group (53% in GWVs, 39% in era controls), but analysis of nonparticipants and participants reveals no differences in hypertension or diabetes
Smith et al., 2003 (Vol. 4)	DoD hospitalization study (1991-2000); analysis of health outcomes and exposure to nerve agents	99,614 active-duty military considered exposed vs 318,458 nonexposed, according to revised DoD exposure model	First hospitalization for any disease of the circulatory system (ICD-9-CM codes 390-459); hospitalization for cardiac dysrhythmia	Circulatory system diseases: RR 1.07 (95% CI 1.01-1.13); Cardiac dysrhythmia: RR 1.23 (95% CI 1.04-1.44)		Restricted to DoD hospitals; restricted to hospitalizations for only Gulf War veterans who remained on active duty after the war; no adjustment for confounding exposures
Gray et al., 1996 (Update)	Retrospective cohort, hospitalizations from August 1991 through September 1993	547,076 active-duty GWVs, 618,335 NDVs	Hospital-discharge diagnoses of circulatory system disease in DoD hospital system (ICD-9 classification)	OR about 0.90-0.95 (95% CI 0.85-1.05) across all 3 years, 1991-1993. Exact values not given	Prewar hospitalization, sex, age, race, service branch, marital status, rank, length of service, salary, occupation	Very short follow-up period; no outpatient data; restriction to DoD hospitals, and thus to persons remaining on active duty after the war; no adjustment for potential confounders such as smoking
Gray et al., 2000 (Update)	Retrospective cohort, hospitalizations from August 1991 through December 1994	652,979 GWVs, 652,922 randomly selected NDVs 182,164 DoD hospitalizations; 16,030 VA hospitalizations; 5185 COSHPD hospitalizations	Hospital-discharge diagnoses of circulatory system disease in DoD, VA, and COSHPD hospital systems	Circulatory system disease: DoD PMR 0.94 (95% CI 0.91-0.98); VA PMR 0.85 (95% CI 0.76-0.93); COSHPD PMR 0.98 (95% CI 0.82-1.14)	Age, sex, race (only for DoD PMR) Age, sex (for VA and COSHPD PMR)	Able to assess only illnesses that resulted in hospitalization; possible undetected confounders PMR has lower sensitivity than a comparison of hospitalization rates would have

Study	Design	Population	Outcomes	Results	Adjustments	Comments
Smith et al., 2002 (Update)	DoD hospitalizations 1991-1999; exposure modeling for oil-well fire smoke	405,142 active-duty GWVs who were in theater during the time of Kuwaiti oil-well fires	Hospitalization for diseases of the circulatory system and for ischemic heart disease specifically	Significant decrease in risk ratio for exposed to oil-well fire smoke vs nonexposed in 3 of 5 exposure categories Lower risk of ischemic heart disease in all exposed vs nonexposed (RR 0.82, 95% CI 0.68-0.99)	Adjusted for "influential covariates," defined as demographic or deployment variables with p values less than 0.15	Objective measure of disease not subject to recall bias; no issues with self-selection; however, only DoD hospitals, only active duty, no adjustment for potential confounders such as smoking
Smith et al., 2006 (Update)	Retrospective cohort study (cohort data from DMDC)	Active-duty personnel with a single deployment to: Gulf War theater (n = 455,465); Southwest Asia peacekeeping mission, 1991-1998 (n = 249,047); Bosnia, 1995-1998 (n = 44,341)	Postdeployment hospitalization events (1991-2000) for an ICD-9-CM diagnosis of a disease of the circulatory system (390-459)	Compared to GWVs, veterans of Bosnia showed reduced risk (HR 0.70, 95% CI 0.59-0.83), and veterans of Southwest Asia showed similar risk (HR 1.06, 95% CI 0.97-1.16)	Sex, age, marital status, pay grade, race/ethnicity, service branch, occupation, and predeployment hospitalization; time-dependent covariate to account for changing hospitalization methods, diagnostic criteria, and procedures	Lower hazard ratio observed in veterans of Bosnia may be partially explained by shorter follow-up period Limitations: active-duty personnel only; hospitalizations at DoD facilities only
Kang and Bullman, 2001 (Update)	Cross-sectional, mortality 1991-1997	621,902 GWVs, 746,248 NDVs	Mortality and vital status determined with VA BIRLS database and SSA Master Beneficiary Record database	Men RR 0.90 (95% CI 0.81-1.01) Women RR 0.96 (95% CI 0.55-1.69)	Age, race, service branch, type of unit, marital status	Study had good power to detect small increases in risk; limited by relying on death certificates rather than medical records and no adjustment for pre-deployment health status or confounders such as smoking

Study	Design	Population	Outcomes	Results	Adjustments	Comments
Bullman et al., 2005 (Update)	Retrospective cohort; followup from March 1991 through 2000	100,487 US Army GWVs exposed to chemical warfare agents at Khamisiyah; 224,980 nonexposed Army GWVs (derived from Kang and Bullman, 2001); exposure determined from the DoD (2000) plume model	Association of exposure to chemical warfare agents and mortality due to diseases of the circulatory system, determined through BIRLS, SSA; COD data from NDI	1.76% exposed vs 1.88% nonexposed (RR 0.89, 95% CI 0.74-1.06)	Age, race, sex, rank, unit component	Possible exposure misclassification, possible bias due to healthy warrior effect
Statistics Canada, 2005 (Update)	Retrospective cohort study (Cohort based on Goss Gilroy, 1998)	5117 Canadian GWVs; 6093 Canadian NDVs, frequency matched for age, sex, and military duty status	Mortality due to diseases of the circulatory system determined from the CMD and CCD	MRR 0.49 (95% CI 0.17-1.40)	Age, sex, rank, marital status	Limitations: Small sample size results in low statistical power; short follow-up; young age of cohort; no information on confounding factors such as smoking Approximately 2200 members of the deployed cohort were present in the Persian Gulf during the period of fighting
Macfarlane et al., 2005 (Update)	Cohort; 13-year follow-up	51,753 UK GWVs and 50,808 NDVs, randomly selected, matched by age, sex, service branch, rank; also fitness for active service in the Army and Royal Air Force	Mortality due to diseases of the circulatory system	MRR 0.87 (95% CI 0.66-1.14)		Complete and long-term follow-up; cohort of moderate size; potentially other uncontrolled confounders such as smoking

Study	Design	Population	Outcomes	Results	Adjustments	Comments
DASA, 2008 (Update)	Summary statistics of causes of death from April 1, 1991, to December 31, 2007	UK GWVs (n = 53,409) vs era veterans (n = 54,143)	Mortality due to diseases of the circulatory system	MRR 0.87 (95% CI 0.70-1.07)	Age	Roughly the same cohort as MacFarlane et al., 2005
Ishoy et al., 1999b (Update)	Cross-sectional	686 Danish peacekeepers deployed to gulf in 1990-1997 vs 231 age- and sex-matched armed forces nondeployed controls	Blood pressure measured by physician	Deployed vs nondeployed: Systolic: 127 (sd = 12) vs 126 (sd = 11) mmHg Diastolic: 78 (sd = 9) vs 76 (sd = 10) mmHg		Participation rate 83.6% deployed, 57.8% nondeployed
Sim et al., 2003 (Update)	Cross-sectional, mailed questionnaire and clinical examination	1371 male and 30 female Australian GWVs; 1368 male and 32 female NDVs	Blood pressure measured by a physician	High-normal blood pressure, males: OR 1.1 (95% CI 0.9-1.3) Hypertension, males: OR 1.1 (95% CI 0.9-1.4); females: similar prevalence (3%) in both groups	Service type, rank, age, education, marital status	High participation in deployed veterans (male 81%, female 79%), but low participation in control group (male 57%, female 44%) possibly leading to participation bias

NOTES: BIRLS = Beneficiary Identification Records Locator Subsystem (VA); BMI = body mass index; CCD = Canadian Cancer Database; CI = confidence interval; CMD = Canadian Mortality Database; COD = cause of death; COSHPD = California Office of Statewide Health Planning and Development; DMDC = Defense Manpower Data Center; DoD = Department of Defense; GWV = Gulf War veteran; HR = adjusted hazard ratio; MI = myocardial infarction; mmHg = millimeters of mercury; MRR = mortality rate ratio; NDI = National Death Index; NDV = nondeployed veteran; OR = adjusted odds ratio; PHQ = Patient Health Questionnaire; PMR = patient medical record; RR = adjusted risk ratio; sd = standard deviation; SSA = Social Security Administration; VA = Department of Veterans Affairs.

DISEASES OF THE RESPIRATORY SYSTEM

Respiratory conditions such as asthma, bronchitis, chronic obstructive pulmonary disease, and various symptoms consistent with respiratory disease, such as wheezing and shortness of breath, have consistently been self-reported more frequently by deployed Gulf War veterans than controls. Exposures of concern in the theater include smoke from oil-well fires, high levels of ambient dust, pesticide sprays, and nerve gas exposure. A primary study met the committee's criteria for methodological rigor (Chapter 2) and used objective measures of pulmonary function or death from respiratory disease. In a secondary study, the determination of a respiratory illness was based on veterans' self-reports of symptoms or self-reported physician-diagnosed conditions. Primary studies are summarized in Table 4-8.

Summary of *Volume 4*

Primary Studies

The Volume 4 committee identified five primary studies that undertook to explore the association between pulmonary conditions and deployment to the Gulf War. Two of these studies were analysis of data from the 1995 National Health Survey of Gulf War Era Veterans and Their Families (Kang et al., 2000) conducted by the VA on 1061 Gulf War veterans and 1128 nondeployed veterans. This population was derived from a cohort of randomly selected participants from the previous 1995 study who had completed the earlier mailed questionnaire on self-reports of health conditions. Eisen et al. (2005) reported on the prevalence of self-reported asthma, bronchitis, and emphysema and found no significant differences between the two groups after adjusting for smoking and demographic variables. In a further study that applied spirometry and symptom interviews to a random selection of 1036 Gulf War deployed veterans compared with 1103 nondeployed US veterans, Karlinsky et al. (2004) found that only a history of smoking and wheezing among the respiratory outcomes studied were significantly elevated in the deployed veterans. No significant difference in the number of self-reported physicians' visits or hospitalizations for respiratory disorders was seen between the groups. Spirometric measurements also showed no significant difference between the two groups. The study did not report participation rate. The study also looked at the effect of potential exposure to the Khamisiyah nerve gas releases by selectively comparing veterans deployed into the geographic areas potentially affected by the release. No significant differences were noted in the measured pulmonary functions of these veterans when compared to nondeployed controls or veterans who were unlikely to have been exposed to the nerve gas.

Gray et al. (1999a) also found that between 527 Gulf War Seabees and 970 nondeployed Seabees, pulmonary function parameters (force vital capacity [FVC] and forced expiratory volume in 1 second [FEV_1]) showed no significant difference between the two groups, whereas respiratory symptoms (cough: OR 1.8, 95% CI 1.2-2.8; shortness of breath: OR 4.0; 95% CI 2.2-7.3) were significantly more common among deployed veterans compared with nondeployed veterans after adjustment for age, height, race, and smoking status.

Two studies of non-US Gulf War era veterans included an examination of respiratory outcomes. Australian Gulf War veterans were studied by Kelsall et al. (2004b) for respiratory outcomes. The prevalence of respiratory symptoms such as wheezing, chest tightness, cough, and dyspnea was higher (ORs ranged from 1.2-1.8; 95% CIs ranged from 0.9 to 2.3) among 1456 deployed veterans than among 1588 nondeployed veterans. Self-reported physician diagnosis of respiratory diseases such as asthma, chronic bronchitis, and emphysema was also higher in deployed veterans but not significant except for chronic bronchitis (OR 1.9, 95% CI 1.2-3.1), and pulmonary function were similar between the two groups. Danish peacekeepers, both military and nonmilitary, deployed to the gulf after the end of the conflict were studied by Ishoy and colleagues (1999b). They found that that the respiratory symptom of shortness of breath were more common among 686 deployed personnel when compared to a 231 professionally matched group of nondeployed subjects (14% vs 3.5%, $p < 0.001$). However, no significant difference was found on pulmonary function testing (FVC, FEV_1, peak flow) between the two groups.

Several primary studies examined the association between exposure to smoke from the Kuwaiti oil-well fires and respiratory outcomes. Cowan et al. (2002) conducted a case-control study examining the effect of exposure to oil-well fire smoke using exposure estimates based on troop locations and National Oceanographic and Atmospheric Administration (NOAA) modeling. They found that the risk of physician-diagnosed asthma increased with increasing exposure categories after controlling for sex, age, race, rank, smoking history, and self-reported exposure. They did not use pulmonary function tests and did not distinguish preexisting asthma from new onset asthma. A large population-based study of 1560 Iowa veterans found no association between modeled oil-well fire exposure and the risk of asthma or bronchitis as defined by interview questions about wheezing and chest tightness and cough (Lange et al., 2002). However, when the risk of asthma or bronchitis was compared to self-reports of exposure to oil-well fires a significant association was found with increasing self-reported exposure.

Smith and colleagues (2002) studied post war hospitalizations and estimates of exposure to oil-well fire smoke based on troop location and NOAA modeling. Among 405,142 active-duty veterans, no association was found between modeled exposures and hospitalizations for asthma or acute or chronic bronchitis. A modest but non significant increase in risk for hospitalizations for emphysema was associated with exposure (RR 1.36, 95% CI 0.62-2.98).

Secondary Studies

The Volume 4 committee reviewed numerous multiple secondary studies, most of which relied on self-reported respiratory symptoms. Most of the studies consistently found increased self-reports of respiratory symptoms and illness among Gulf Was veterans compared with nondeployed counterparts. This finding was true both for US studies (Eisen et al., 2005; Gray et al., 2002; Iowa Persian Gulf Study Group, 1997; Kang et al., 2000; Kroenke et al., 1998; Petruccelli et al., 1999; Steele, 2000) as well as studies of veterans from the United Kingdom (Cherry et al., 2001b; Nisenbaum et al., 2004; Simmons et al., 2004; Unwin et al., 1999), Denmark (Ishoy et al., 1999b), Australia (Kelsall et al., 2004b), and Canada (Goss Gilroy, 1998).

Secondary studies that focused on exposure to oil-well fires were relatively few. One found an increase in respiratory symptoms associated with self-reports of exposure to oil-well fire smoke (Proctor et al., 1998). A prospective study of British veterans deployed to Kuwait found no significant changes in $FEF_{25\%-75\%}$[3] across across a period of presumed oil-well fire smoke exposure; however, the exposure appears to have been low (Coombe and Drysdale, 1993). Two ecological studies of asthma hospitalizations among Kuwaiti residents found no significant difference after the conflict (Abul et al., 2001; Al-Khalaf, 1998).

[3]$FEF_{25\%-75\%}$ = Forced expiratory flow, midexpiratory phase.

Two studies addressed the potential association between nerve agent exposure and respiratory illness. Gray et al. (1999b) found a slightly increased risk of hospitalizations for respiratory illness to be associated with modeled exposure to the Khamisiyah detonation based on the 1997 modeling, while Karlinsky et al. (2004) found no association between pulmonary function test and DoD modeling from 2000.

Updated and Supplemental Literature

Primary Studies

The Update committee identified three additional primary studies of respiratory outcomes and the Gulf War combat experience.

In a study by Smith et al. (2006), three cohorts were defined and followed for hospitalizations from their exposure window until hospitalization, separation from the military, or December 31, 2000, whichever came first. The investigators used Cox hazard modeling and looked at hospitalizations for 14 ICD-9 categories of diagnosis. The cohorts represented Gulf War veterans, veterans deployed to Southwest Asia after the war, and veterans deployed to the Bosnian conflict. The study found a nonsignificant increase in respiratory disease hospitalizations for veterans deployed to Southwest Asia after the Gulf War as compared to Gulf War veterans (OR 1.08, 95% CI 1.00-1.16). Bosnian veterans had a significant decrease in respiratory disease hospitalizations when compared to Gulf War veterans (OR 0.73, 95% CI 0.63-0.84).

A study by MacFarlane et al. (2000) identified 53,462 UK Gulf War veterans who had served in the gulf between September 1990 and June 1991. A 53,462 member reference group composed of Gulf War era nondeployed UK veterans was assembled. The study selected the referent cohort through a stratified randomized sample of era vets matched on age, sex, rank, service branch, and level of fitness. Mortality as of March 31, 1999, was determined by use of a National Health Service central registry that was coded using ICD-9 codes. The study found 376 deaths among deployed and 352 deaths among nondeployed vets. At the time of mortality ascertainment, 1485 and 2257 were lost to follow-up in the cohorts respectively. There were no excess deaths due to diseases of the respiratory system found in either cohort. An update of the same cohort through 2004 (Macfarlane et al., 2005) again found no significant excess in deaths related to respiratory disease among Gulf War veterans versus nondeployed veterans.

Bullman et al. (2005) examined the relationship between estimated exposure to chemical munitions destruction (sarin gas) at Khamisiyah in 1991 with cause-specific mortality of Gulf War veterans through December 31, 2000. Using the DoD's 2000 sarin plume exposure model (Rostker, 2000), 100,487 deployed military personnel were identified as potentially exposed, and 224,980 were considered unexposed. The authors reported no increase in mortality risk due to respiratory diseases among exposed veterans as compared to unexposed veterans (RR 1.03, 95% CI 0.62-1.72). Similarly, no increased risk for respiratory disease mortality was observed when the authors divided the exposed group into persons exposed for either 1 or 2 days for comparison with the unexposed group.

Secondary Studies

Four secondary studies not previously reviewed were identified that addressed respiratory illness among Gulf War veterans and relied on self-reports.

Steele (2000) conducted a telephone survey of veterans who were Kansas residents and had served during the Gulf War. Of 2211 locatable and eligible veterans, 2030 agreed to participate (92%). Fifty were eliminated because their self-reported deployment status could not be verified. A total of 1548 Gulf War deployed veterans and 482 nondeployed veterans were interviewed about the presence of physician-diagnosed or physician-treated disorders with new onset after the Gulf War. Respiratory disorders were more commonly reported among deployed than nondeployed. Gulf War deployed veterans were twice as likely to report suffering from asthma (OR 2.08, 95% CI 1.02-4.26) and were almost 5 times as likely to report suffering from lung disease (OR 4.77, 95% CI 1.14-20.04). The study adjusted for sex, age, income and education level and suffered from a slight differential participation rate between groups (93% in deployed veterans vs 88% nondeployed veterans).

Proctor et al. (2001a) compared responses to questionnaires between 148 Gulf War deployed veterans of the Fort Deven's cohort, and 50 Germany deployed veterans. The authors found that Gulf War deployed veterans reported more chronic respiratory allergies (16% vs 13%) and more chronic lung problems (11.8% vs 6.5 %). Neither of these differences reached statistical significance, and no adjustments were made in the comparisons.

McCauley et al. (2002), using a telephone survey, interviewed three groups of US Gulf War veterans with different deployment experiences. These included Gulf War deployed veterans in proximity to the Khamisiyah detonations, veterans deployed to the gulf during the war but not in proximity to the Khamisiyah detonations, and veterans who were on active duty during, but not deployed to, the Gulf War. The authors found a nonsignificant excess in self-reported diagnosis of lung disease among deployed versus nondeployed veterans (OR 1.8, 95% CI 0.8-4.1) and no excess among Khamisiyah exposed versus Khamisiyah nonexposed veterans (OR 0.3, 95% CI 0.2-0.8).

In a mailed symptom survey to a sample of veterans from the National Health Survey of the Gulf War Era Veterans and Their Families conducted in 1995 (Kang et al., 2000), Kang et al. (2009) found a significant excess of self-reports of physician-diagnosed emphysema or chronic bronchitis and asthma among 6111 randomly surveyed Gulf War veterans when compared to 3859 nondeployed era veterans. The study suffered from a very low response rate (34% overall) and lacked a mechanism for verification of self-reports.

Statistics Canada (2005) conducted a mortality follow-up study of Canadian Gulf War veterans and compared them to a reference group of randomly selected Canadian veterans eligible but not deployed to the Gulf War and to the general Canadian population. There were 5117 members in the deployed cohort and 6093 members in the nondeployed population. Probabilistic matching of the military records of the cohorts to mortality records from the Canadian Mortality Data Base was conducted. The study authors estimated the study power to be 80% to find a 60% increase in total mortality; however, there were insufficient deaths from respiratory disease (ICD-9, code 460-519) to make a meaningful comparison between veteran cohorts or with the general population.

Kang and Bullman (1996) examined standardized mortality rates (SMRs) for multiple causes of death among Gulf War veterans up to September 1993 compared to the general US population and to nondeployed veterans. They found a significant decrease in deaths due to respiratory illness (SMR 0.14, 95% CI 0.07-0.23) when Gulf War veterans were compared to the US population and a slight but insignificant increase when compared to nondeployed veterans. These observations were based on very small numbers including only 14 deaths in both the deployed and nondeployed groups. A second study updated the same cohort for mortality outcomes up to December 31, 1997, using the same methods (Kang and Bullman, 2001). Again, no significant differences were noted between deployed and nondeployed veterans for respiratory causes of mortality. Again, both veteran cohorts showed significantly lower mortality for respiratory outcomes when compared to the general US population.

Summary and Conclusions

Studies based on self reported symptoms and self reported diagnoses related to respiratory disease have inconsistently but frequently shown an excess among Gulf War veterans. However there appears to be no increase in respiratory disease among Gulf War veterans when examined with objective measures of disease. Pulmonary function studies and mortality studies have shown no significant excess of lung function abnormalities or of death due to respiratory disease among Gulf War veterans.

> **Therefore, the committee concludes that there is insufficient/inadequate evidence to determine whether an association exists between deployment to the Gulf War and respiratory disease. The committee also concludes that there is limited/suggestive evidence of no association between deployment to the Gulf War and decreased lung function in the first 10 years after the war.**

TABLE 4-8 Respiratory System Diseases

Study	Design	Population	Outcomes	Results	Adjustments	Comments
Eisen et al., 2005 (Vol. 4)	Population-based, cross-sectional, prevalence, medical evaluation	1061 US deployed vs 1128 nondeployed	Self-reported asthma, bronchitis, or emphysema; obstructive lung disease (history of disease or symptoms plus use of bronchodilators or 15% improvement in FEV_1 after bronchodilator use)	Asthma, bronchitis, or emphysema: OR 1.07 (95% CI 0.65-1.77) Obstructive lung disease: OR 0.91 (95% CI 0.52-1.59)	Age, sex, race, years of education, smoking, duty type, service branch, rank	Low participation rates, especially among nondeployed
Karlinsky et al., 2004 (Vol. 4)	Cross-sectional, medical evaluation	1036 US deployed vs 1103 nondeployed	PFT results classified into five categories: normal, nonreversible obstruction, reversible obstruction, restrictive, small-airways obstruction	No association of PFT-based classifications with deployment status, nor with exposure to nerve agents at Khamisiyah based on 2002 DoD exposure models		No adjustment for smoking or other confounders; description of sampling strategy inadequate to evaluate bias; no explanation of "matching" or control of matching in analysis
Gray et al., 1999a (Vol. 4)	Cross-sectional, medical evaluation	527 Gulf War veterans vs 970 nondeployed from 14 US Navy Seabees commands	Cough; shortness of breath; FVC (L); FEV_1 (L)	Cough : OR 1.8 (95% CI 1.2-2.8) Shortness of breath: OR 4.0 (95% CI 2.2-7.3) FVC (L): 4.96 vs 4.99, $p = 0.77$ FEV_1 (L): 4.05 vs 4.04, $p = 0.81$	Age, height, race, smoking status	No use of modeled oil-fire exposures
Kelsall et al., 2004b (Vol. 4)	Cross-sectional, medical evaluation	1456 Australian deployed vs 1588 nondeployed	Asthma; bronchitis; $FEV_1/FVC\% < 70\%$	Asthma: OR 1.2 (95% CI 0.8-1.8); Bronchitis: OR 1.9 (95% CI 1.2-3.1); $FEV_1/FVC\% < 70\%$: OR 0.8 (95% CI 0.5-1.1);	Service type, rank, age, education, marital status	Generally well done; substantial potential for selection bias (response rates: deployed 81%, comparison 57%); no

Study	Design	Population	Outcomes	Results	Adjustments	Comments
				FVC, but not FEV_1, associated with self-report of oil-fire exposure		use of modeled oil-fire exposures
Ishoy et al., 1999b (Vol. 4)	Cross-sectional, population-based, medical evaluation	686 peace-keeping Danish deployed to Gulf War theater vs 231 nondeployed controls	Shortness of breath; FVC; FEV_1; peak flow	14% vs 3.5% Percent of predicted: 100.7 vs 100.7, NS 95.6 vs 96.4, NS 94.0 vs 92.8, NS	None	Appropriate population-based controls but differential participation: 84% deployed vs 58% nondeployed; smoking histories similar in deployed and nondeployed
Smith et al., 2006 (Update)	Hospitalizations cohort study (cohort data from DMDC)	Active-duty personnel with a single deployment to: Gulf War theater (n = 455,465); Southwest Asia peacekeeping mission, 1991-1998 (n = 249,047); Bosnia, 1995-1998 (n = 44,341)	Postdeployment hospitalization events (1991-2000) for an ICD-9-CM diagnosis of respiratory disease (140-208), and for testicular cancer specifically	Veterans of Bosnia compared to GWV: HR 0.73 (95% CI 0.63-0.84) Veterans of Southwest Asia compared to GWV: HR 1.08 (95% CI 1.00-1.16)	Sex, age, marital status, pay grade, race/ethnicity, service branch, occupation, and predeployment hospitalization; time-dependent covariate to account for changing hospitalization methods, diagnostic criteria, and procedures	Active-duty personnel only; hospitalizations at DoD facilities only
Macfarlane et al., 2000, 2005 (Update)	Cohort study	2000: 53,462 UK GWVs vs 53,450 nondeployed UK veterans 2005: 51,753 UK GWVs and 50,808 nondeployed UK veterans	Mortality (1991-1999/2004) due to diseases of the respiratory system	2000: 3 deaths in GWVs compared to 3 deaths in control group, MRR 1.0 (95% CI 0.1-7.5) 2005: 9 deaths in GWVs compared to 6 deaths in control group, MRR 1.64 (95% CI 0.58-4.66)	Matching by sex, age, branch, fitness for service	

Study	Design	Population	Outcomes	Results	Adjustments	Comments
Studies of respiratory outcomes specifically associated with modeled oil-well fire exposure						
Cowan et al., 2002 (Vol. 4)	Case-control study of exposure to smoke from oil-well fires; DoD registry, Army only	873 with asthma vs 2464 controls	Physician-assigned diagnosis of asthma 3-6 years after war	Self-reported exposure: OR 1.56 (95% CI 1.23-1.97) Cumulative modeled exposure: OR 1.24 (95% CI 1.00-1.55) for intermediate cumulative modeled exposure; OR 1.40 (95% CI 1.11-1.75) for high exposure. Number of days at > 65 $\mu g/m^3$: OR 1.22 (95% CI 0.99-1.51) for 1-5 days; OR 1.41 (95% CI 1.12-1.77) for 6-30 days	Sex, age, race, military rank, smoking history, self-reported exposure	Effect seen in former smokers and never-smokers, but not current smokers. Key strength: modeled exposure rather than only self-reported exposure. Limitations: self-selected population; no specified criteria for asthma diagnosis and no pulmonary function data; pre-exposure asthma status unknown
Lange et al., 2002 (Vol. 4)	Cross-sectional study of exposure to smoke from oil-well fires; derived from cohort study	1560 Iowa veterans	Asthma symptoms; bronchitis symptoms; structured interviews conducted 5 years after the war	For modeled exposure, adjusted ORs for quartiles of exposure, 0.77-1.26 with no dose-response relationship; for self-reported exposure, asthma ORs 1.77-2.83, bronchitis ORs 2.14-4.78	Sex, age, race, military rank, smoking history, military service, level of preparedness for war	Key strengths: modeled exposure rather than only self-reported exposure, population-based sample. Key limitation: symptom-based case definition of bronchitis and asthma
Smith et al., 2002 (Vol. 4)	DoD hospitalizations 1991-1999; exposure modeling for oil-well fire smoke	405,142 active-duty Gulf War veterans	ICD-9-CM codes for: Asthma Acute bronchitis Chronic bronchitis Emphysema Respiratory conditions due to chemical fumes and vapors Other respiratory	Exposed vs nonexposed: RR 0.90 (95% CI 0.74-1.10) RR 1.09 (95% CI 0.62-1.90) RR 0.78 (95% CI 0.38-1.57) RR 1.36 (95% CI 0.62-2.98) RR 0.71 (95% CI 0.23-2.17) RR 1.45 (95% CI 0.86-2.46)	"Influential predictors" of $p < 0.15$ included in analyses	Objective measure of disease not subject to recall bias; no issues with self-selection; however, only DoD hospitals, only active duty, no information on smoking or other exposures that may be

Study	Design	Population	Outcomes	Results	Adjustments	Comments
			diseases			related to respiratory symptoms, most adults with asthma or chronic bronchitis have never been hospitalized for that condition
Study of respiratory outcomes specifically associated with exposure to Khamisiyah nerve agent						
Gray et al., 1999b (Vol. 4)	DoD hospitalizations 1991-1995, exposure to nerve agents at Khamisiyah based on 1997 DoD exposure models	Not exposed (n = 224,804), uncertain low-dose exposure (n = 75,717), exposed (n = 48,770)	Respiratory system disease (vs not exposed): Uncertain low dose < 0.013 mg-min/m^3 0.013-0.097 mg-min/m^3 0.097-0.514 mg-min/m^3	 OR 0.92 (95% CI (0.85-0.99) OR 0.90 (95% CI 0.77-1.04) OR 0.89 (95% CI 0.79-1.02) OR 1.26 (95% CI 1.05-1.51)	Sex, age group, prewar hospitalization, race, service type, marital status, pay grade, occupation	See Smith et al., 2002. Probable substantial exposure misclassification as models were revised, lack of a clear dose-response pattern, little biologic plausibility given that no effect was seen for nervous system diseases
Bullman et al., 2005 (Update)	Cohort mortality study; follow-up from March 1991 through 2000	100,487 US Army GWVs exposed to chemical warfare agents at Khamisiyah; 224,980 nonexposed army GWVs; exposure determined from the DoD plume model (Rostker, 2000)	Association of exposure to chemical warfare agents and respiratory disease mortality, determined through BIRLS, SSA; COD data from NDI	Exposed vs unexposed RR 1.03 (95% CI 0.62-1.72)	Age, race, sex, rank, unit component	Limitations: short latency, possible exposure misclassification

NOTE: BIRLS = Beneficiary Identification and Records Locator Subsystem (VA); CI = confidence interval; COD = cause of death; DMDC = Defense Manpower Data Center; FEV_1 = forced expiratory volume in the first second of expiration; FVC = forced vital capacity; GWV = Gulf War veteran; HR = adjusted hazard ratio; NDI = National Death Index; NS = not significant; OR = adjusted odds ratio; PFT = pulmonary function test; RR = adjusted risk ratio; SSA = Social Security Administration.

DISEASES OF THE DIGESTIVE SYSTEM

Digestive disorders may be functional (Drossman, 2006; Drossman et al., 2006), structural, or in some cases combinations of both (Grover et al., 2009). The functional gastrointestinal (GI) disorders (FGIDs), such as irritable bowel syndrome (IBS) or functional dyspepsia, are syndromes—that is, recurrent or prolonged clusters of symptoms that occur together. They result from known disturbances in GI functioning and central dysregulation of this GI function and should be differentiated from psychiatric multisymptom syndromes (for example, somatization disorder) that are determined by central amplification of normal somatic and visceral neural signaling (Drossman et al., 2002, 2006). The FGIDs range in severity from occasional mild episodes to more persistent and disabling symptoms with impaired health-related quality of life. These disorders fit a biopsychosocial construct (Drossman, 1998) and are understood as brain–gut axis dysfunction where psychosocial factors may disrupt gut functioning and vice versa (Jones et al., 2006). Genetic or early environmental predisposing factors including family enablement of illness behaviors (Levy et al., 2000) or early trauma or abuse history (Drossman et al., 1995), in many cases coupled with exposure to acute GI infection (Spiller and Campbell, 2006), can precipitate or exacerbate the clinical expression of FGIDs, causing them to manifest as disturbed motility (that is, constipation, diarrhea, nausea, vomiting), or visceral hypersensitivity (that is, pain, bloating, abdominal fullness). The symptoms can be sustained or perpetuated in the presence of psychological comorbidities including PTSD, anxiety, and depression; maladaptive coping style; or impaired social networks (Creed et al., 2006; Drossman et al., 2002; Levy et al., 2006).

Relevant to this review is the concept of postinfectious IBS, where the FGID is triggered by exposure to infectious agents, which normally cause acute gastroenteritis, but with coexistent stress, in this case deployment to the Gulf War, the symptoms are sustained (Drossman, 1999; Dunlop et al., 2003; McKeown et al., 2006; Spiller and Campbell, 2006). In a recently completed study using the Defense Medical Surveillance System, 31,866 cases of active-duty soldiers with FGIDs registered between 1999 and 2007 were matched to non-FGID active-duty controls. Researchers found a highly significant association of prior infectious gastroenteritis (greatest effect for bacterial gastroenteritis) to those with FGIDs (all $p < 0.001$), including functional diarrhea (OR 6.28), IBS (OR 3.72), functional constipation (OR 2.15), and functional dyspepsia (OR 2.39), and 28.8% of the active duty personnel studied still received care for the FGID 2 years after initial diagnosis. Thus there is a strong association of prior acute gastroenteritis (Riddle et al., 2009).

The pathophysiology of the FGIDs relate specifically to dysregulation of neural pathways between the brain and gut (that is, the brain–gut axis) that produce motility and sensory disturbances (visceral hypersensitivity), dysregulation of the hypothalamic-pituitary adrenal axis, altered corticolimbic pain modulation, and inflammation of the bowel mucosa associated with altered bacterial flora pain modulation, and inflammation of the bowel mucosa associated with altered bacterial flora (Drossman, 2006; Drossman et al., 2002; Kassinen et al., 2007).

The diagnosis of a functional GI disorder is made by fulfilling standardized symptom-based criteria (Rome criteria) for a minimal period of time, usually 6 months (Drossman, 2006). These criteria have not been used in published studies of Gulf War veterans with the exception of one physiological study (Dunphy et al., 2003). However, recently there have been several research abstracts published using Rome III criteria that describe increased incidence rates of

IBS after wartime exposure (Tuteja et al., 2008; Wurzelmann et al., 2008) as well as one published study of increased adult Rome III-diagnosed IBS incidence rates that related to severe early-life wartime exposure during World War II (Klooker et al., 2009).

GI diseases, sometimes called "organic" or structural diseases, such as peptic ulcer and inflammatory bowel disease (that is, ulcerative colitis and Crohn's disease), are characterized by morphological abnormalities seen on x-ray, endoscopy, or through laboratory tests. For example, with Crohn's disease the intestine may be inflamed and have ulcerations, strictures, fistulas, or abscesses. The diagnoses of these diseases need to be validated by medical records since some physicians may place an organic label on the patient's symptoms (such as gastritis or peptic ulcer) but without proper morphological correlation. Such labeling will confound the diagnosis of these diseases when surveys are used, particularly when the data are based on the individual's recollection of a physician's diagnosis.

For the purposes of this section, the committee defined primary studies by their methodological rigor (see Chapter 2) and outcome assessment requiring sufficiently valid symptom clusters consistent with a functional GI diagnosis, or in the case of structural diseases, physical examination. The primary studies are summarized in Table 4-9.

Summary of *Volume 4*

Primary Studies

In *Volume 4*, three studies were identified that met that committee's criteria for primary studies: Eisen et al. (2005), who conducted a survey and physical examinations, and two hospitalization studies by Gray et al. (1996, 2002).

Ten years after the Gulf War, in the National Health Survey of Gulf War Era Veterans and Their Families, a nationally representative population-based study, the VA conducted medical evaluations to determine the prevalence of common diseases in deployed veterans (Eisen et al., 2005). In 1999-2001, 1061 deployed and 1128 nondeployed veterans were evaluated at several VA centers. The veterans had been randomly selected from 11,441 deployed and 9476 nondeployed veterans who had participated in a 1995 VA survey (Kang et al., 2000) that used a self-report questionnaire. Dyspepsia was diagnosed through in-person interviews according to two criteria: a history or symptoms of dyspepsia (frequent heartburn and recurrent abdominal pain) and use of antacids, histamine-2 receptor blockers, or other medications to treat dyspepsia. The prevalence of dyspepsia was 9.1% and 6.0% in deployed and nondeployed veterans, respectively (OR 1.87, 95% CI 1.16-2.99). Reports of gastritis were 5.9% and 4.2%, respectively (OR 1.57, 95% CI 0.88-2.78). Study limitations for these outcomes are: dyspepsia was diagnosed crudely as recurrent abdominal pain or frequent heartburn, which is more commonly associated with gastroesophageal reflux disease; IBS, a more common functional GI disorder, was not evaluated; and despite three recruitment waves, participation was only 53% of eligible Gulf War and 39% of eligible nondeployed veterans.

A study by Gray et al. (1996) showed no excess hospitalizations in DoD hospitals for digestive system disorders, as broadly defined by a range of ICD codes, from 1991 to 1993. That study compared hospitalizations of almost 550,000 Gulf War veterans and almost 620,000 nondeployed veterans who remained on active duty until 1993. Another further hospitalization study conducted by Gray et al. (2000) covered the years 1991-1994 and examined DoD, VA, and California hospitals. The study examined hospitalizations at nonfederal hospitals in California to eliminate potential bias related to veterans seeking care outside DoD and VA facilities.

Proportional morbidity ratios (PMRs) of hospital-discharge diagnoses (14 diagnostic categories from ICD-9) in Gulf War deployed and nondeployed veterans were compared. Hospitalizations for digestive system diseases for deployed versus nondeployed veterans were increased in VA hospitals (PMR 1.12, 95% CI 1.05-1.18) and in California hospitals (PMR 1.11, 95% CI 0.97-1.24), but not in DoD hospitals (PMR 0.98, 95% CI 0.96-0.99). The limitation of these studies is their inability to capture any but the most severe digestive system disorders (most would be treated on an outpatient basis).

Secondary Studies

In *Volume 4*, two studies were identified as secondary: Sostek et al. (1996) and Ishoy et al. (1999a,b). Sostek et al. is discussed in the section "Updated and Supplemental Literature." Ishoy et al. (1999a,b) analyzed self-reported GI symptoms in relation to Gulf War exposures among deployed Danish Gulf War veterans and nondeployed controls. Eight of 14 GI symptoms were reported significantly more frequently by veterans than by controls but only the prevalence of recurrent diarrhea for 1 year and rumbling in the stomach more than two times per week remained significant after adjustment.

Updated and Supplemental Epidemiologic Literature

Other primary and secondary studies were identified by the Update committee. A primary study by Sostek et al. (1996) focused on evaluating the prevalence and spectrum of GI complaints in a group of 57 Gulf War deployed National Guard veterans and 44 nondeployed veteran controls. Notably, the self-reporting of medical, including GI, symptoms occurring before the war was low (0-9%) and not different between groups. However, after the war, Gulf War veterans reported qualitatively and quantitatively markedly higher rates ($p \leq 0.001$) of GI symptoms than the nondeployed veterans, which persisted many years after deployment: intra- or supraumbilically located abdominal pain (70% vs 9%); excessive gas (74% vs 23%); abdominal pain with increased or watery bowel movements (44% vs 5%); loose or > 3 stools per day (74% vs 18%); incomplete rectal evacuation (60% vs 7%), and decreased appetite (42% vs 7%), and about 80% remained symptomatic after the war. Postwar comparisons showed less significant differences ($p = 0.05$) between deployed veterans and controls in other GI symptoms: relief of pain with bowel movements (47% vs 16%), postprandial pain (46% vs 14%), mucus in the stools (19% vs 0%), rectal pain with bowel movements (26% vs 5%), nausea and vomiting (23% vs 2%), and heartburn (33% vs 7%). However, these individuals also reported high frequencies of other non-GI symptoms, suggesting that there may be a tendency to report physical symptoms in general. The frequency of blood in the stool was low and not significantly different between groups, and this may likely reflect local sources such as hemorrhoids. Histopathological assessment of colonic biopsies many years after deployment in the symptomatic Gulf War veterans showed that 6 out of 15 had mild chronic inflammation of the lamina propria, a finding that by current standards would be considered a feature of IBS possibly originating from infectious exposure (Chadwick et al., 2002; Dunlop et al., 2003). This finding has also been reported in 53 Gulf War veterans being evaluated by endoscopy and biopsy for chronic GI complaints (Lang and Saylor, 1995). The strength of this study is the histopathological evidence for inflammation suggestive of postinfectious IBS. In addition, the survey questions were highly specific for functional GI disorders as they reflect physiological disturbance of the gut (for example, pain relieved by defecation, sense of incomplete evacuation) and together are more than sufficient to meet the Rome III criteria for IBS and possibly other functional GI disorders (Drossman, 2006; Longstreth, 2006; Longstreth et al., 2006). For these reasons this study is considered to be primary.

An update of previous data by Gray and colleagues (2002) was a survey of nearly 12,000 active-duty Seabees, from 14 commands, still on active duty for at least 3 years after the Gulf War. The study subjects were queried about self-reported physician-diagnosed illnesses, symptoms, and exposures. IBS was one of the physician-diagnosed illnesses listed on the survey. Deployed Gulf War Seabees were much more likely than nondeployed Seabees to report being diagnosed with irritable bowel syndrome (2.48% vs 0.81%, OR 3.57, 95% CI 2.22-5.73). Irritable bowel syndrome was one of a cluster of four physician-diagnosed conditions—along with PTSD, chronic fatigue syndrome, and multiple chemical sensitivity syndrome—found to be more prevalent among Gulf War deployed Seabees than nondeployed Seabees, and these four conditions were highly associated with one another. Among the deployed Seabees, being diagnosed with one of these four conditions also was associated with reporting many other symptoms (16 other symptoms) whereas other deployed Seabees not reporting any of these four conditions had fewer (6) other symptoms. Because the focus of this study was to cluster symptoms and conditions that might shed light on a unique Gulf War illness, the analysis undertook no further evaluation of GI conditions in isolation.

Numerous studies have queried deployed and nondeployed US Gulf War veterans about gastrointestinal or stomach symptoms generally (Lindem et al., 2003a,b,c; Steele, 2000); they have also been asked about a number of specific gastrointestinal symptoms such as gas (Fukuda et al., 1998; Proctor et al., 1998), bloating (Fukuda et al., 1998), cramps (Fukuda et al., 1998; Proctor et al., 1998; Steele, 2000), abdominal pain (Fukuda et al., 1998; Knoke et al., 2000; Steele, 2000); diarrhea (Fukuda et al., 1998; Kang et al., 2000; Knoke et al., 2000; Proctor et al., 1998; Steele, 2000), constipation (Knoke et al., 2000; Proctor et al., 1998), loose bowel movements (Knoke and Gray, 1998), and nausea or upset stomach (Kroenke et al., 1998; Proctor et al., 1998; Steele, 2000). In all of these studies deployed veterans reported more GI symptoms than their nondeployed counterparts.

Kang et al. (2000) asked Gulf War veterans about whether they had any of three specific digestive conditions: gastritis, enteritis, or colitis. The sample included active-duty, reserve, and National Guard personnel as well as an oversampling of female veterans who were in the military between September 1990 and May 1991. The prevalence of gastritis was more than doubled in the deployed veterans compared with the nondeployed veterans (25% vs 12%). In 2004-2005, Kang et al. (2009) conducted a follow-up study of the 15,000 deployed and 15,000 nondeployed veterans originally surveyed in 1995 (Kang et al., 2000). Veterans were asked via a mailed questionnaire if their doctor had ever told them they had any of 23 medical conditions, including gastritis and irritable bowel syndrome. Both gastritis and IBS were among the top five medical conditions with the greatest relative risk; the relative risk was 1.52 (95% CI 1.40-1.65) for gastritis and 1.50 (95% CI 1.35-1.66) for IBS, adjusted for age, sex, race, body mass index, current cigarette smoking, rank, branch of service, and unit component. This study is limited by the use of a self-report survey, and indeed gastritis using symptom reports is more likely to be functional dyspepsia. Because the questionnaire items were not sufficiently detailed to make a diagnosis of a functional digestive disorder (via Rome criteria) or to identify structural disorders by endoscopy, this study is considered to be secondary.

Surveys of deployed Gulf War troops from other countries showed similar results to those of the Danish veterans (Ishoy et al., 1999a,b). UK Gulf War veterans self-reported more diarrhea, feeling bloated, stomach pain, heartburn, constipation, vomiting (Cherry et al., 2001a); flatulence, or burping (Unwin et al., 1999); and digestive, stomach, and intestinal disorders (Simmons et al., 2004) than nondeployed veterans. Australian Gulf War veterans also self-reported more moderate to severe flatulence or burping (OR 1.6, 95% CI 1.3-2.1), indigestion (OR 1.7, 95% CI 1.3-2.3), diarrhea (OR 2.4, 95% CI 1.6-3.5), stomach cramps (OR 2.2, 95% CI 1.5-3.3), constipation (OR 1.8, 95% CI 1.0-3.0), and nausea (OR 2.5, 95% CI 1.4-4.5). Although the Australian study used a postal questionnaire to initially ask veterans about having received a physician's diagnosis of or treatment for a medical condition, the veterans were later asked in person about their responses by a physician. The physician then determined whether the diagnoses or treatments reported on the questionnaire and discussed with the patient were a possible or probable diagnosis based on the veterans' responses. Based on this approach (which added a level of medical judgment to the self-reports but did not verify the self-reported diagnoses with additional testing such as an endoscopy or x-ray), compared with nondeployed veterans, deployed veterans were more likely to have a possible or probable diagnosis of stomach or duodenal ulcers (OR 1.6, 95% CI 1.1-2.75) and irritable bowel syndrome (OR 2.4, 95% CI 1.4-4.3) (Sim et al., 2003). Canadian Gulf War veterans reported more digestion problems other than stomach ulcers that did nondeployed Canadian veterans (13.4% vs 6.6%) (Goss Gilroy, 1998).

A recent systematic review evaluated the risk of developing painful conditions among Gulf War deployment versus nondeployed veterans. Using six studies (Cherry et al., 2001a; Gray et al., 2002; Kang et al., 2000; Knoke et al., 2000; Sostek et al., 1996; Steele, 2000). Thomas et al. (2006) found that pain from various conditions was more likely to occur in deployed veterans, and the most significant effect was seen with abdominal pain (OR 3.23, 95% CI 2.31-4.51).

In summary, numerous studies indicate that Gulf War veterans self-report more GI symptoms than nondeployed veterans. Most of these studies are limited because their methods are insufficient to determine a clear association between deployment and the onset of a functional disorder by standard Rome criteria (Drossman et al., 2006) or of a structural disorder (Drossman and Ringel, 2004). Furthermore, the diagnosis of structural diseases should be validated by medical records because physicians not infrequently place an organic label on a patient's symptoms (for example, gastritis or peptic ulcer) without performing diagnostic studies, and this will confound the diagnosis in a survey, particularly if the data are based on the subjects' recollections of physicians' diagnoses.

Other studies have evaluated hospitalizations and mortality of Gulf War veterans for digestive diseases. To avoid criticism when comparing deployed personnel with nondeployed personnel as may have occurred in the Gray et al. (1996, 2000) hospitalization studies (creating a "healthy deployer" effect), Smith et al. (2006) compared postdeployment hospitalizations for active-duty military personnel deployed to the Gulf War, deployed to southwest Asia after the war, or deployed to Bosnia. Hospitalizations were based on ICD-9 discharge diagnoses from military hospitals from August 1, 1990, to December 31, 2000. Active-duty personnel deployed to Bosnia were at reduced risk of hospitalization for digestive system diseases or conditions compared with Gulf War veterans (HR 0.60, 95% CI 0.54-0.67). There was no difference in hospitalizations for digestive system diseases between those deployed during the Gulf War and those deployed to the region after the war (HR 0.99, 95% CI 0.94-1.05). Hazard ratios were adjusted for sex, age, marital status, pay grade, ethnicity/race, service branch, occupation, and predeployment hospitalization.

Two studies assessed mortality in UK Gulf War veterans from diseases of the digestive system (DASA, 2009; Macfarlane et al., 2005). Macfarlane et al. (2005) assessed mortality of the UK Gulf War (51,753) and era (50,808) veteran cohorts from April 1, 1991, to June 30, 2004. Based on data from the National Health Service, the Gulf War veterans experienced fewer deaths from digestive diseases than the era cohort (mortality rate ratio 0.77, 95% CI 0.40-1.46), adjusted for age. The UK Defence Analytical Services Agency (DASA) published summary statistics on causes of deaths in Gulf War veterans between April 1, 1991, and December 31, 2007 (DASA, 2009). Mortality rates for the 53,409 Gulf War veterans were compared with the 53,143 era veterans. The adjusted mortality rate ratio for diseases of the digestive system was 0.71 (95% CI 0.46-1.11).

Finally, one study is notable for using specific Rome III criteria for the diagnosis of irritable bowel syndrome in war-time situations. Tuteja et al. (2008) studied 247 Gulf War deployed and nondeployed veterans from Salt Lake City who were in the reserves or National Guard and deployed between 1990-1991. It was found that there was an increased reporting of IBS from before deployment (5.8%) to during deployment (38.9%; $p = 0.03$) and this continued after deployment 18 years later (33.6%). Similar significant findings were seen with symptoms of diarrhea, constipation, and bloating. Furthermore, a history of an enteric infection was a risk factor for developing IBS (OR 3.6, 95% CI 1.9-6.9) now called postinfectious IBS. These data are presently available in abstract form only, and therefore this study is considered to be secondary.

Summary and Conclusions

There were many reports of gastrointestinal disturbances in Gulf War deployed veterans and the symptoms have persisted during the 19 years since the war. Notably all studies are in the direction favoring a greater prevalence of various GI symptoms and primarily functional GI disorders including IBS and dyspepsia.

Several of the papers attempted to link the symptoms to various exposures including side effects from nerve agent prophylaxis, using contaminated water, and burning of animal waste, but support from this is also limited and nonconfirmatory. More compelling is the emerging evidence for exposure to enteric pathogens during deployment leading to the development of postinfectious IBS. These data have been strengthened in recent years as a result of several lines of evidence:

- The incidence of acquiring an acute gastroenteritis among deployed veterans is higher than nondeployed veterans, over 50% in some series (IOM, 2007).
- Deployed veterans or other individuals experiencing war trauma who are exposed to an infectious gastroenteritis are at greater risk to be later diagnosed with IBS (Pulling et al., 2008; Riddle et al., 2009; Tuteja et al., 2008).
- Deployed veterans that have IBS symptoms have increased microscopic inflammatory changes in the bowel mucosa which can result from prior mucosal infection (Lang and Saylor, 1995; Sostek et al., 1996).
- Microscopic inflammation in IBS is associated with increased cytokine activity and mast cell degranulation that produces visceral hypersensitivity and abdominal pain (Barbara et al., 2004; Chadwick et al., 2002).

- Postinfectious IBS symptoms are facilitated by psychological distress via central nervous system (such as the hypothalamic-pituitary adrenal axis) effects on mucosal inflammation and enhanced pain via anterior cingulate cortex activation (Barbara et al., 2008; Drossman, 1999; Dunlop et al., 2003; Gwee et al., 1999).

Furthermore there is a large body of physiological data in IBS including among Gulf War veterans that demonstrate altered physiological functioning (such as diarrhea and constipation caused by altered migrating motor complexes and high-amplitude propagated contractions) that separates this condition from mere symptom reporting tendency (somatization). One study showed lowered visceral sensitivity, pain intensity, and anxiety in relation to rectal distention and cutaneous hand stimulation among Gulf War veterans compared to nondeployed veterans and civilians (Dunlop et al., 2003). Another study showed altered autonomic activity and lowered pain thresholds in response to acute physical and psychological stress (Murray et al., 2004) and an association of altered gastrointestinal motility and GI symptoms when IBS subjects are administered CRF, a stress hormone (Fukudo et al., 1998). A full review of this area can be found elsewhere (Kellow et al., 2006a,b).

The data on organic disorders are scanty and negative. See Table 4-9 for a summary of the primary studies reviewed above.

There are some limitations in the epidemiological body of evidence, mostly related to methods of effect assessment. One is that with the exception of two published abstracts, the self-reporting of GI symptoms did not fulfill the criteria for diagnosing a functional GI disorder, although in at least one published case series the diagnoses can be inferred (Sostek et al., 1996). In addition, existing studies in the deployed military population cannot yet determine the degree to which the gastrointestinal symptoms are specific to IBS and other FGIDs or are part of a larger spectrum of illness (that is, multisystem disease; see also the section on multisymptom illnesses in this chapter). Within civilian populations persons with these disorders exist on a spectrum where mild to moderate symptoms are limited to the GI tract, but more severe illness is associated with increased comorbidities. Therefore, the committee recommends that further studies in a deployed military population be undertaken to determine the presence of medical and psychosocial comorbidities in those with FGIDs. Finally, the committee concludes that there was also a lack of adequate medical diagnostic testing to identify a GI structural disease.

Nevertheless, taken together, the overall pattern of symptoms found in the few primary and numerous secondary studies confirms an association between deployment to the Gulf War and functional GI symptoms, including abdominal pain, diarrhea, nausea, and vomiting, and a few studies exist that provide presumptive data to allow standardized diagnosis of functional GI disorders. These studies are strengthened by physiological and mechanistic data in war veterans with IBS, and particular reference is made to the emerging evidence for preexisting acute gastroenteritis as a predictive factor in postinfectious IBS and dyspepsia. The committee recommends that further studies be conducted to determine the role of prior acute gastroenteritis among deployed soldiers in the development of FGIDs. Thus, the association of deployment-related stress with GI symptoms is accepted, the association with functional GI disorders is supported but not complete, and an association with structural GI diseases cannot be determined.

The committee concludes that there is sufficient evidence for an association between deployment to the Gulf War and gastrointestinal symptoms consistent with functional GI disorders such as irritable bowel syndrome and functional dyspepsia. The committee also concludes that there is inadequate/insufficient

evidence to determine whether an association exists between deployment to the Gulf War and the development of structural gastrointestinal diseases.

TABLE 4-9 Digestive System Diseases

Study	Study Design	Population	Outcomes	Results	Adjustments	Comments
Eisen et al., 2005 (Vol. 4)	Cross-sectional, prevalence	1061 GWVs, 1128 NDVs	Physician evaluation, questionnaire for dyspepsia; GI symptoms and medical conditions reported from earlier survey	Dyspepsia (OR 1.87, 95% CI 1.16-2.99); self-reported gastritis (OR 1.57, 95% CI 0.88-2.78)	Age, sex, race, smoking, duty type, service branch, rank, years of education	Study limited by low participation rate, length of time since war; weak diagnostic criteria
Gray et al., 1996 (Vol. 4)	Retrospective cohort study (hospitalization records)	DoD hospitals: 547,076 GWVs; 618,335 NDVs	Digestive system diseases	All ORs < 1.0	Hospitalization rates and rate ratios adjusted for age, sex; multiple logistic-regression models adjusted for all observed demographic differences between groups	Study data reflect only hospitalization experience of persons who remained on active duty through September 1993
Gray et al., 2000 (Vol. 4)	Retrospective cohort study (hospitalization records)	GWVs (August 1990-July 1992, n = 652,979) and NDVs (n = 652,922) stratified by California residence, service, and service branch of all nondeployed veterans (n = 2,912,737)	Digestive system diseases	VA hospitals: PMR 1.12 (95% CI 1.05-1.18); DoD hospitals: PMR 0.98 (95% CI 0.96-0.99); COSHPD hospitals: PMR 1.11 (95% CI 0.97-1.24)	Hospitalization records were matched on sex, age	Findings might be influenced by chance or by potential confounders, including health registry participation
Sosteck et al., 1996 (Update)	Cross-sectional, prevalence	57 male GWVs, 44 NDVs of National Guard unit	Questionnaire about GI and non-GI symptoms with recall before, during, after Gulf War period	Prevalence of GI symptoms: abdominal pain 70% vs 9%; diarrhea 74% vs 18%; incomplete rectal evacuation 60% vs 7%; gas 74% vs 23%; decreased appetite 42% vs 7% (all p < 0.001)		Response rate 74%; limitations include small sample (recall before, during, after Gulf War), questionnaire (at time of assessment)

Study	Study Design	Population	Outcomes	Results	Adjustments	Comments
Gray et al., 2002 (Update)	Retrospective, case-control	US Navy Seabees: 3831 GWVs, 4933 veterans deployed elsewhere, 3104 NDVs	Self-reported physician diagnoses, self-reported symptoms from postal questionnaire	Gulf War Seabees vs nondeployed: self-reported peptic ulcer disease (OR 3.11, 95% CI 1.67-5.78); self-reported IBS (OR 3.57, 95% CI 2.22-5.73); new GI disease diagnosed since September 1990 (OR 2.10, 95 % CI 1.39-3.17); clustering of CFS, PTSD, MCS, IBS: Seabees who had one averaged 13-18 other symptoms, Seabees without and averaged only 6 other symptoms	Age, sex, active-duty or reserve status, race or ethnicity, current smoking, current alcohol drinking	Study limited by recall bias, IBS not analyzed exclusively, response rate 70%, large sample

NOTE: CFS = chronic fatigue syndrome; CI = confidence interval, COSHPD = California Office of Statewide Health Planning and Development; DIS = Diagnostic Interview Schedule; DoD = Department of Defense; GI = gastrointestinal; GWV = Gulf War veteran; IBS = irritable bowel syndrome; MCS = multiple chemical sensitivity; MMR = adjusted mortality ratio; NDV = nondeployed Gulf War veterans; OR = odds ratio; PCL-C = PTSD Checklist-Civilian, PMR = proportional morbidity ratio; PTSD = posttraumatic stress disorder; SF-36 = Short form 36; VA = Department of Veterans Affairs.

SKIN DISEASES

Skin conditions, particularly rashes, are among the most frequent health problems reported by Gulf War veterans (Murphy et al., 1999). Rash usually refers to *dermatitis*, an umbrella term covering several subtypes, including atopic dermatitis, contact dermatitis, seborrheic dermatitis, and psoriasis. During the Gulf War, troops were exposed to several toxicants that could cause allergic skin reactions, including pesticides and solvents.

In reviewing studies that included dermatologic symptoms and diseases, the committee defined a primary study according to methodological rigor (Chapter 2) and use of a dermatologic examination to diagnose or verify a skin disorder. In a secondary study, the determination of a dermatologic effect was based on veterans' self-reports of symptoms or self-reported physician-diagnosed conditions. Primary studies for skin disorders are summarized in Table 4-10. Skin cancers are discussed in the section on cancer.

Summary of *Volume 4*

Primary Studies

To determine the link between deployment to the Gulf War and dermatologic diseases, the Volume 4 committee identified two primary studies: Eisen et al. (2005) who used a large, nationally representative study of US Gulf War veterans; and Higgins et al. (2002) who conducted in-person dermatologic evaluations of UK Gulf War deployed veterans (111 disabled and 98 nondisabled) and 133 disabled veterans not deployed to the Gulf War. These studies were conducted 10 and 8 years after the Gulf War, respectively. Eisen et al. (2005) used medical evaluation data derived from the 1995 VA National Health Survey of Gulf War Era Veterans and their Families (Kang et al., 2000). A dermatologist used teledermatology, at least two digital photographs, and the results of a standardized history and physical examination to assign dermatologic conditions into two categories: group 1 consisted of freckles, seborrheic keratoses, moles, cherry hemangiomas, skin tags, and scars; group 2 consisted of dermatologic diagnoses not included in group 1. The prevalence of group 1 diagnoses did not differ between deployed and nondeployed veterans (OR 0.87, 95% CI 0.68-1.12); the prevalence of a diagnosis of one or more group 2 skin conditions was 34.6% in deployed veterans and 26.8% in nondeployed veterans (OR 1.38, 95% CI 1.06-1.80). The most common group 2 skin conditions among deployed veterans were onychomycosis (4.1%) and folliculitis (4.0%). After adjustment of individual group 2 skin conditions, two skin conditions in this group were diagnosed more frequently ($p = 0.02$) in deployed than in nondeployed veterans: verruca vulgaris (warts) (OR 4.02, 95% CI 1.28-12.6) and atopic dermatitis (OR 8.1, 95% CI 2.4-27.7).

In the cross-sectional study by Higgins et al. (2002) the prevalence of any skin condition was 47.7% in disabled Gulf War veterans, 36.7% in nondisabled Gulf War veterans, and 42.8% in disabled nondeployed veterans, as determined on physical examination by a dermatologist. The investigators found no differences among groups in any dermatologic conditions other than seborrheic dermatitis: 7.2% in disabled deployed veterans and 9.2% in nondisabled deployed veterans versus 2.3% in disabled nondeployed veterans.

Secondary Studies

The Volume 4 committee identified two large well-designed studies of Gulf War veterans that were considered secondary studies because they lacked a dermatologic examination or were imprecise regarding specific dermatologic diagnoses: Kang et al. (2000) and Proctor et al. (1998). In the first phase of the VA National Health Survey of Gulf War Era Veterans and Their Families, Kang et al. (2000) compared 11,441 deployed veterans with 9476 nondeployed veterans identified by the DMDC. Dermatitis other than eczema and psoriasis was among the five most frequently reported medical conditions diagnosed by a physician in the preceding 12 months. The skin conditions reported by the deployed and nondeployed veterans were eczema or psoriasis (7.7% vs 4.4%; rate difference 3.34, 95% CI 3.26-3.42), other dermatitis (25.1% vs 12.0%; rate difference 13.16, 95% CI 13.04-13.28), and diseases of the hair or scalp or hair loss (16.9% vs 7.2; rate difference 9.65, 95% CI 9.55-9.75). A sample of participants were later evaluated by clinical examination in the Eisen et al. study (2005). Proctor et al. (1998) assessed the prevalence of dermatologic conditions—such as rashes, eczema, and skin allergies—in US veterans. The estimated prevalence was 15.5% for the 186 Gulf War deployed veterans from the Fort Devens cohort, 11.7% for the 66 deployed veterans from the New Orleans cohort, and 1.9% for the 48 veterans deployed to Germany during the Gulf War.

Updated and Supplemental Literature

Primary Studies

The Update committee identified one new primary study: Ishoy et al. (1999b). This study reported on Danish peacekeepers deployed to the Persian Gulf area during 1990-1997. The 686 deployed veterans and 231 nondeployed age-, sex-, and profession-matched veterans each received a medical examination and were interviewed for a full medical history by a physician based on a previously administered questionnaire. Veterans indicated whether any medical condition had its onset before or after deployment to the gulf. The examinations found that the prevalence of the following conditions with onset during or after deployment or August 1990 was higher in deployed veterans than in nondeployed veterans: eczema (15.0% vs 3.0%, $p < 0.001$), retarded wound healing (6.0% vs 1.7%, $p < 0.01$), other skin problems (17.1% vs 5.2%, $p < 0.001$), hair loss or hair disease (4.2% vs 0.9%, $p < 0.01$), and sweaty, clammy, or damp hands (7.9% vs 3.9%, $p < 0.05$). There were no significant differences in the prevalence of psoriasis and nettle rash between deployed and nondeployed troops. Although the examination process used to verify the veteran's actual skin conditions at the time of the interview by the physician is somewhat unclear in the report, the use of a physician to discuss the veterans' responses to the questionnaire provides support for the designation of this report as primary.

Secondary Studies

The Update committee also reassessed the two primary studies from *Volume 4* and determined that the Eisen study was a primary study based on a dermatologist's diagnosis of two specific skin disorders: vulgaris (warts) and atopic dermatitis. However, for the Higgins et al. (2002) study, the committee also found that based on its study design that compared disabled deployed and disabled nondeployed veterans, as well as the lack of an appropriate comparison group (that is nondeployed nondisabled veterans serving in the same era), this study could not be considered a primary study.

Several large cohort studies conducted in other countries reported similar findings in Gulf War veterans based on self-reports via questionnaires. Based on the lack of a physician's examination or diagnosis, these studies are considered to be secondary. The population-based survey of UK deployed veterans found the prevalence of dermatitis to be 21%, a rate higher than that in two control groups: one dispatched to Bosnia (OR 1.6, 95% CI 1.3-2.0) and the other era controls (OR 1.6, 95% CI 1.4-1.9) (Unwin et al., 1999). A higher prevalence of the following physician-diagnosed skin conditions was also reported in 1456 deployed veterans compared with 1588 nondeployed veterans in an Australian population-based study by Kelsall et al. (2004a): moderate to severe rash and skin irritation (OR 2.0, 95% CI 1.6-2.5); dermatitis (OR 1.8, 95% CI 1.3-2.6); and skin diseases other than dermatitis, skin cancer, eczema, or psoriasis (OR 1.3, 95% CI 1.1-1.7).

Several additional secondary studies were identified that indicated that the prevalence of generally nonspecified skin diseases or conditions in deployed Gulf War veterans was greater than in nondeployed veterans, but all of these studies relied on self-reports:

- Goss Gilroy (1998)—Skin allergies or other skin conditions in Canadian veterans.
- Cherry et al. (2001a)—Skin rashes, sweating, itching skin, hair loss, boils, or abscesses in UK veterans.
- Simmons et al. (2004)—Skin allergies in UK veterans (OR 3.3, 95% CI 3.0-3.7).
- Steele (2000)—Physician-diagnosed or treated skin conditions other than skin cancer (OR 3.83, 95% CI 2.50-5.87); rashes (OR 5.73, 95% CI 3.41-9.62); moderate or multiple skin symptoms (OR 4.09, 95% CI 2.53-6.63) in Kansas veterans.
- Wolfe et al. (1998)—Akin rashes, eczema, skin allergies in veterans from Massachusetts and Louisiana.
- Proctor et al. (2001a)—Skin rash (14.0% vs 4.3%).
- Gray et al. (1999a)—Rash (OR 4.3, 95% CI 2.8-6.5).

A more recent secondary study is that of Kang et al. (2009), who in 2004-2005 conducted a follow-up study of the 15,000 deployed and 15,000 nondeployed veterans originally surveyed in the 1995 National Health Survey of Gulf War Era Veterans and Their Families (Kang et al., 2000). A mailed questionnaire asked veterans if their doctor had ever told them they had any of 23 medical conditions, including dermatitis or any other skin trouble. The relative risk for skin problems was 1.41 (95% CI 1.32-1.51) adjusted for age, sex, race, body mass index, current cigarette smoking, rank, branch of service, and unit component.

Three studies examined hospitalizations of Gulf War veterans for skin disorders. Gray et al. (1996) found no excess hospitalizations in 1991-1993 of Gulf War veterans compared with other veterans for skin diseases, as broadly defined by a range of ICD codes. That study compared hospitalizations at DoD facilities of almost 550,000 Gulf War veterans and almost 620,000 nondeployed veterans. The multivariate ORs ranged from about 0.97 in 1991 to almost 1.0 in 1993 (actual values and confidence intervals not given). An expansion of this study to capture veterans who may have left the military was conducted by Gray et al. (2000). This study covered the years 1991-1994 and examined records from DoD, VA, and California hospitals. Proportional morbidity ratios (PMRs) of hospital-discharge diagnoses for skin diseases in Gulf War deployed and nondeployed veterans were compared. PMRs for hospitalization for skin disease were not increased for Gulf War veterans in DoD hospitals (PMR 1.01, 95% CI 0.97-1.05), VA hospitals (PMR 1.14, 95% CI 1.00-1.27), or California hospitals (PMR 0.84, 95% CI

0.54-1.14. Smith et al. (2006) compared postdeployment hospitalizations from August 1, 1990, to December 31, 2000, for active-duty military personnel deployed to the Gulf War, deployed to southwest Asia after the war, or deployed to Bosnia. Active-duty personnel deployed to Bosnia were at reduced risk of hospitalization for skin diseases or conditions compared with Gulf War veterans (HR 0.57, 95% CI 0.46-0.71). There was no difference in hospitalizations for skin diseases between those deployed during the Gulf War and those deployed to the region after the war (HR 0.99, 95% CI 0.88-1.11). The limitation of these studies is their inability to capture any but the most severe skin diseases as most would be treated on an outpatient basis.

Summary and Conclusions

The committee placed the greatest weight on studies that included medical evaluation and identification of specific dermatologic diagnoses. Both primary studies showed a higher prevalence of some skin diseases or conditions in deployed than in nondeployed Gulf War veterans. A nationally representative study of US Gulf War veterans found a relationship between deployment and atopic dermatitis and verruca vulgaris (warts) but not other skin conditions (Eisen et al., 2005), and a Danish study found increased prevalence of eczema and other unspecified skin conditions in deployed veterans (Ishoy et al., 1999b).

Secondary studies are largely consistent with the primary studies but lack specificity regarding dermatologic outcomes or rely only on self-reported symptoms or physician-diagnosed dermatologic conditions. Three secondary studies are somewhat more specific in reporting a greater prevalence of eczema or psoriasis in deployed veterans (Kang et al., 2000; Proctor et al., 1998; Wolfe et al., 1998).

In summary, there is a high frequency of self-reports of various types of rash and other skin conditions among deployed versus nondeployed veterans, and, in general, these reports are confirmed by dermatologic examination. Overall, very few studies have rigorously assessed the prevalence of skin conditions in Gulf War veterans, and results are mixed, with increases for some skin conditions but not for others. Furthermore, there is no consistency across these studies, which suggests that the findings could be occurring by chance. Finally, most of the studies are weak in design and limited by self-selection and possible reporting bias.

On the basis of the few studies of dermatologic conditions, unrelated skin conditions occur more frequently among Gulf War deployed veterans, but the findings as to specific skin conditions are not consistent among the studies. See Table 4-10 for a summary of the primary papers that the committee considered for dermatologic outcomes.

The committee concludes that there is inadequate/insufficient evidence of an association between deployment to the Gulf War and skin disorders.

TABLE 4-10 Skin Diseases

Reference	Design	Population	Outcomes	Results	Adjustments	Comments
Eisen et al., 2005 (Vol. 4)	Population-based, cross-sectional, prevalence, medical evaluation	1061 US deployed and 1128 nondeployed	Atopic dermatitis and verruca vulgaris (warts)	Atopic dermatitis: 1.2% vs 0.3% (OR 8.1, 95% CI 2.4-27.7); verruca vulgaris (warts): 1.6% vs 0.6% (OR 4.02, 95% CI 1.28-12.6)	Age, sex, race, years of education, smoking, duty type, service branch, rank	Low participation rates, especially among nondeployed
Higgins et al., 2002 (Vol. 4)	Prospective case-comparison study	111 disabled and 98 nondisabled UK GWVs; 133 disabled NDV controls (54 deployed to Bosnia and 79 nondeployed era controls) (population randomly sampled from Ismail et al., 2002, cohort)	Skin conditions	No significant difference in prevalence of all skin conditions combined: Disabled GWVs: 47.7% Nondisabled GWVs: 36.7% Disabled NDVs: 42.8% Sebhorrheic dermatitis: 8.1% in disabled deployed vs 2.3% in disabled nondeployed ($p = 0.06$)	Age, sex, rank, smoking, and alcohol	Response rates: Disabled GWVs: 67% Nondisabled GWVs: 62% Disabled Bosnia: 55% Disabled NDVs: 43%
Ishoy et al., 1999b (Update)	Cross-sectional, prevalence	686 Danish peacekeepers deployed to gulf in 1990-1997 vs 231 age- and sex-matched armed forces nondeployed controls	Health examination by physician, self-report questionnaire	Prevalence of skin conditions with onset after gulf: eczema 15.0% vs 3.0%, $p < 0.001$; retarded wound healing 6.0% vs 1.7%, $p < 0.01$; other forms of skin problems 17.1% vs 5.2%, $p < 0.001$; hair loss or hair disease 4.2% vs 0.9%, $p < 0.01$; sweaty, clammy, or damp hands 7.9% vs 3.9%, $p < 0.05$		Participation rate 83.6% deployed, 57.8% nondeployed; lack of information on adjustment for confounders in multivariate analysis

NOTES: CI = confidence interval; GWV = Gulf War veteran; NDV = nondeployed veteran; OR = adjusted odds ratio.

DISEASES OF THE MUSCULOSKELETAL SYSTEM

Arthritis is the most common form of joint disease. Several powerful risk factors are major trauma, repetitive joint use, and age. Arthritis is diagnosed according to a combination of clinical features and radiographic findings. Arthralgia, which is a self-reported symptom of arthritis, refers to painful joints. In the absence of other clinical features and radiographic findings, arthralgias are not necessarily diagnostic of arthritis. Some disorders such as fibromyalgia are considered separately in this report. Reports of musculoskeletal symptoms, such as lower back pain (lumbago), muscle stiffness, and joint stiffness, which have not been diagnosed as a medical condition, are discussed in the section on multisymptom illness. Primary studies of musculoskeletal diseases are summarized in Table 4-11.

Summary of *Volume 4*

Primary Studies

Arthralgias were one of 12 primary health outcome measures studied by Eisen and colleagues (2005). They conducted medical evaluations in phase III of VA's nationally representative, population-based study of Gulf War Veterans. From 1999-2001, 1061 deployed and 1128 nondeployed veterans were evaluated. They had been randomly selected from 11,441 deployed and 9476 nondeployed veterans who had participated in the phase I questionnaire in 1995 (Kang et al., 2000). Researchers were blinded to deployment status. Arthralgias were defined as persistent and clinically significant bone or joint symptoms with or without joint effusion, and treatment with anti-inflammatory agents, narcotic pain medications, or nonnarcotic pain medications. There was no significant difference in arthralgias between deployed and nondeployed veterans (OR 1.15, 95% CI 0.70-1.89). One study limitation was that despite three recruitment waves, the participation rate in the Eisen et al. (2005) study was low: only 53% of Gulf War veterans and 39% of nondeployed veterans participated. To determine nonparticipation bias, the authors obtained previously collected findings on participants and nonparticipants from the DMDC and gathered sociodemographic and self-reported health findings from the 1995 VA study (Kang et al., 2000). Both deployed and nondeployed participants were more likely than nonparticipants to report arthritis of any kind.

Secondary Studies

Two other studies examined differences in prevalence of arthritis, but they relied on self-reporting. Kang et al. (2000), using a stratified random-sampling method, compared data from the DMDC on 693,826 Gulf War veterans and 800,680 nondeployed veterans, and asked about arthritis as a self-reported condition. They found a significant difference in such reporting between deployed and nondeployed veterans (22.5% vs 16.7%, rate difference of 5.87, 95% CI 5.74-6.00). Gray et al. (2002) looked at 3831 Gulf War deployed veterans, 4933 veterans deployed elsewhere, and 3104 nondeployed Seabees. The authors found increased reporting of arthritis among Gulf War than deployed compared with Seabees deployed elsewhere (5.87% vs 4.42%). The latter, in turn, were similar to other nondeployed Seabees (4.42% vs 4.38%). The OR for Gulf War veterans versus veterans deployed elsewhere was 1.44 (95% CI 1.17-1.76), and that for Gulf War deployed versus nondeployed veterans was 1.63 (95% CI 1.29-2.08).

Updated and Supplemental Literature

Primary Studies

The new primary studies identified by the committee consisted of hospitalization studies that had discharge diagnoses of some form of musculoskeletal disease. Specific diagnoses were not provided in any of the studies.

Gray et al. (1996) used a retrospective cohort approach to compare hospitalization discharge diagnoses for 547,076 Gulf War deployed and 618,335 nondeployed active-duty personnel at DoD medical facilities. Hospitalizations for 14 ICD-9-CM diagnostic categories, which included "musculoskeletal system diseases," were assessed across three time periods following the war: August 1, 1991, to December 31, 1991; January 1, 1992, to December 31, 1992; and January 1, 1993, to September 30, 1993. Hospitalizations for musculoskeletal system diseases were not increased among the Gulf War deployed personnel versus nondeployed for 1991 or 1992, and were only marginally increased (OR about 1.01, exact value not given; 95% CI included 1.0) for 1993. This study is limited, however, because of the relatively short follow-up, the lack of outpatient data, restriction to DoD hospitals, restriction to hospitalizations of those who remained on active duty after the war, and limited adjustment for potential confounders.

A later publication expanded the Gray et al. (1996) study to include hospitalizations for reserve and separated military personnel over the same three time periods. This study also included discharge diagnoses for hospital stays from DoD hospitals, the VA system, and the California Office of Statewide Health Planning and Development for the years 1991-1994 (Gray et al., 2000). Because the total number of deployed and nondeployed veterans was not available, the researchers calculated proportional morbidity ratios (PMRs). The PMRs for musculoskeletal system diseases for the DoD hospitals, the VA hospitals, and the California hospitals were 1.01 (95% CI 0.99-1.02), 0.86 (95% CI 0.81-0.91), and 0.79 (95% CI 0.64-0.93), respectively. This analysis is limited since it did not include outpatient diagnoses, it could not determine hospitalization rates, and it did not allow adjustment for confounding.

Musculoskeletal system diseases were examined in an additional study comparing hospitalization rates in DoD hospitals through 2000 in three cohorts of veterans: Gulf War veterans, veterans deployed to southwest Asia after the Gulf War, and veterans deployed to Bosnia (Smith et al., 2006). After adjustment for sex, age, marital status, pay grade, race/ethnicity, service branch, occupation, and predeployment hospitalizations, the rate of hospitalizations for musculoskeletal system diseases (identified according to ICD-9-CM discharge codes) was slightly increased in the southwest Asia deployed veterans compared with the Gulf War veterans (HR 1.06, 95% CI 1.01-1.12) and decreased for the Bosnia deployed veterans compared with the Gulf War veterans (HR 0.78, 95% CI 0.71-0.86).

Gray et al. (1999b) assessed hospitalizations for Gulf War veterans potentially exposed to the nerve agents sarin and cyclosarin following the Khamisiyah demolition. Discharge diagnoses from DoD hospitals between March 1991 and September 1995 were examined for 349,291 Army Gulf War active-duty veterans. Plume estimates were overlaid on military unit locations to classify the veterans as no exposure, uncertain low exposure, and three levels of possible subclinical exposures. There was no increased risk of hospitalization for musculoskeletal system diseases for any of the exposure groups (risk ratios all less than 1.0). A follow-up to this study (Smith et al., 2003) examined DoD hospitalization data for active-duty personnel through December 2000. Comparing 99,614 exposed veterans to 318,458 nonexposed veterans, the adjusted risk ratio for hospitalization for musculoskeletal system diseases was 0.99 (95% CI 0.96-1.02). Exposure was based on the 2000 Khamisiyah gaseous hazard area modeling done by the DoD.

A similar assessment of DoD hospitalizations between August 1991 through July 1991 for 405,142 active-duty Gulf War veterans who had been exposed to smoke from the Kuwaiti oil-well fires compared with nonexposed veterans was conducted by Smith et al. (2002). Exposure to particulate matter from the fires was estimated based on meteorological data, diffusion modeling, and troop location data; seven exposure levels were developed ranging from no exposure to an average daily exposure of > 260 μg/m^3 for more than 50 days. No increased risk of hospitalization for musculoskeletal system diseases was seen for any of the exposure groups (risk ratios all less than 1.0).

Secondary Study

The committee identified one secondary study that reported on musculoskeletal diseases in Gulf War veterans. Bourdette et al. (2001) conducted physical examinations of 443 Gulf War deployed veterans residing in the northeast United States, 244 of whom met the authors' definition of unexplained illness and 113 of whom did not meet the case definition served as controls. The prevalence of osteoarthritis was similar between cases and controls, and there were no reports of autoimmune or inflammatory rheumatic diseases. The authors noted that four veterans were diagnosed with spondyloarthropathy, but they did not indicate whether these veterans were cases or controls.

Summary and Conclusion

Among those examined, there was no significant difference in arthralgias, a surrogate for arthritis, but data on self-reports indicate that arthritis was more common among those deployed to the gulf. The data, however, suffer from the problem of self-reporting of a common condition that can be easily confused with other symptoms without a thorough diagnosis by a physician. There appears to be no significant increase in the prevalence of arthralgias among veterans who underwent a medical examination.

The hospitalization studies reviewed by the committee also showed no increased risk of hospitalization for musculoskeletal system diseases among Gulf War deployed veterans compared with their nondeployed counterparts. Possible exposure to oil-well fire smoke and nerve agents from the Khamisiyah demolition also failed to result in increased hospitalizations. The committee notes, however, that many musculoskeletal diseases, such as arthritis, do not typically require hospitalization and are more likely to be treated on an outpatient basis.

Therefore, the committee concludes that there is insufficient/inadequate evidence of an association between deployment to the Gulf War and musculoskeletal system diseases.

TABLE 4-11 Musculoskeletal Diseases

Study	Design	Population	Outcomes	Results	Adjustments	Comments
Eisen et al., 2005 (Vol. 4)	Population-based, cross-sectional, prevalence, medical evaluation	1061 deployed vs 1128 nondeployed	Persistent and clinically significant bone or joint symptoms with or without joint effusion, and treatment with anti-inflammatory agents, narcotic pain medications, or nonnarcotic pain medications	Prevalence: 6.4% vs 6.8% (OR 1.15, 95% CI 0.70-1.89)	Age, sex, race, years of education, smoking, duty type, service branch, rank	Low participation rates, especially among nondeployed
Gray et al., 1996 (Update)	Retrospective cohort, hospitalizations from August 1991 through September 1993	547,076 active-duty GWVs, 618,335 NDVs	Hospital-discharge diagnoses of musculoskeletal system diseases in DoD hospital system	Exact values not given 1991: OR < 1.0 (95% CI < 1.0); 1992: OR < 1.0 (95% CI < 1.0) 1993, OR about 1.01 (95% CI 0.9-1.15)	Prewar hospitalization, sex, age, race, service branch, marital status, rank, length of service, salary, occupation	Short follow-up period; no outpatient data; restriction to DoD hospitals, and thus to persons remaining on active duty after the war; no adjustment for other potential confounders
Gray et al., 2000 (Update)	Retrospective cohort, hospitalizations from August 1991 through December 1994	652,979 GWVs, 652,922 randomly selected NDVs 182,164 DoD hospitalizations; 16,030 VA hospitalizations; 5185 COSHPD hospitalizations	Hospital-discharge diagnoses of musculoskeletal system diseases in DoD, VA, and COSHPD hospital systems	DoD PMR 1.01 (95% CI 0.99-1.02) VA PMR 0.86 (95% CI 0.81-0.91) COSHPD PMR 0.79 (95% CI 0.64-0.93)	Age, sex, race (only for DoD PMR)	Able to assess only illnesses that resulted in hospitalization; possible undetected confounders PMR has lower sensitivity than a comparison of hospitalization rates would have

Study	Design	Population	Outcomes	Results	Adjustments	Comments
Smith et al., 2006 (Update)	Retrospective cohort study (cohort data from DMDC)	Active-duty personnel with a single deployment to: Gulf War theater (n = 455,465); southwest Asia peacekeeping mission, 1991-1998 (n = 249,047); Bosnia, 1995-1998 (n = 44,341)	Postdeployment hospitalization events (1991-2000) for an ICD-9-CM diagnosis of a musculoskeletal system disease (ICD-9 codes 710-739)	Compared to GWVs, veterans of Bosnia showed reduced risk (HR 0.78, 95% CI 0.71-0,86), veterans of southwest Asia at slightly increased risk (HR 1.06, 95% CI 1.01-1.12)	Sex, age, marital status, pay grade, race/ethnicity, service branch, occupation, and predeployment hospitalization; time-dependent covariate to account for changing hospitalization methods, diagnostic criteria, and procedures	Limitations: active-duty personnel only; hospitalizations at DoD facilities only
Smith et al., 2002 (Update)	DoD hospitalizations 1991-1999; exposure modeling for oil-well fire smoke	405,142 active-duty Gulf War veterans who were in theater during the time of Kuwaiti oil-well fires	Hospitalization for musculoskeletal system diseases (ICD-9-CM codes 710-739)	No association between exposure and musculoskeletal system diseases across all exposure levels	Adjusted for "influential covariates," defined as demographic or deployment variables with p values less than 0.15	Objective measure of disease not subject to recall bias; no issues with self-selection; however, only DoD hospitals, only active duty, no adjustment for potential confounders such as smoking
Gray et al., 1999b (Vol. 4)	DoD hospitalizations 1991-1995, exposure to nerve agents at Khamisiyah based on 1997 DoD exposure models	Not exposed (n = 224,804), uncertain low-dose exposure (n = 75,717), exposed (n = 48,770)	Musculoskeletal system disease (vs not exposed): Uncertain low dose; < 0.013 mg-min/m^3; 0.013-0.097 mg-min/m^3; 0.097-0.514 mg-min/m^3	 OR 0.90 (95% CI 0.86-0.94) OR 0.90 (95% CI 0.83-0.98) OR 0.90 (95% CI 0.83-0.96) OR 0.98 (95% CI 0.87-1.09)	Sex, age group, prewar hospitalization, race, service type, marital status, pay grade, occupation	See Smith et al. (2002); also, probable substantial exposure misclassification as models were revised, lack of a clear dose-response pattern, little biologic plausibility given that no effect was seen for nervous system diseases

Study	Design	Population	Outcomes	Results	Adjustments	Comments
Smith et al., 2003 (Update)	DoD hospitalization study (1991-2000); analysis of health outcomes and exposure to nerve agents (follow-up of Gray et al., 1999b)	99,614 active-duty military considered exposed vs 318,458 nonexposed, according to revised DoD exposure model	First hospitalization for any musculoskeletal system disease (ICD-9-CM codes 710-739)	Exposed vs unexposed: RR 0.99 (95% CI 0.96-1.02)		Restricted to DoD hospitals; restricted to hospitalizations for only Gulf War veterans who remained on active duty after the war; no adjustment for confounding exposures

NOTE: CI = confidence interval; COSHPD = California Office of Statewide Health Planning and Development; DMDC = Defense Manpower Data Center; DoD = Department of Defense; GWV = Gulf War veteran; HR = hazard ratio; NDV = nondeployed veteran; OR = odds ratio; PMR = proportional mortality ratio; RR = risk ratio; VA = Department of Veterans Affairs.

FIBROMYALGIA AND CHRONIC WIDESPREAD PAIN

Fibromyalgia is characterized by widespread muscle and skeletal pain in combination with point tenderness at numerous soft tissue sites, according to the American College of Rheumatology (ACR) (Wolfe et al., 1990). Fibromyalgia cannot be confirmed through pathologic or laboratory tests, and thus diagnosis is dependent upon clinical examination. The case definition requires both widespread pain (pain on both sides of the body, above and below the waist, and including axial skeletal pain) lasting for at least 3 months and pain (not just tenderness) in at least 11 of 18 tender point sites on palpation with an approximate force of 4 kg. The presence of a second clinical disorder does not exclude a diagnosis of fibromyalgia. Other symptoms of fibromyalgia include fatigue, sleep disturbance, morning stiffness, and cognitive impairment, but those are not sensitive and specific enough to use for classification (Wolfe et al., 1990). Early characterization of the condition as an inflammation of muscle (hence the label fibrositis) has not been borne out through research (Goldenberg et al., 1990). There are no widely accepted causative factors for fibromyalgia, but in the general population its prevalence is about 3.4% in women and 0.5% in men, making it one of the more common rheumatologic disorders (Wolfe et al., 1995). Prevalence of fibromyalgia increases with age (Wolfe et al., 1995), and on the basis of longitudinal studies, the course is chronic but variable in intensity (Wolfe et al., 1997). It should be noted that the existence of fibromyalgia as a distinct disease entity is considered controversial by some expert commentators (Nimnuan et al., 2001; Pearce, 2004).

Summary of *Volume 4*

Primary Studies

The Volume 4 committee considered as primary only those studies that based diagnosis of fibromyalgia on symptom reporting and physical examination, rather than only on symptom-reporting alone. In phase III of VA's national population-based study, Eisen et al. (2005) examined the prevalence of fibromyalgia in Gulf War deployed veterans (n = 1061) compared to a nondeployed era veteran control group (n = 1128). The cohorts were randomly selected from 11,441 deployed and 9476 nondeployed veterans, who had participated in the phase I questionnaire in 1995 (Kang et al., 2000). The authors conducted medical evaluations from 1999-2001, and based diagnosis of fibromyalgia on the ACR criteria (Wolfe et al., 1990). Self-reported diagnoses of fibrositis or fibromyalgia did not vary between deployed and nondeployed veterans (0.6% and 0.8% respectively; adjusted OR 1.21, 95% CI 0.36-4.10). However, fibromyalgia diagnosed on the basis of physical examination was present in 2.0% of deployed and 1.2% of nondeployed veterans (adjusted OR 2.32, 95% CI 1.02-5.27). Strengths of the study include the population-based sampling strategy, blinding of evaluating physicians, and use of validated diagnostic criteria based on physical examination. Limitations include the potential for substantial selection bias due to modest participation rates (53% of Gulf War veterans and 39% of nondeployed veterans).

Smith and colleagues (2000) examined the association of hospitalizations for fibromyalgia between 1991 and 1997 with deployment status among 551,841 deployed and 1,478,704 nondeployed active-duty personnel. The study found higher risk of fibromyalgia hospitalization among the deployed group (RR 1.23, 95% CI 1.05-1.43). However, survival curves suggest that the higher observed risk results from a spike in hospitalizations due to the

DoD Comprehensive Clinical Evaluation Program (CCEP), which ran for 1 year between 1994 and 1995 in an attempt to provide evaluation and treatment for all Gulf War veterans who believed they were suffering a medical condition related to their deployment. Deployed veterans who participated in the CCEP had more than 26 times the risk of being hospitalized for fibromyalgia than did nonparticipants. By comparison, the authors found that for the 3-year period prior to the CCEP, the rate of hospitalization for fibromyalgia was similar between Gulf War veterans and their nondeployed contemporaries (RR 0.92, 95% CI 0.74-1.13). The Smith et al. study has the advantage of a large, population-based sample and good statistical power for the detection of an effect. Its major limitations are the inclusion of only active-duty personnel, changes in hospitalization rates for fibromyalgia in association with the practices of the CCEP, and the fact that few cases of fibromyalgia are severe enough to warrant hospitalization. The findings on fibromyalgia are summarized in Table 4-12.

Secondary Studies

The Iowa study (Iowa Persian Gulf Study Group, 1997) surveyed 1896 deployed and 1799 nondeployed Iowa veterans. No physical examinations were conducted; fibromyalgia was assessed from the symptom criteria described by Wolfe and colleagues (Wolfe et al., 1995). Symptoms of fibromyalgia were present in 18.2% and 23.8% of deployed regular military and National Guard veterans, respectively, and 9.2% and 13.2% of nondeployed regular military and National Guard veterans, respectively, with an adjusted prevalence difference of 9.3% (95% CI 7.3-11.2). Steele (2000) conducted a similar telephone interview study among 1545 deployed and 435 nondeployed Kansas Gulf War veterans. Of the deployed and nondeployed veterans, 2% (n = 24) and less than 0.5% (n = 2), respectively, reported having received a physician's diagnosis of fibromyalgia with new onset between 1990 and 1998 (adjusted OR 3.69, 95% CI 0.86-15.84).

A survey of the entire cohort of Canadian Gulf War deployed veterans (Goss Gilroy, 1998) found that they were more likely than nondeployed veterans—group-matched to cases on sex, age, and regular versus reserve status—to report symptoms of fibromyalgia (16% vs 10%; adjusted OR 1.81, 95% CI 1.55-2.13).

Bourdette et al. (2001) studied 244 Oregon and Washington Gulf War veterans who had unexplained illness after clinical evaluation to exclude "explainable" illness. Of these veterans, 50 (20.8%) fulfilled the ACR criteria for fibromyalgia. The study's main limitations are its lack of a nondeployed comparison group and lack of clarity about the nature of the clinical examination for fibromyalgia.

Updated and Supplemental Literature

Primary Studies

The Update committee identified only one new primary paper that looked specifically at CWP in deployed and nondeployed Gulf War veterans. A random sample of a population-based cohort of regular military and National Guard and reserve veterans (Iowa Persian Gulf Study Group, 1997), 1896 deployed and 1799 nondeployed, who listed Iowa as their home state at the time of enlistment were surveyed in 1995-1996. Veterans were identified through the DMDC. The study was conducted through structured telephone interviews to determine the prevalence of CWP on the basis of responses to the SF-36. Gulf War veterans reported significantly more bodily pain than did nondeployed veterans ($p < 0.01$). In a follow-up study of a subset of this cohort 5 years after the baseline survey, Ang et al. (2006) conducted in-person follow-up examinations of 370 Gulf War veterans who had not met the case definition of CWP at baseline. The goal of the follow-up study was to identify predictors of delayed-onset CWP. Of the 370 veterans, 69 (18.6%) had met the classification criteria for CWP at the follow-up evaluation: 51 in the deployed group and 18 in the nondeployed group. According to a logistic multiple-regression model, CWP was significantly associated with perceived life stress (based on responses to the Brief Life Stress Questionnaire) at the time of the Gulf War, whether military related or not (OR 1.4, 95% CI 1.0-2.0), and with perceived life stress in the 6 months after returning home (OR 1.3, 95% CI 1.0-1.8). CWP also correlated with combat exposure during deployment (OR 1.5, 95% CI 1.1-2.0) although not specifically with deployment to the gulf itself (OR 1.1, 95% CI 0.6-2.0). Symptoms of alcohol use at the 5-year baseline survey were protective for CWP at 10 years (OR 0.2, 95% CI 0.1-0.6, $p = 0.0039$). The authors used the Expanded Combat Exposure Scale in the baseline survey and reported that for every 5-point increase in combat exposure score, there was a 50% increase in the likelihood that a veteran would develop CWP. Although the study had the advantage of using an in-person evaluation for the medical diagnosis of CWP and had a relatively large population of deployed and nondeployed veterans, there was a possibility of recall bias for life and deployment stressors reported 5 years after the conflict, and only veterans from Iowa were evaluated. Furthermore, only veterans who did not meet the CWP criteria at baseline were considered for the follow-up evaluation; veterans who may have developed CWP during the first 5 years after the conflict were not included in the follow-up examination.

Secondary Studies

Using data from the Iowa Persian Gulf Study Group (1997), Forman-Hoffman et al. (2007) analyzed information from the structured telephone interview conducted with 1896 deployed veterans and 1799 nondeployed veterans in 1995-1996. CWP was based on the following criteria: the veteran reported having fibromyalgia or fibrositis in the previous 12 months or reported overall body pain that occurred almost every day for at least 3 months during the previous 12 months, and had body pain in the 24 hours before the interview. The deployed veterans reported significantly more symptoms of CWP than did nondeployed veterans (OR 2.03, 95% CI 1.60-2.58); the OR was adjusted for age, sex, race, rank, branch of service, military status, smoking, and current income.

Stimpson et al. (2006) surveyed UK veterans who had served only in the Gulf War ($n = 2959$), only in Bosnia ($n = 2052$), or both in the Gulf War and in Bosnia ($n = 570$), and a comparison era group of veterans who had not been deployed to either the Gulf War or Bosnia ($n = 2614$) for self-reports of CWP. A mailed questionnaire containing a pain manikin to ascertain the pattern and intensity of pain was sent to 12,592 male and female veterans in 1997; the response rate for the three groups was 60-70%. Data from the shaded manikins were used to determine whether the pain pattern met the ACR definition of CWP. The prevalence of reporting of CWP in the Gulf War deployed group (16.8%) and the Gulf War and Bosnia deployed group (15.8%), but not in the Bosnia only deployed group (7.6%), was significantly higher ($p < 0.0001$) than that in the era group (8.5%). Veterans who reported pain in one limb were also 30 times more likely to report pain in the symmetrically opposite limb rather than a second limb on the same side of the body; the authors found this suggestive of "systemic pain" rather than pain from an injury. Although the sample was large, the study is limited by a lack of physical examination and a lack of indication as to whether the veterans had sustained injuries during deployment or were using pain medication at the time of the survey.

A similar study by Cherry et al. (2001a,b) 6-8 years after the Gulf War also used a pain manikin to identify whether and where veterans had experienced pain for at least 24 hours in the preceding month. Among the 9588 male and female UK Gulf War veterans in all service branches, 12.2% reported widespread pain on a manikin compared with 6.5% of 4790 nondeployed veterans; widespread pain was considered to be present if the manikin showed axial skeletal and contralateral body pain. CWP was associated with exposure to insect repellent, medical attention, and side effects of nerve-agent prophylaxis.

Several studies have reviewed the presence of chronic pain in veterans, but the definition of chronic pain varied with the study (Hyams et al., 1996; Kuzma and Black, 2006; Thomas et al., 2006). Kuzma and Black (2006) noted that many studies of Gulf War veterans reported increased pain symptoms that could be clustered into CWP, but the terminology used in the studies was not consistent and included joint pain and general aches and pain; these pain clusters may or may not have met the ACR criteria for CWP.

Summary and Conclusion

The diagnosis of fibromyalgia is based entirely on symptoms and physical examination; there are no pathologic or laboratory tests with which to confirm it. Among the available cross-sectional studies that include both Gulf War deployed and nondeployed veterans, only Eisen and colleagues (2005) used the full ACR case definition of fibromyalgia, including criteria based on physical examination. The study by Smith and colleagues (2000) found no association between Gulf War deployment and hospitalization for fibromyalgia. That finding does not appear inconsistent with positive findings in the Eisen et al. study, in that few cases of fibromyalgia are severe enough to warrant hospitalization. Notably, the prevalence of a diagnosis of fibromyalgia in the Eisen et al. study is about 300 times the prevalence of hospitalization for fibromyalgia in the Smith et al. study. Two secondary studies from Iowa and Canada both found significantly increased fibromyalgia symptoms among deployed veterans compared with nondeployed veterans, but lacked a physical examination to enable the use of the full criteria for diagnosis. In conclusion, largely on the basis of the Eisen et al. study, which used the criteria of the ACR for diagnosis of fibromyalgia but could have been subject to unrecognized selection bias, there is a higher prevalence of fibromyalgia among deployed Gulf War veterans than among nondeployed veterans.

The committee reviewed one primary study and three secondary studies on Gulf War deployment and CWP. Although each of the studies found a higher prevalence of CWP in deployed than nondeployed veterans, all had considerable limitations. In Ang et al. (2006), the prevalence of CWP was found to increase both with increased combat exposure and with increased perception of life stress at the time of deployment; the study is limited in that only veterans with no pain 5 years after the conflict were evaluated 10 years after the conflict. The Stimpson et al. study (2006) also found an increase in CWP associated with deployment. The other two secondary studies also showed more CWP in deployed than in nondeployed veterans.

The committee concludes that there is limited but suggestive evidence of an association between deployment to the Gulf War and both fibromyalgia and chronic widespread pain.

TABLE 4-12 Fibromyalgia and Chronic Widespread Pain

Study	Design	Population	Outcomes	Results	Adjustments	Comments
Eisen et al., 2005 (Vol. 4)	Population-based, cross-sectional, prevalence, medical evaluation	1061 deployed, 1128 nondeployed	Symptoms and physical examination using criteria of American College of Rheumatology (Wolfe et al., 1990)	Prevalence: 2.0% vs 1.2%, OR 2.32 (95% CI 1.02-5.27)	Age, sex, race, years of education, cigarette smoking, duty type, service branch, rank	Uses gold standard for diagnosis of fibromyalgia; low participation rates, especially among nondeployed
Smith et al., 2000 (Vol. 4)	Postwar hospitalization study	551,841 deployed, 1,478,704 nondeployed	Hospitalization (1991-1997); Cox proportional-hazards models ICD-9 codes for fibromyalgia (729.1)	RR 1.23 (95% CI 1.05-1.43); however, survival curves indicate excess due to hospitalization only for purposes of evaluation during the CCEP; before CCEP: RR 0.92 (95% CI 0.74-1.13)	Sex, age, branch of service	No increase after accounting for CCEP effect; limited to active duty; most cases of fibromyalgia are not severe enough to warrant hospitalization
Ang et al., 2006 (Update)	Cohort of veterans from IPGWSG	370 veterans who were free of CWP at 5 years were examined 10 years after war: 267 GWVs, 103 NDVs	Structured telephone interview about 5 years after the war; in-person follow-up medical examination 10 years after war of 370 veterans who did not report chronic widespread pain 5 years after war	Neither deployment to nor time in gulf significantly correlated with CWP: OR 1.1, 95% CI 0.6-2.0 and OR 1.0, 95% CI 0.7-13.0, respectively; combat exposure correlated: OR 1.5, 95% CI 1.1-2.0; perception of stress due to military experience at time of war correlated more significantly with CWP: OR 1.6, 95% CI 1.1-2.3, $p = 0.0084$	Controls matched for age, sex, branch of service	Potential for recall bias; only veterans who were free of CWP at 5 years were assessed 10 years after war

NOTE: CCEP = Comprehensive Clinical Evaluation Program; CI = confidence interval; CWP = chronic widespread pain; GWV = Gulf War veteran; IPGWSG = Iowa Persian Gulf War Study Group; NDV = nondeployed veteran; OR = odds ratio; RR = risk ratio.

DISEASES OF THE GENITOURINARY SYSTEM

Genitourinary outcomes were not addressed separately in *Volume 4* of the *Gulf War and Health* series. Major conditions in this group include kidney disease, urolithiasis ("kidney stones"), urinary tract infections, prostatitis, and sexual difficulties. Gynecologic outcomes including abnormal cervical pathology and inflammatory disease of the ovary have also been assessed in studies of Gulf War veterans and are discussed in this section. Cancers of the genitourinary system such as testicular cancer are not addressed in this section, but are discussed in the section on cancer. Table 4-13 summarizes the findings of primary studies of genitourinary system diseases.

Genitourinary Outcomes

Updated and Supplemental Literature

Primary Studies

Frommelt et al. (2000) used existing clinical records on Papanicolaou (Pap) smears to assess differences in cervical pathology among female Gulf War veterans. The authors evaluated Pap smear results from a cohort of 6715 Air Force women who served on active duty between August 7, 1990, and March 1, 1991, and had routine Pap smears conducted in 1994. A subset also had Pap smear data available for 1995 and/or 1996. Pap smear test results evaluated by the Armed Forces Institute of Pathology, which is the cytology laboratory used by 28 military treatment facilities, were collected for 1446 female Gulf War veterans and 5269 female veterans who were not deployed to the gulf. Overall, there were no observed differences in cervical pathology between the two groups. Among veterans aged 26-30 years, a diagnosis of "other than within normal limits" occurred more frequently among Gulf War veterans (11.5%) compared to nondeployed veterans (6.6%) ($p = 0.013$) in 1994, but no differences were detected among other age groups ranging from 20 and younger to over 50 years of age. The data were too sparse in 1995 and 1996 to conduct age-stratified analyses. The authors suggest there is no biologically plausible evidence to support an age-specific association between Gulf War service and abnormal cervical cytology.

McDiarmid and colleagues have followed a small cohort of 77 survivors of friendly-fire accidents who were exposed to depleted uranium (DU). The researchers conducted biennial clinical exams for uranium-related health effects. Clinical assessments included numerous urinary and serum markers of renal function as well as semen analyses and neuroendocrine measures as indicators of reproductive health (McDiarmid et al., 2000, 2001, 2004, 2006, 2007a,b, 2009). Over the 16 years of follow-up, biomarkers of renal function have not differed meaningfully (statistically or clinically) between those with low (< 0.1 microgram U/g creatinine) and high (≥ 0.1 microgram U/g creatinine) DU exposure. Similarly, no adverse DU effects on semen parameters or serum concentrations of testosterone, leutinizing hormone, or follicle-stimulating hormone have been observed. The comparisons, however, were based on small numbers (n = 35 for the 2007 exam) and did not control for potential confounders.

Secondary Studies

Several large-scale surveys addressed self-reported genitourinary conditions among Gulf War deployed and nondeployed military personnel. For the purpose of this review, these studies are considered secondary, mostly because of the lack of objective medical measures.

The first wave of the National Survey of Gulf War Veterans and Their Families conducted in 1995 sampled 15,000 Gulf War deployed veterans and 15,000 nondeployed era veterans (Kang et al., 2000). Responses from 11,441 Gulf War veterans (75% response) and 9476 Gulf War Era veterans (64% response) were used to estimate the population prevalence of chronic medical conditions within the previous 12 months. Gulf War veterans reported bladder infections (difference in prevalence proportions 1.54%, 95% CI 1.49-1.59) and "any disease of the genital organs" (difference in prevalence proportion 2.51%, 95% CI 2.45-2.57) slightly more frequently than nondeployed veterans. A follow-up survey was conducted in this same population in 2005 (Kang et al., 2009). The prevalence of self-reported conditions 14 years after the war was re-examined among 6111 Gulf War veterans (40% response) and 3859 Gulf War era veterans (27% response). Consistent with the previous findings in this cohort, an increased prevalence of bladder infections (prevalence ratio 1.32, 95% CI 1.17-1.49) and "any disease of the genital organs" (prevalence ratio 1.23, 95% CI 1.10-1.38) was observed among Gulf War veterans.

In a 1997-1999 study of all US Navy Seabees (Gray et al., 2002), deployment was associated with increased self-reports of physician-diagnosed conditions (with onset after August 1991) including impotence (OR 3.06, 95% CI 1.95-4.83), prostatitis (OR 1.54, 95% CI 1.07-2.21), and urinary tract infection (OR 2.50, 95% CI 1.83-3.44), but not kidney disease or kidney stones. A total of 11,868 (62.6%) of 18,945 Seabees responded to the mailed questionnaire: 3831 Gulf War deployed, 4933 deployed elsewhere, and 3104 nondeployed Seabees.

A survey of UK veterans conducted between 1998 and 2001 compared self-reported health outcomes among 23,358 male Gulf War veterans (53% response) and 17,730 male Gulf War era veterans (42% response) (Simmons et al., 2004). Reports of new medical conditions since 1990 were collected using open-ended questions and coded into 36 categories based loosely on ICD-10 classifications. The prevalence of genitourinary system disorders was higher among Gulf War veterans (OR 1.8, 95% CI 1.5-2.1). More specifically this category consisted of genital system and bladder problems (OR 2.2, 95% CI 1.7-2.7) and kidney disease or symptoms (OR 1.5, 95% CI 1.2-1.9). The subgroup of "genital system and bladder problems" included 13 reports of "burning semen" among Gulf War veterans and 1 among nondeployed veterans (0.1% vs 0.0%).

Proctor et al. (1998) compared the frequency of self-reported symptoms classified into nine groups of body systems. Using responses to a 52-item symptom checklist, the prevalence of genitourinary symptoms was evaluated among 186 Gulf War veterans from the New England area, 66 Gulf War veterans from the New Orleans area, and 48 Gulf War era veterans deployed to Germany. The Gulf War deployed veterans reported a higher prevalence of individual genitourinary symptoms, which included frequent urination and pain during intercourse, when compared to the group deployed to Germany. The frequency of each symptom was reported on a scale of 0-4 (0 = no symptom, 1 = rarely, 2 = some, 1-2 times/week, 3 = often, several times/week, 4 = very often, almost every day), and the frequencies were also summed to create "body-system symptom" scores for each system. Of the nine symptom categories assessed, genitourinary system symptom scores were the only system scores that were not statistically increased among either group of Gulf War veterans when compared to the Germany deployed veterans. The study was limited by small numbers and the potential for differential recall.

Unwin et al. (1999) conducted a 1997-1998 survey of male Gulf War veterans (n = 2735), nondeployed veterans (n = 2422), and servicemembers deployed to Bosnia (n = 2393) (65% response rate). Participants were asked to respond to a questionnaire that inquired about the presence of 50 symptoms and 39 medical disorders during the previous month. Gulf War veterans who had been deployed had an increased prevalence of sexual problems compared with nondeployed (OR 3.2, 95% CI 2.4-4.2) and with Bosnia deployed (OR 2.2, 95% CI 1.5-3.1). Gulf War deployed veterans also had a greater prevalence of disease of the genital organs than either comparison group (deployed vs nondeployed: OR 1.5, 95% CI 1.1-2.2; deployed vs Bosnia deployed: OR 1.6, 95% CI 1.1-2.4).

In a 1998 phone survey of Kansas veterans, the 1548 deployed Gulf War veterans were more likely than 482 nondeployed veterans to report that they or their partner felt a burning sensation after sex (OR 3.75, 95%CI 1.88-7.49) (Steele, 2000). This condition was reported by 8% of Gulf War veterans and 2% of nondeployed veterans. The Iowa Persian Gulf Study Group (1997) also compared self-reported medical conditions between deployed and nondeployed Iowa veterans within the regular military and within the National Guard or reserve. Gulf War veterans in the National Guard or reserves reported a higher prevalence of symptoms of sexual discomfort for their female partner (prevalence difference 3.6, 95% CI 2.3-4.8) compared with their nondeployed counterparts. No differences in sexual discomfort were reported for the respondents themselves. Sexual discomfort was not associated with Gulf War deployment among members of the regular military.

Self-reported genitourinary and reproductive problems were also assessed among Gulf War veterans according to their potential exposure to sarin or cyclosarin at the Khamisiyah demolition (Page et al., 2005). In the National Health Survey of Gulf War Era Veterans Study, the prevalence of genitourinary conditions including frequent or painful urination (OR 0.91, 95% CI 0.70-1.19), bladder infection (OR 0.98, 95% CI 0.80-1.20), and any disease of the genital organs (OR 0.94, 95% CI 0.76-1.17) was similar among the exposed and unexposed Gulf War veterans. Sexual difficulties such as painful sexual intercourse (OR 1.16, 95% CI 0.81-1.65) or impotence/other sexual problems (OR 0.85, 95% CI 0.65-1.12) were also similar between the two groups.

Pierce (1997) assessed the effects of Gulf War service on women's health by administering two surveys to a stratified sample of all women serving in the US Air Force during the Gulf War, including active-duty personnel, reserve, and National Guard. For the first survey, 153 Gulf War deployed veterans and 331 women deployed elsewhere (92% response) reported gynecologic, reproductive, and general medical conditions for which they had sought medical care since joining the Armed Forces. The prevalence of abnormal Pap smears and genital herpes did not differ by deployment status at this time. However, when asked 2 years later (87% response) about conditions experienced in the previous 12 months, Gulf War deployed veterans reported an increased prevalence of abnormal Pap smears (10.4% vs 4.9%, $p < 0.036$). Among the deployed veterans, no statistical differences in the prevalence of abnormal Pap smears were observed by duration of deployment. The results of a later survey conducted in a larger sample (n = 1164) of the same female veteran population showed that Gulf War deployed veterans were more likely to report 29 of 48 symptoms when compared to women deployed elsewhere (Pierce, 2005). Among the symptoms reported more frequently by deployed veterans "urinary urgency and frequency" was the only genitourinary condition identified in the report. This condition was reported by 16% of Gulf War deployed veterans compared with 11% of women deployed elsewhere ($p < 0.05$).

Hospitalization for Genitourinary System Diseases

Updated and Supplemental Literature

Primary Studies

Of the six postwar hospitalization studies that assessed diseases of the genitourinary system, three compared the hospitalization experiences between Gulf War deployed and nondeployed veterans and three examined the effects of environmental exposures to nerve agents or oil-well fires within Gulf War veterans. Most studies were restricted to active-duty personnel treated in DoD hospitals and evaluated the broad outcome of "diseases of the genitourinary system."

Gray et al. (1996) examined DoD hospitalizations among 547,076 Gulf War veterans and 618,335 Gulf War era veterans across three post-war time periods encompassing August 1991 through September 1993 (that is, 1991, 1992, 1993). Discharge diagnoses for 14 ICD-9-CM categories of hospitalization including "diseases of the genitourinary system" were assessed. Only subjects on active-duty were included in the cohort. The odds of hospitalization for genitourinary conditions were slightly higher for Gulf War veterans in the 5 months (1991) following the war (OR about 1.8, exact number not given, 95% CI greater than 1.0), but similar patterns were not observed in 1992 or 1993 (ORs less than 1.0 for both years). When specific diagnoses within this category were examined, the observed association was attributed to inflammatory disease of the ovary, fallopian tube, pelvic cellular tissue, and peritoneum (standardized rate ratio [SRR] 1.35, 95% CI 1.11-1.65) and infertility among females (SRR 1.59, 95% CI 1.19-2.11), redundant prepuce and phimosis among males (a diagnosis typically associated with elective circumcision) (SRR 1.59, 95% CI 1.22-2.07), and other disorders of the breast among males and females (SRR 1.30, 95% CI 1.03-1.63). The authors suggest these patterns were consistent with elective hospitalization deferred until after the war. Conditions with latency periods greater than the 2-year observation period would be missed in this study of active-duty personnel, along with outcomes occurring in individuals who did not remain on active duty following the war.

In an effort to address the limitations of studies restricted to active-duty personnel, Gray et al. (2000) compared hospitalizations for Gulf War deployed veterans and nondeployed veterans within three hospital systems providing care for active-duty, reserve, and former military personnel. Hospitalization data for the 14 major ICD-9-CM diagnostic categories were collected from DoD, VA, and COSHPD hospital systems for the period of August 1, 1991, through December 31, 1994. The lack of denominator data on the population eligible for hospitalization in the VA and COSHPD systems precluded the calculation of hospitalization rates. Thus, proportional morbidity ratios were estimated within each hospital system. The authors acknowledge PMRs may be less sensitive than hospitalization rates for detecting differences in hospitalizations between deployed and nondeployed groups. During the four years following the war, deployed veterans had similar or lower proportions of hospitalizations for "diseases of the genitourinary system" than nondeployed veterans in all hospital systems (DoD PMR 1.01. 95% CI 0.98-1.03; VA PMR 0.96, 95% CI 0.87-1.05; COSHPD PMR 0.80, 95% CI 0.59-1.00). Study limitations include the inability to assess less severe outcomes and limited control for confounding.

Smith et al. (2006) compared the postdeployment hospitalizations of 455,465 Gulf War veterans with servicemembers deployed for peacekeeping missions in southwest Asia (n = 249,047) and Bosnia (n = 44,341). DoD hospitalizations for 14 ICD-9-CM diagnostic categories were identified for active-duty personnel through the end of 2000. To account for differences in existing illness before deployment, the models were adjusted for predeployment hospitalization. When compared to those deployed to the Gulf War, hospitalization rates for genitourinary system diseases were similar for those deployed to southwest Asia (HR 1.00, 95% CI 0.92-1.09) and lower for those deployed to Bosnia (HR 0.60, 95% CI 0.51-0.70). Similar patterns were observed when hospitalization for the specific diagnosis of nephritis was considered. The authors reasoned that the lower hospitalization rates among personnel deployed to Bosnia reflect differences in access to care while in theater. Limitations consisted of restriction to DoD hospitals, no inclusion of outpatient data, and the exclusion of personnel who did not remain on active duty.

DoD hospitalizations among 405,142 Gulf War deployed personnel were assessed in relation to exposure to smoke from oil-well fires (Smith et al., 2002). Hospitalizations through July 31, 1999 (8-year observation period) were identified for active-duty personnel who were in the Gulf War theater of operations during the Kuwaiti oil-well fires (February 2, 1991, to October 31, 1991) and did not remain in the region after the war. Exposure to oil-well fire smoke was determined by whether troop unit location was within the smoke plume area defined by the Hybrid Single-Particle Lagrangian Integrated Trajectories model. Seven categories of smoke plume exposure were created using combinations of average daily dose (none, 1-260 $\mu g/m^3$, > 260 $\mu g/m^3$) and duration of exposure (1-25 days, 26-50, and > 50 days). Risk of hospitalization for genitourinary system diseases was not increased at any level of smoke plume exposure. The rate ratio for the most highly exposed group (average daily exposure > 260 $\mu g/m^3$ for > 50 days) compared to the nonexposed group was 0.95 (described as not significant, confidence interval not reported). The limitations noted above for Gray et al. (1996) and Smith et al. (2006) apply to this study as well.

Smith et al. (2003) updated results of a previous analysis (Gray et al., 1999b) by comparing hospitalizations among 431,762 Gulf War deployed personnel who were and were not likely to have been exposed to nerve agents released by the Khamisiyah demolition. The more recent study improved exposure estimates by applying the revised meteorologic-dispersion models and updated unit location data to estimate exposure to sarin and cyclosarin (Winkenwerder, 2002). The study also incorporated 5 additional years of hospitalization data to extend the observation period to almost 10 years. DoD hospitalization data for 15 major ICD-9-CM diagnostic categories were collected through December 31, 2000. Postwar hospitalizations for genitourinary system diseases were similar among military personnel who were and were not exposed to gaseous nerve agents resulting from the demolition of chemical weapons at Khamisiyah (rate ratio 0.96, 95% CI 0.91-1.00). The results for genitourinary system diseases were consistent with the finding previously reported in Gray et al. (1999b). Like Gray et al. (1996) and Smith et al. (2006), this study did not include outpatient visits, only addressed hospitalizations in DoD facilities during active-duty status, and had limited ability to control for potential confounding by behavioral or other environmental factors.

Summary and Conclusions

Based on a single study using clinical confirmation of Pap smear results among female veterans, current evidence does not support an association between Gulf War deployment and cervical pathology. Of note, however, a secondary study of self-reported Pap smear results was not consistent with these findings. Similarly, the results of large-scale surveys addressing other self-reported genitourinary conditions have been largely inconsistent with the results of the cause-specific hospitalization studies. In the 10 secondary studies assessing the effects of Gulf War deployment on self-reported genitourinary outcomes, the prevalence of various self-reported genitourinary conditions was greater among Gulf War deployed veterans compared to nondeployed veterans. Exposure to nerve agents released by the Khamisiyah demolition, however, does not appear to be related to increased reporting of genitourinary conditions among Gulf War veterans. However, this evidence is also limited to a single study. Depleted uranium exposure also does not appear to alter biomarkers of renal function or semen parameters. The specific conditions being evaluated in surveys of Gulf War veterans have varied across studies, generally addressing frequency of urination, urinary tract infections, sexual problems, or broadly defined "disease of the genital organs." Furthermore, secondary studies addressing deployment and genitourinary conditions are limited by self-reported outcomes, lack of clinical confirmation, potential recall bias, and generally poor response rates. However, the consistency with which sexual problems are reported more frequently among Gulf War veterans is notable, given assessment of such conditions is generally limited to symptom reporting. The discrepancies between hospitalization studies and survey studies of genitourinary outcomes may reflect variation in the severity and types of genitourinary outcomes ascertained by the different approaches; differences in active-duty, reserve, and former military personnel; the influence of reporting and selection biases; or the role of chance.

The results of hospitalization studies suggest that excess hospitalization due to diseases of the genitourinary system did not occur among active-duty Gulf War veterans within the 10 years following the war. There is also some suggestion that postwar hospitalizations for genitourinary conditions were similar among Gulf War deployed veterans who were and were not exposed to nerve agents or oil-well fire smoke. The results, however, are not generalizable to the entire cohort of Gulf War veterans since most studies were restricted to personnel remaining on active duty during the observation period. Furthermore, by limiting such studies of genitourinary outcomes to hospitalizations, conditions that are not severe enough to require inpatient care are not assessed. Combining all genitourinary conditions into a single broad diagnostic category of "diseases of the genitourinary system" may also have limited the ability to detect associations with more specific, but etiologically distinct, outcomes.

The committee concludes there is limited/suggestive evidence of no association between Gulf War deployment and hospitalization for genitourinary diseases.

The committee concludes there is limited/suggestive evidence of an increased prevalence of self-reported sexual difficulties among Gulf War veterans.

The committee concludes there is inadequate/insufficient evidence to determine whether an association exists between Gulf War deployment and other specific conditions of the genitourinary system.

TABLE 4-13 Diseases of the Genitourinary System

Study	Design	Population	Outcomes	Results	Adjustments	Comments
Frommelt et al., 2000 (Update)	Retrospective cohort	1446 female GWVs and 5269 female NDVs with routine Pap smears conducted in 1994	Pap smear results	Nonnormal diagnosis more frequent in deployed veterans (11.5%) compared to controls (6.6%) in 26-30 year old age group ($p = 0.013$); no significant difference in occurrence of nonnormal diagnoses detected in any other age group	5-year age groups (20-50, over 50), marital status, race, rank	
McDiarmid et al., 2009 (Update)	Case series (Follow-up of McDiarmid et al., 2000, 2001, 2004, 2005, 2006, and 2007; see IOM, 2008, for detailed summary)	35 GWVs exposed to DU during friendly-fire incidents in 1991, divided into low- and high-exposure groups; examined in April-June 2007, 16-year follow-up	Urinary and serum markers, semen analyses, neuroendocrine measures	Biomarkers of renal function do not differ meaningfully (statistically or clinically) between low and high exposure to DU after 16 years of follow-up		Very small cohort, no control for potential confounders
Gray et al., 1996 (Update)	Retrospective cohort, DoD hospitalizations from August 1991 through September 1993	547,076 active-duty GWVs, 618,335 NDVs	Hospital-discharge diagnoses of a disease of the genitourinary system in DoD hospital system (ICD-9 classification)	Any genitourinary disease (exact values not given) 1991: OR about 1.1 (95% CI 1.0-1.15); 1992 and 1993: ORs about 1.0 (95% CI 0.95-1.05) Inflammatory disease of ovary, fallopian tube, pelvic cellular tissue, and peritoneum: RR 1.35 (95% CI 1.11-1.63) Other disorders of the breast: RR 1.30 (95% CI 1.03-1.63) Redundant prepuce and phimosis: OR 1.59 (95% CI 1.22-2.07) Infertility, female: RR 1.59 (95% CI 1.19-2.11)	Prewar hospitalization, sex, age, race, service branch, marital status, rank, length of service, salary, occupation	Very short follow-up period; no outpatient data; restriction to DoD hospitals, and thus to persons remaining on active duty after the war; no adjustment for potential confounders such as smoking

Study	Design	Population	Outcomes	Results	Adjustments	Comments
Gray et al., 2000 (Update)	Retrospective cohort, hospitalizations from August 1991 through December 1994	652,979 GWVs, 652,922 randomly selected NDVs 182,164 DoD hospitalizations; 16,030 VA hospitalizations; 5,185 COSHPD hospitalizations	Hospital-discharge diagnoses of a disease of the genitourinary system in DoD, VA, and COSHPD hospital systems	DoD PMR 1.01 (95% CI 0.98-1.03); VA PMR 0.96 (95% CI 0.87-0.1.05); COSHPD PMR 0.80 (95% CI 0.59-1.00)	Age, sex, race (only for DoD PMR)	Able to assess only illnesses that resulted in hospitalization; possible undetected confounders PMR has lower sensitivity than a comparison of hospitalization rates would have
Smith et al., 2006 (Update)	Retrospective cohort study of DoD hospitalizations (cohort data from DMDC)	Active-duty personnel with a single deployment to: Gulf War theater (n = 455,465); southwest Asia peacekeeping mission, 1991-1998 (n = 249,047); Bosnia, 1995-1998 (n = 44,341)	Postdeployment hospitalization events (1991-2000) for an ICD-9-CM diagnosis of a disease of the genitourinary system (580-629) and nephritis specifically	Compared to GWVs, veterans of Bosnia showed reduced risk (HR 0.60, 95% CI 0.51-0.70), and veterans of southwest Asia showed similar risk (HR 1.00, 95% CI 0.92-1.09) Nephritis, Bosnia: HR 0.47 (95% CI 0.20-1.08); SW Asia: HR 1.30 (95% CI 0.84-2.01)	Sex, age, marital status, pay grade, race/ethnicity, service branch, occupation, and predeployment hospitalization; time-dependent covariate to account for changing hospitalization methods, diagnostic criteria, and procedures	Lower hazard ratio observed in veterans of Bosnia may be partially explained by better access to care in theater Limitations: active-duty personnel only; hospitalizations at DoD facilities only; no outpatient data
Smith et al., 2002 (Update)	Retrospective cohort study of DoD hospitalizations 1991-1999; exposure modeling for oil-well fire smoke	405,142 active-duty Gulf War veterans who were in theater during the time of Kuwaiti oil-well fires	Hospitalization for diseases of the genitourinary system	Risk was not increased at any level of smoke plume exposure	Adjusted for "influential covariates," defined as demographic or deployment variables with p values less than 0.15	Objective measure of disease not subject to recall bias; no issues with self-selection; however, only DoD hospitals, only active duty, no adjustment for other potential confounders

Study	Design	Population	Outcomes	Results	Adjustments	Comments
Smith et al., 2003 (Update)	Retrospective cohort study of DoD hospitalizations (1991-2000); analysis of health outcomes and exposure to nerve agents (follow-up of Gray et al. 1999b)	99,614 active-duty military considered exposed vs 318,458 nonexposed, according to revised DoD exposure model	Hospitalization for any disease of the genitourinary system (ICD-9-CM codes 580-629)	RR 0.96 (95% CI 0.91-1.00)		Restricted to DoD hospitals; restricted to hospitalizations for only Gulf War veterans who remained on active duty after the war; no adjustment for confounding exposures

NOTE: CI = confidence interval; COSHPD = California Office of Statewide Health Planning and Development; DMDC = Defense Manpower Data Center; DoD = Department of Defense; DU = depleted uranium; GWV = Gulf War veteran; HR = adjusted hazard ratio; MRR = mortality rate ratio; NDV = nondeployed veteran; OR = adjusted odds ratio; PHQ = Patient Health Questionnaire; PMR = patient medical record; RR = adjusted risk ratio; VA = Department of Veterans Affairs.

ADVERSE REPRODUCTIVE AND PERINATAL OUTCOMES

This section evaluates the findings on birth defects in the offspring of veterans, adverse pregnancy outcomes, infertility, and sexual problems. As appropriate, the major results from each study are addressed by whether the father or the mother served in the gulf and by outcome. Table 4-14 summarizes all the primary studies on adverse reproductive and perinatal outcomes reviewed by the committee.

Birth Defects

Birth defects occur in about 3% of live births. The numerous types of serious or disabling birth defects include structural defects, chromosomal abnormalities, and birth defect syndromes (California Birth Defects Monitoring Program, 2009). Because of that diversity, epidemiologists attempting to calculate whether birth defects are increased in a particular group such as deployed veterans, sometimes encounter the problem of making multiple comparisons; that is, the greater the number or the more types of comparisons, the greater the likelihood that one or more of them will appear significant when no true differences exists. Several statistical techniques are used to adjust for, or minimize, the problem of multiple comparisons, but they are not foolproof.

Summary of *Volume 4*

Primary Studies

In the most comprehensive population-based study, Araneta et al. (2003) identified birth defects among infants of military personnel born from January 1, 1989, to December 31, 1993, from population-based birth defect registries in six states: Arizona, Hawaii, Iowa, and selected counties of Arkansas, California, and Georgia (metropolitan Atlanta). They compared the prevalence of 48 selected congenital anomalies diagnosed from birth to the age of 1 year between Gulf War veterans' and nondeployed veterans' infants conceived before the war; between Gulf War veterans' and nondeployed veterans' infants conceived during or after the war; and between infants conceived by Gulf War veterans before and after the war. The authors performed separate analyses on the basis of whether the mother or the father was engaged in military service. If both parents were in the military then the birth was categorized as an infant of a military mother. The study found higher prevalence of three cardiac defects (tricuspid valve insufficiency, aortic valve stenosis, and coarctation of the aorta), and one kidney defect (renal agenesis and hypoplasia) among infants conceived after the war to Gulf War veteran fathers. There also was a higher prevalence of hypospadias (malformation of the urethra and urethral groove), a genitourinary defect among sons conceived postwar to Gulf War veteran mothers compared to their nondeployed counterparts. Aortic valve stenosis, coarctation of aorta, and renal angenesis and hypoplasia were also elevated among infants conceived among the Gulf War veteran fathers postwar compared to those conceived prewar. There was only 1 birth defect recorded among 142 births conceived prewar to Gulf War veteran mothers, and this precludes comparisons with this group.

This study is particularly informative because it relies on active surveillance systems to identify medically confirmed outcomes diagnosed through the first year, rather than at birth, and uses information from population registries, as opposed to information from voluntary participation by study subjects. Because both nonmilitary and military hospitals participated in the registries in all states except California (nonmilitary only), births among reservists, National Guard, and former military personnel were eligible, as well as among those on active duty. The study also included comparisons of births to Gulf War veterans before and after deployment. One limitation is that the study relied on availability of unique personal identifiers in military and birth certificate data, which leads to the possibility that some military offspring might be missed among the cases, and that would make the observed prevalence more conservative than the actual. Another is the study's low power to assess individual defects that are rare. The authors also published the results of the pilot study of their method, which was performed in only Hawaii (Araneta et al., 2000); because the data are incorporated in the larger six-state study, they are not reviewed separately here.

Anecdotal reports raised the possibility of increased prevalence of Goldenhar syndrome, a rare craniofacial abnormality, among children of Gulf War veterans. External features of the syndrome are ear abnormalities, such as microtia, anotia, and preauricular tags. In a case-control study performed by Werler et al. (2005), birth records of infants born with the malformation hemifacial microsomia were examined to determine whether there was an association between Gulf War service of the parents and the birth defect. Hemifacial microsomia was identified in 232 cases from craniofacial clinics in 26 cities and matched to 832 controls by pediatrician and child's age. Mothers of case subjects and controls were interviewed by telephone in 1996-2002 to identify pregnancy exposures, including military service, particularly in the Gulf War, of the mother or father 5-11 years before the child's birth. Of the cases, four mothers and 30 fathers had served in the military, as had 10 control mothers and 100 control fathers; of those, four case parents (all in the Army) and 23 control parents (including nine in the Army) had served in the Gulf War. The association with Army service overall was significant (OR 2.4, 95% CI 1.4-4.2), but the association with having served in the Gulf War was not (OR 0.8, 95% CI 0.3-2.3). Study limitations include self-reported military service, small numbers of exposed and limited control for potential confounding. The study by Werler et al. (2005) was described in *Volume 4*, but the primary or secondary status of the paper was not classified. For the purpose of this review, the study was considered primary.

Secondary Studies

Additional studies of birth defects are considered secondary either because they rely on self-reports (and thus introduce potential recall bias), because they rely exclusively on birth records from military hospitals and are likely to incompletely ascertain malformations, or because they consider only groups of birth defects. Studying groups of birth defects, although useful in identifying patterns, makes it difficult to determine which specific defects may be increased.

Cowan et al. (1997) examined routinely collected data on all live births in 135 military hospitals in 1991-1993 to compare the frequency of birth defects in children of active-duty Gulf War veterans and nondeployed active-duty veterans. Information on 33,998 infants born to Gulf War deployed veterans (30,151 men and 3847 women) and 41,463 born to nondeployed veterans (32,638 men and 8825 women) was reviewed. The prevalence of any birth defect (that is, any ICD-9-CM code related to congenital malformations) was 7.45% for deployed veterans and 7.59% for nondeployed veterans (RR 0.98, 95% CI 0.93-1.03). There was no significant association between service in the Gulf War and the prevalence of any birth defect for male veterans (OR 0.97, 95% CI 0.91-1.03) or female veterans (OR 1.07, 95% CI 0.94-1.22) after adjustment for mother's age at delivery, race or ethnicity, and marital status of parent at the time of the Gulf War. The unadjusted OR for having an infant with severe birth defects was 1.03

(95% CI 0.92-1.15) for male active-duty veterans, 0.92 (95% CI 0.71-1.20) for female active-duty veterans, and 1.00 (95% CI 0.90-1.10) for men and women combined. The authors note that when the adjusted ORs were calculated, no associations were seen, but they did not provide the data. When birth defects were evaluated by ICD-9-CM diagnostic groupings for the five most common severe anomalies, no statistical increases in associations were observed for male or female veterans. A limitation of the study is that it examined data only from live births to active-duty personnel in military hospitals. It is likely that higher risk pregnancies were referred to civilian hospitals. Since not all congenital malformations are evident at birth, some outcomes may have been underascertained when relying on hospital birth records.

A population-based study of male Canadian veterans (Goss Gilroy, 1998) surveyed deployed and nondeployed veterans for self-reported birth defects. Overall, deployed veterans reported a higher prevalence of birth defects (a combined category that included births before, during, and after the Gulf War). Birth defects that occurred at similar frequencies included urogenital and kidney defects.

Two additional secondary studies assessed broad groups of birth defects. In a population-based survey in the United States, Kang et al. (2001) observed an excess prevalence of self-reported "likely birth defects" and specifically "moderate to severe defects" among infants of Gulf War deployed fathers and mothers compared with nondeployed fathers and mothers. Most defects were isolated anomalies, and no clear patterns were found. First pregnancies ending after June 30, 1991, were considered in this analysis. The observed number of birth defects among children (liveborn and stillborn) born after deployment to National Guard personnel in two units in southeast Mississippi was not greater than expected on the basis of population-based registries (Penman et al., 1996).

Updated and Supplemental Literature

Primary Studies

Doyle et al. (2004) was considered secondary in *Volume 4*, but it is considered primary in this review, primarily due to medical confirmation of self-reported outcomes. Doyle and colleagues (2004) evaluated the prevalence of self-reported birth defects among the offspring of all UK veterans (male and female) deployed to the gulf and among the offspring of nondeployed veterans who responded to a postal questionnaire. Response rates were higher among the Gulf War veterans (53% of men, 72% of women) than the comparison group (42% of men, 60% of women). The authors considered pregnancies conceived after deployment (after January 1, 1991, for nondeployed veterans) through November 8, 1997. Medical confirmation was requested for all fetal deaths at 16 weeks or more or of unknown gestation and for liveborn children in whom a congenital abnormality, serious childhood medical condition, or death was reported. Among infants conceived by fathers deployed to the gulf compared with infants of fathers not deployed, the OR for any malformation was 1.5 (95% CI 1.3-1.7). Elevated ORs were observed specifically for malformations of the genital system, urinary system, musculoskeletal system, and cranial neural crest; for "other" malformations of the digestive system; for "other" nonchromosomal malformations; and for metabolic and single-gene defects. The ORs for urinary system and musculoskeletal system defects remained increased when the cases were restricted to the 55% that had clinical confirmation. No significant associations with birth defects were found for infants of mothers deployed to the gulf, although the analyses were limited by small numbers.

Secondary Studies

Three additional studies were identified that evaluated the effect of deployment on birth defects (Ishoy et al., 2001a; Kelsall et al., 2007; Verret et al., 2008), although none met the criteria for primary studies. In addition to the criteria for secondary studies described above, studies were considered secondary if too few birth defect cases were identified to make meaningful comparisons. Thus, Araneta et al. (1997), which was previously described but not classified as either primary or secondary in *Volume 4*, is considered secondary in this review.

In a study of Goldenhar syndrome, DoD hospital discharge data were used to identify all infants born to active-duty personnel after the Gulf War (or December 31, 1990, for nondeployed veterans) through September 30, 1993 (Araneta et al., 1997). In the population of 75,414 infants, five cases born to Gulf War veteran fathers and two cases born to nondeployed fathers were identified (Araneta et al., 1997). Given the small numbers, it is difficult to determine whether an excess risk is associated with service in the gulf.

A study of Danish veterans assessed self-reported "congenital disease or malformations" for children born to male veterans after 1991 (Ishoy et al., 2001a). The prevalence of congenital malformations was 2.1% among the 661 peacekeepers and 2.8% among the 215 nondeployed veterans. The difference between the groups was not significant.

Kelsall et al. (2007) surveyed Australian Gulf War veterans (n = 1424) and nondeployed (n = 1548) Australian Defense Force personnel in 2000-2002 to compare self-reported birth defects and other reproductive outcomes. No association was observed between a father's Gulf War deployment and any reported birth defect (OR 1.0, 95% CI 0.6-1.6). Evaluations of specific malformations were not reported. Birth defects data were collected for live births only, which would exclude the most severe malformations. Additional limitations include poor response among nondeployed veterans and lack of control for maternal factors.

When compared to 10-year prevalence data from the Paris Registry of Congenital Malformations, the prevalence of major anomalies did not differ between French Gulf War veterans and the general French population, with the exception of Down syndrome which occurred less frequently among veterans (prevalence ratio 0.36, 95% CI 0.13-0.78) (Verret et al., 2008). Within the same publication, the authors also report the results of a nested case-control study conducted within the cohort of French Gulf War veterans to assess the effects of Gulf War-related exposures on all birth defects combined. No associations were observed for self-reported exposures to the smoke of oil-well fires, sandstorms, chemical alarms, or pesticides. According to the authors, an effort was made to minimize recall bias by restricting controls to veterans with at least one symptom-related hospitalization. However, the inclusion criterion was not applied equally to the cases. Because control selection was plausibly related to exposure, the results of the case-control analyses were subject to selection bias.

Summary and Conclusions

Primarily on the basis of the Araneta et al. (2004) and Doyle et al. (2004) studies, because of the availability of medical confirmation in those studies, there is some suggestion of increased risk of birth defects among offspring of Gulf War veterans. However, with the possible exception of urinary tract abnormalities, the specific defects with increased prevalence in the two studies were not consistent. Furthermore, the association between deployment and urinary tract abnormalities was not consistent when considering parent-specific exposures. That is, the association observed in Araneta et al. (2004) was specific to maternal deployment, and the association observed in Doyle et al. (2004) was confined to paternal deployment. Overall, studies of Gulf War service and congenital malformations have been limited because specific birth defects are relatively rare, multiple comparisons were performed, and sample sizes were small when divided by timing of exposure (before or after conception) and whether the mother or the father was exposed. Thus, overall there is no consistent pattern of higher prevalence of birth defects among offspring of male or female Gulf War veterans, and no single defect, except urinary tract abnormalities, has been found in more than one well-designed study.

> **The committee concludes there is inadequate/insufficient evidence to determine whether an association exists between deployment to the Gulf War and specific birth defects.**

Adverse Pregnancy Outcomes

Studies of adverse pregnancy outcomes have evaluated the prevalence of spontaneous abortions, stillbirths, ectopic pregnancies, preterm births, low birth weight and macrosomia in the pregnancies of Gulf War deployed and nondeployed men and women.

Summary of *Volume 4*

Primary Studies

Only one study of adverse pregnancy outcomes used hospital-discharge records, rather than relying exclusively on self-reported outcomes. Araneta and colleagues (2004) recruited women admitted to military hospitals for pregnancy-related diagnoses (including livebirths, stillbirths, spontaneous and induced abortions, ectopic pregnancies, and pregnancy-related complications) from August 2, 1990, to May 31, 1992. Reproductive outcomes were collected from surveys administered in 1997 and 1998 to the 3825 US women with pregnancy-related hospital admissions. Of the 1110 respondents with complete data, there were 415 predeployment and in-theater conceptions among Gulf War veterans (referred to as "Gulf War-exposed pregnancies"), 298 postwar conceptions among Gulf War veterans, and 427 conceptions among nondeployed women from deployed units. Self-reported outcomes were confirmed by hospital discharge data. The odds of spontaneous abortions (OR 2.9, 95% CI 1.9-4.6) and ectopic pregnancies (OR 7.7, 95% CI 3.0-19.8) were higher among Gulf War veterans' postwar conceptions compared to conceptions among nondeployed women. The frequency of these outcomes among so called Gulf War-exposed conceptions was also increased compared to pregnancies among nondeployed veterans, but not in a significant way. Because only military hospitals were included, only information on active-duty personnel was available. The authors also acknowledge that deployment status, which was based on deployment dates for each military unit, may have been misclassified for pregnant women whose deployment orders were cancelled or delayed due to pregnancy. Furthermore, spontaneous abortions were not completely ascertained, given a substantial proportion of losses occur before pregnancies are clinically recognized (Wilcox et al., 1988).

Secondary Studies

Doyle and colleagues (2004) also studied self-reported miscarriages and stillbirths among Gulf War deployed fathers and mothers. The authors assessed clinically confirmed reports of congenital malformations. However, similar efforts to evaluate clinically confirmed reports of miscarriages and stillbirths were not described, and the outcomes assessed were limited to self-reports. Thus, when considering the analysis of other adverse pregnancy outcomes, the study is considered secondary. Response rates were 53% for male Gulf War veterans, 72% for female Gulf War veterans, 42% for male nondeployed veterans and 60% for female nondeployed veterans. The authors observed no effect of Gulf War service on miscarriages reported by female veterans. The number of stillbirths among females was too small for meaningful assessment. There was a 40% increase in the odds of miscarriage among pregnancies reported by male Gulf War veterans compared with their nondeployed counterparts (OR 1.4, 95% CI 1.3-1.5), and the effect was stronger for early miscarriages (OR 1.5, 95% CI 1.3-1.6). However, in the Nuclear Industry Family Study, Maconochie et al. (1999) found evidence of underreporting of miscarriages among the nonexposed workers. The potential selection bias could explain the associations observed among the Gulf War veterans, if there was selective participation related to pregnancy outcome.

In the Kang et al. (2001) study described above, adverse pregnancy outcomes, including spontaneous abortions, stillbirths and preterm births, were compared between Gulf War deployed and nondeployed veteran mothers and fathers. There was an excess prevalence of self-reported spontaneous abortions (OR 1.62, 95% CI 1.32-1.99) among pregnancies conceived by Gulf War deployed fathers. Stillbirths were also reported more frequently among deployed fathers (OR 1.65, 95% CI 0.91-2.98), but this difference was not significant. Among veteran mothers, the odds of spontaneous abortion were modestly increased for those deployed to the Gulf War, but the 95% confidence interval did not exclude the null value (OR 1.35, 95% CI 0.97-1.89). No differences for preterm birth or infant death were observed among males or females. The limitations of this study include self-reported outcomes and differential participation rates for deployed (75% response) and nondeployed (65% response) veterans.

Updated and Supplemental Literature

Five additional secondary studies evaluating the effect of deployment on adverse pregnancy outcomes were identified (Ishoy et al., 2001a; Kang et al., 2009; Kelsall et al., 2007; Verret et al., 2008; Wells et al., 2006). All of these studies were based on self-reported data.

Interview data from 661 male Danish peacekeepers who served in the gulf in 1990-1997 and 215 male Danish military personnel who were not deployed to the gulf revealed no differences in prevalence of spontaneous abortions, live births, or infant deaths (Ishoy et al., 2001a). In addition to self-reported outcomes, the study did not control for the influence of important confounders.

One of the largest studies of reproductive outcomes in female Gulf War veterans was conducted by Wells et al. (2006). In this 1996-1997 survey of 8742 married male and female US Gulf War era veterans, no associations between deployment status and number of pregnancies reported between 1991 and 1995 were observed for males or females. Among the 2159 men and 2233 women reporting one or more pregnancies during this 4-year period, Gulf War deployment status was not associated with an increased odds of miscarriage, stillbirth, ectopic pregnancy, low birth weight, or macrosomic (> 4000 g) births among females. Among males, a weak, marginal association was observed between Gulf War deployment and miscarriage (OR 1.24, 95% CI 0.96-1.61), but no associations with other adverse pregnancy outcomes were observed. Limitations of this study include self-reported outcomes, poor response rate (51%), and limited information on maternal risk factors. Thus, the results may be susceptible to recall bias, selection bias, and confounding.

In the Australian veteran cohort described above, Kelsall et al. (2007) assessed the self-reported outcomes of pregnancies occurring in 1991 or later among 1424 Gulf War veterans

(80.5% response) and 1548 nondeployed military personnel (56.8% response). Among the male participants of this survey conducted between August 2000 and April 2002, deployment was not associated with miscarriages/stillbirths, pregnancy terminations, low birth weight, or preterm birth.

In a cross-sectional survey on the reproductive health of French Gulf War veterans (Verret et al., 2008), a nondeployed comparison group was not included in the study population. Thus, the effects of deployment on reproductive outcomes were not assessed in this population. According to the authors, the frequencies of reproductive characteristics, which included postdeployment miscarriage and stillbirth, were similar to frequencies in the general French population. Statistical comparisons, however, were not provided.

After conducting a 2000 follow-up survey to the 1995 National Health Survey of Gulf War Era Veterans and Their Families, Kang et al. (2009) reported the prevalence of selected self-reported reproductive characteristics among female Gulf War and Gulf War era veterans. Gulf War veterans reported an excess prevalence of "serious problems with mood before period" (OR 1.28, 95% CI 1.13-1.45) but no difference in having given birth within the last 6 months (OR 2.11, 95% CI 0.89-5.04) or having had a miscarriage in the last 6 months (OR 0.42, 95% CI 0.15-1.17). Comparison of births and miscarriages, however, were based on small numbers.

Summary and Conclusions

Although the results from the Araneta et al. (2004) study, which had hospital discharge data available, are suggestive of an increased risk of spontaneous abortions and ectopic pregnancies, the results may not be generalizable to deployed women who left the service or to pregnancy-related admissions to nonmilitary hospitals. These findings for spontaneous abortion were not replicated in the four secondary studies of female veterans, which used self-reported outcome data. Similarly, only one secondary study assessed ectopic pregnancies and observed no differences by deployment status among male or female veterans. Among males, no consistent associations with Gulf War deployment were observed for spontaneous abortion, preterm birth or low birth weight, although three studies reported modest increases in self-reported miscarriages among deployed males.

The committee concludes there is inadequate/insufficient evidence to determine whether an association exists between deployment to the Gulf War and adverse pregnancy outcomes such as miscarriage, stillbirth, preterm birth, and low birth weight.

Fertility

Studies of fertility problems have assessed semen parameters, hospitalization for infertility or genitourinary system diseases, self-reported difficulties achieving a pregnancy, and serum concentrations of reproductive hormones in males. Infertility is typically defined as trying to conceive unsuccessfully for 12 months or more after discontinuing contraception, although the quality of the outcome measurement has varied across studies and has included inference from self-reported disorders of infertility or sperm abnormalities, reports of "having difficulty getting pregnant," reports of consulting a doctor after trying unsuccessfully for more than 1 year, and seeking treatment for childlessness.

Summary of *Volume 4*

Primary Studies

In the study by Ishoy et al. (2001a), 661 Danish peacekeepers who served in the gulf in 1990-1997 and 215 Danish military personnel who were not deployed to the gulf completed a clinical exam and a health interview that included questions about reproductive health and sexual problems. A clinical evaluation of serum concentrations of reproductive hormones—including luteinizing hormone, follicle-stimulating hormone, serum hormone-binding globulin, inhibin B and testosterone—found no significant differences between the deployed and nondeployed veterans. Furthermore, no differences in self-reported infertility, defined as "treatment due to childlessness after August 1990" were observed.

A group of 10,465 UK Gulf War veterans and 7376 nondeployed veterans (drawn from the same population as the Doyle et al. study described above) who fathered or tried to father children after the war and before August 1997 reported excess prevalence of infertility (defined as consulting a doctor after trying unsuccessfully for more than 1 year) compared to their nondeployed counterparts (OR 1.38, 95% CI 1.20-1.60) (Maconochie et al., 2004). The prevalence of type 1 infertility (never achieving pregnancy; OR 1.41, 95% CI 1.05-1.89) and type II infertility (never achieving a live birth; OR 1.50, 95% CI 1.18-1.89) were also significantly higher. Furthermore, more Gulf War veterans than nondeployed veterans experienced time to conception for planned pregnancies of more than 1 year (OR 1.18, 95% CI 1.04-1.34). Although the authors attempted to verify self-reported infertility, clinical diagnostic information was received from the subject's physician for only one-third of those reporting fertility problems. Additional limitations include low response rates (53% for deployed veterans and 42% for nondeployed veterans), possible recall bias, and lack of information on partners' fertility status.

Updated and Supplemental Literature

Primary Studies

Semen characteristics and neuroendocrine parameters have been assessed biennually in a small cohort of Gulf War veterans exposed to depleted uranium (DU) as a result of friendly-fire accidents (McDiarmid et al., 2000, 2001, 2004, 2007a,b, 2009). When comparing groups with high and low urinary uranium concentrations, no adverse DU effects on semen parameters or serum concentrations of testosterone, leutinizing hormone (LH), or follicle-stimulating hormone (FSH) have been observed up to 16 years after the initial exposure. Although serum prolactin concentrations have not been statistically different for the low and high uranium groups, prolactin concentrations in both groups were above normal limits in recent evaluations (McDiarmid et al., 2006, 2009). Up to 77 DU-exposed Gulf War veterans have been evaluated in this cohort over time, but only a small subset of individuals have been assessed at each time point. For example, 35 members underwent clinical evaluation during the most recent 2007 follow-up, with only 17 of those providing semen samples (McDiarmid et al., 2009). Thus, comparisons are based on small numbers and do not adjust for potential confounders.

Secondary Studies

Gray and colleagues (1996) conducted a hospitalization study (1991-1993) in which they compared almost 550,000 Gulf War veterans with almost 620,000 nondeployed veterans across three time periods following the war (1991, 1992, 1993). The study found increased hospitalizations, in 1991 only, for the broad category "genitourinary system diseases," When specific diagnoses within this category were examined, the observed association was attributed to infertility among females (OR 1.59, 95% CI 1.19-2.11), inflammatory disease of the ovary, fallopian tube, pelvic cellular tissue, and peritoneium (OR 1.35, 95% CI 1.11-1.63), redundant prepuce and phimosis among males (a diagnosis typically associated with elective circumcision) (OR 1.59, 95% CI 1.22-2.07), and other disorders of the breast among males and females (OR 1.30, 95% CI 1.03-1.63). The authors suggest these patterns were consistent with elective hospitalizations deferred until after the war. The major limitation of this study is the focus on DoD hospitalizations, which would miss hospitalizations of individuals who did not remain on active duty following the war. Furthermore, conditions associated with infertility would rarely require hospitalization, which is the predominant reason for classifying this study as secondary.

Three additional secondary studies addressed self-reported fertility problems among veterans who served in the Gulf War. All but one study assessed these conditions in males.

Using mailed questionnaires to survey Gulf War deployed and nondeployed male Australian veterans, Kelsall et al. (2007) found that before 1991 deployed veterans were no more likely than nondeployed veterans to report difficulties getting pregnant after trying for at least 12 months. Deployment, however, was associated with experiencing fertility difficulties for the first time in 1991 or later (OR 1.4, 95% CI 1.0-1.8). Of those reporting fertility problems in 1991 or later, the deployed veterans were more likely to have subsequently fathered a child. Verret et al. (2008) examined the prevalence of self-reported infertility (inferred from disorders of infertility or sperm abnormalities) and other reproductive outcomes in the cross-sectional study of French Gulf War veterans. Infertility was reported by 0.9% of the 5638 male veterans, but the lack of a comparison group hindered the assessment of the effect of Gulf War deployment on this condition.

In Kang et al. (2009), a higher proportion of female Gulf War veterans (9.9%) than Gulf War era veterans (4.3%) reported "having difficulty getting pregnant" (OR 2.2, 95% CI 1.50-3.22).

Summary and Conclusions

There is no evidence of significant differences in concentrations of male reproductive hormones between Gulf War veterans and nondeployed veterans. However, this question has been addressed by only one study. When semen parameters and reproductive hormones were compared within a DU-exposed cohort of Gulf War veterans, no differences were detected between those with high and low DU exposure. Although changes in hormonal concentrations and semen characteristics are reproductive outcomes of interest, they are not definitive indicators of infertility (with the exception of azoospermia). For the most part, studies of Gulf War deployment and infertility have relied on self-reports that give rise to a substantial opportunity for recall bias. Furthermore, studies have rarely examined this question among female veterans. Although it appears that problems with fertility are reported more frequently among Gulf War veterans compared to their nondeployed counterparts, cautious interpretation is warranted given the small number of available studies, all of which are susceptible to reporting bias and selective participation.

The committee concludes there is inadequate/insufficient evidence to determine whether an association exists between deployment to the Gulf War and fertility problems.

Sexual Dysfunction

Studies of self-reported sexual dysfunction have included reports of decreased libido, erectile dysfunction, discomfort or pain during intercourse, and a burning sensation after sex. One primary study was discussed in *Volume 4.* The committee identified no new primary studies of sexual dysfunction in Gulf War veterans but did consider seven secondary studies.

Summary of *Volume 4*

When Ishoy et al. (2001b) asked Danish military personnel whether they experienced any sexual problems (decreased libido or nonorganic erectile dysfunction) that they attributed to service in the gulf, self-reported sexual problems were higher among Gulf War veterans (12%) than among controls (3.7%) for an age-adjusted OR of 2.9 (95% CI 1.4-6.0, p = 0.003). Self-reported sexual problems were "clinically validated by the examining physician during the interview." The deployed veterans were more likely to report sexual problems if they had seen killed or wounded people (p = 0.002), watched a friend or colleague being threatened or shot at (p = 0.02), or been threatened with arms themselves (p = 0.04) than if they had not had these experiences.

Updated and Supplemental Literature

Proctor et al. (1998) compared self-reported symptoms from random stratified samples of 186 Gulf War veterans from the New England area, 66 Gulf War veterans from the New Orleans area, and 48 Gulf War era veterans deployed to Germany. Using a 52-item symptom checklist administered between 1994 and 1996, the prevalence of self-reported pain during intercourse was 2.4% among the New England veterans, 1.9% among the New Orleans veterans, and 0% among the veterans not deployed to the gulf. The odds ratio comparing Gulf War deployed and nondeployed groups could not be calculated because the prevalence in the reference group was zero. Of note, the Gulf War deployed group reported a higher prevalence of all but one of the 52 symptoms (excessive sweating) when compared to the group deployed to Germany.

Simmons et al. (2004) used a mail questionnaire to survey all UK Gulf War veterans and demographically similar veterans who had served at the same time but were not deployed to the gulf. Of the 42,818 male veterans who responded (48% response) between 1998 and 2001, 24,379 had been deployed and 18,439 had not. Sexual dysfunction or a lack of sexual drive was reported by 0.8% and 0.2% of the deployed and nondeployed veterans, respectively, for an OR of 4.6 (95% CI 3.2-6.6, p < 0.001) adjusted for age and service status at the time of the survey, service and rank at the time of the war, alcohol consumption, and smoking. The prevalence of self-reported "genital system and bladder problems" (OR 2.2, 95% CI 1.7-2.7) was also higher among Gulf War veterans. The category of "genital system and bladder problems" included 13 (0.1%) reports of "burning semen" among Gulf War veterans and 1 (0.0%) among nondeployed veterans.

In the 1997-1999 study of all US Navy Seabees (Gray et al., 2002), 11,868 (62.6%) of 18,945 Seabees responded to a mailed questionnaire. In this study, deployment was associated with self-reports of physician-diagnosed impotence (with onset after August 1991) (OR 3.06, 95% CI 1.95-4.83). Similarly, in a 1997-1998 survey of male Gulf War deployed veterans (n = 2735), nondeployed (n = 2422), and servicemen deployed to Bosnia (n = 2393) (65% response rate), participants were asked to report whether or not they had experienced any of the 50 identified symptoms in the previous month (Unwin et al., 1999). All symptoms, including sexual problems, were reported more frequently among Gulf War deployed veterans when compared to the other groups. The odds ratio for sexual problems was 3.2 (95% CI 2.4-4.2) for deployed versus nondeployed and 2.2 (95% CI 1.5-3.1) for Gulf War deployed veterans versus Bosnia deployed veterans.

In a 1998 phone survey of Kansas veterans, those deployed to the Gulf War were more likely than nondeployed veterans to report that they or their partner felt a burning sensation after sex (OR 3.75, 95% CI 1.88-7.49) (Steele, 2000). The Iowa Persian Gulf Study Group (1997) compared self-reported medical conditions between deployed and nondeployed Iowa veterans within the regular military and within the National Guard or reserve. In this phone survey conducted about 5 years after the Gulf War, symptoms of sexual discomfort were reported for the respondent and his female partner (as reported by the respondent). Gulf War veterans in the National Guard or reserve reported a higher prevalence of symptoms of sexual discomfort for their female partner (prevalence difference 3.6, 95% CI 2.3-4.8) when compared to their nondeployed counterparts. No differences in sexual discomfort were reported for the respondents themselves. Sexual discomfort was not associated with Gulf War deployment among members of the regular military.

The prevalence of selected sexual problems was also assessed among Gulf War veterans according to their potential exposure to sarin or cyclosarin at the Khamisiyah demolition (Page et al., 2005). Among participants in the National Health Survey of Gulf War Era Veterans Study, the prevalence of painful sexual intercourse (OR 1.16, 95% CI 0.81-1.65) or impotence or other sexual problems (OR 0.85, 95% CI 0.65-1.12) did not differ when comparing the exposed and unexposed Gulf War veterans.

Summary and Conclusions

Gulf War veterans consistently report an increased prevalence of sexual problems when compared with nondeployed veterans. The one study assessing exposures specific to Gulf War service reported no association between nerve agent exposure, and reported sexual problems among veterans deployed to the Gulf War. With the exception of a single study that incorporated physician interviews to verify symptom reporting, studies of sexual problems have relied exclusively on survey responses. It is acknowledged that studies assessing the prevalence of sexual problems are generally limited to self-reported symptoms. However, survey studies of self-reported conditions should be interpreted cautiously given concerns about susceptibility to selection and reporting biases.

The committee concludes there is limited/suggestive evidence of an increased prevalence of self-reported sexual difficulties among Gulf War veterans.

TABLE 4-14 Adverse Reproductive and Perinatal Outcomes

Study	Design	Population	Outcomes	Results	Adjustments	Comments
Birth defects						
Araneta et al., 2003 (Vol. 4)	Retrospective cohort, using population-based, birth-defect registries (active surveillance all cases identified from birth to 1 year)	Infants of military personnel born 1/1/1989-12/31/1993 in Arizona, Iowa, Hawaii, and participating counties of Arkansas, California, Georgia to GWV mothers (n = 450) NDV mothers (n = 3966) GWV fathers (n = 11,511) NDV fathers (n = 29,086)	48 birth defects identified by CDC as occurring frequently or of public health importance, excluding pulmonary artery anomalies and adding dextrocardia, chromosomal anomalies (other than trisomies 13, 18, and 21), and Goldenhar syndrome	Postwar conceptions, GWVs vs NDVs (unadjusted RRs): father: tricuspid valve insufficiency, 10/4648 vs 9/11,164 (RR 2.7, 95% CI 1.1-6.6); aortic valve stenosis, 5/4648 vs 2/11,164 (RR 6.0, 95% CI 1.2-31.0); coarctation of aorta, 5/4648 vs 3/11,164 (RR 4.0, 95% CI 0.96-16.8); renal agenesis or hypoplasia, 5/4648 vs 5/11,164 (RR 2.4, 95% CI 0.7-8.3) mother: hypospadias 4/154 vs 4/967 (RR 6.3, 95% CI 1.5-26.3) GWVs postwar vs prewar conceptions (unadjusted RRs): father: aortic valve stenosis 5/4648 vs 0/6863 (RR 16.3, 95% CI 0.9-294); coarctation of aorta, 5/4648 vs 1/6,863 (RR 7.4, 95% CI 0.9-63.3); renal agenesis and hypoplasia, 5/4648 vs 0/6863 (RR 16.3, (95% CI 0.9-294); adjustment did not change results	State, maternal and paternal age, race, marital status, education, plurality, parity, prenatal visits, gestational weight gain, branch of service, military rank, prenatal alcohol exposure, intrauterine growth retardation, low birth weight, small for gestational age, preeclampsia	Limitations: California limited to diagnoses in nonmilitary hospitals; relies on availability of unique personal identifiers in military and birth certificate data, limited power to assess individual defects, multiple comparisons, limited to live births Strengths: population-based, including reservists, National Guard, former military personnel; includes defects diagnosed through first year, medically confirmed as opposed to self-reports, comparisons with prewar experience
Werler et al., 2005 (Vol. 4)	Case-control	HFM cases ≤ 3 years old (born 1996-2002) from craniofacial clinics in 24 US cities (n = 232); controls matched by age and pediatrician (n = 832)	HFM, facial asymmetry, or Goldenhar syndrome and no evidence of Mendelian inherited or chromosomal anomaly	Adjusted ORs: cases vs controls; parental army service, (OR 2.4, 95% CI 1.4-4.2); parental GW army service, (OR 2.8, 95% CI 0.8-9.6); any parental GW service (OR 0.8, 95% CI 0.3-2.3)	Family income, race, BMI in early pregnancy, multiple gestation	Limitations: unmeasured Lifestyle factors Strengths: included cases diagnosed up to of 3 years age

Study	Design	Population	Outcomes	Results	Adjustments	Comments
Doyle et al., 2004 (Update)	Retrospective cohort	All UK GWVs and randomly selected cohort of NDVs. responding to postal questionnaire; conceptions from postdeployment (for NDVs—conceived after 1/1/1991) through 11/8/1997 GWV fathers (n = 16,442) NDV fathers (n = 11,517) GWV mothers (n = 484) NDV mothers (n = 377) External comparison populations: (1) NIFS; (2) annual registered stillbirths in England and Wales, 1991-1998	Fetal death: early and late miscarriage, stillbirth; congenital malformations excluding minor abnormalities among live births; self-report with clinical confirmation attempted for fetal deaths and live births with reported abnormalities	Adjusted ORs: GWVs vs NDVs father: all miscarriages 2829/15,539 vs 1525/10,988 (OR 1.4, 95% CI 1.3-1.5); any congenital malformation, 686/13,191 vs 342/9758 (OR 1.5, 95% CI 1.3-1.7); other malformations of digestive system, 69/13,191 vs 31/9758 (OR 1.6, 95% CI 1.0-2.5); genital system, 45/13,191 vs 19/9758 (OR 1.8, 95% CI 1.0-3.0); urinary system, 103/13,191 vs 48/9758 (OR 1.6, 95% CI 1.1-2.3); musculoskeletal system, 194/13,191 vs 78/9758 (OR 1.8, 95% CI 1.4-2.4); other nonchromosomal malformations, 45/13,191 vs 19/9758 (OR 1.7, 95% CI 1.0-3.0); cranial neural crest, 184/13,191 vs 101/9758 (OR 1.3, 95% CI 1.0-1.7); metabolic and single gene defects, 22/13,191 vs 8/9758 (OR 2.0, 95% CI 0.9-4.8); mothers: no significant associations	Stratum matched on branch of service, sex, age, serving status, rank; ORs adjusted by year of pregnancy end, paternal/maternal pregnancy order, maternal age, service, rank, previous fetal death, multiplicity	Response rates: GWVs: men 53%, women 72%; NDVs: men 42%, women 60% Limitations: poor response rates among men and response rates lower in NDVs, low numbers of miscarriages in NDVs. compared with NIFS population could mean participation and reporting bias; multiple comparisons Strengths: medical confirmation for some cases; fetal deaths as well as live births; external comparison groups to evaluate possible biases
Adverse pregnancy outcomes						
Araneta et al., 2004 (Vol. 4)	Retrospective cohort	Deployed women admitted to military hospitals for pregnancy-related	Self-reported stillbirths, spontaneous abortions, ectopic	Adjusted RRs: mothers: GWV vs NDV postwar conceptions:	Age, race, education, marital status, branch of service, military rank, parity, history	Overall response rate: 50% Limitations: low response rate; no

Study	Design	Population	Outcomes	Results	Adjustments	Comments
		diagnoses (including live births, abortions, ectopic pregnancies, pregnancy-related complications) from 8/2/1990 to 5/31/1992 and who responded to mailed survey: GW-exposed conceptions (n = 415), GW postwar conceptions (n = 298), NDVs (n = 427)	pregnancies, pregnancy-related complications (ICD-9-CM codes 640-676); confirmed by discharge diagnostic data	spontaneous abortions, 68 vs 39 (RR 2.92, 95% CI 1.87-4.56); ectopic pregnancies, 32 vs 6 (RR 7.70, 95% CI 3.00-19.8); GWV vs NDV exposed conceptions: spontaneous abortions, 48 vs 39 (RR 1.44, 95% CI 0.91-2.29); ectopic pregnancies, 10 vs 6 (RR 1.91, 95% CI 0.67-5.46)	of adverse outcome	information on smoking, alcohol, caffeine, other known risk factors for fetal loss; possible limited generalizability due to restriction to military hospital admissions; recall bias Strengths: confirmation with discharge data, assessed GW-exposed and postwar conceptions
Fertility						
Ishoy et al., 2001a (Vol. 4)	Cross-sectional Participation rates: GWVs, 83.6%; NDVs, 57.8%	Danish Gulf War Study, GWVs (n = 661) NDVs (n = 215)	Self-reports of sexual problems (including reduced libido); measured male reproductive hormones: serum concentrations of LH, FSH, testosterone, inhibin B	Male GWVs vs NDVs: self-reported sexual problems, 12.0% vs 3.7% ($p < 0.001$); reproductive hormones, no significant difference; suspected oligospermia, FSH ≥ 10 IU/L, inhibin B ≤ 80 pg/mL, 1.6% vs 1.6%; fertility rates, spontaneous abortion, congenital malformations: no differences	Age; BMI available; stratified on deployment organization, duration of deployment	Limitations: limited control for confounding, small numbers for study of fertility rates, congenital malformations Strengths: measurement of hormones objective and unbiased
Maconochie et al., 2004 (Vol. 4)	Retrospective cohort (same cohort as Doyle et al., 2004)	Male UK veterans fathering or trying to father pregnancies after GW and before 8/97 GWV (n = 10,465) NDV (n = 7376)	Self-reported fertility problems: tried unsuccessfully for > 1 year and consulted doctor; type I infertility: never achieving pregnancy; type II infertility: never achieving live birth;	Adjusted ORs: fertility problems, 732/10,465 vs 370/7376: (OR 1.38, 95% CI 1.20-1.60); type I 259/10,465 vs 122/7376 (OR 1.41, 95% CI 1.05-1.89); type II 356/10,465 vs 166/7376 (OR 1.50, 95% CI 1.18-1.89); time to conception > 1 year for planned pregnancies,	Maternal and paternal age at first infertility consult or post-GW conception, year of first consult or conception, pre-GW pregnancy history, military service and rank, smoking, alcohol,	Response rates: GWVs, 53%; NDVs, 42% Limitations: low response rates, possible recall bias, clinically evaluated only 40% Strengths: attempted clinical evaluation,

Study	Design	Population	Outcomes	Results	Adjustments	Comments
			semen quality; time to conception; attempted clinical confirmation from both partners' physicians	845/9968 vs 528/7408 (OR 1.18, 95% CI 1.04-1.34) (increase in risk stable with time since GW)	pregnancy order	information on nonresponders available
McDiarmid et al., 2009 (Update)	Case series (follow-up of McDiarmid et al., 2000, 2001, 2004, 2005, 2006, and 2007)	35 GWVs exposed to DU during friendly-fire incidents in 1991, divided into low- and high-exposure groups; examined in April-June 2007, 16-year follow-up	Urinary and serum markers, semen analyses, neuroendocrine measures	No adverse DU effects on semen parameters or serum concentrations of testosterone, LH, or FSH Serum prolactin concentrations non-significantly above normal limits in both groups		Very small cohort, no control for potential confounders
Sexual dysfunction						
Ishoy et al., 2001b (Vol. 4)	Cross-sectional (elaboration of findings in Ishoy et al., 2001a)	Danish Gulf War Study: GWVs (n = 661), NDVs (n = 215)	Self-reported sexual problems	Male GWVs vs NDVs: sexual problems (80% decreased libido), 79/661 vs 8/215 (OR 2.9, 95% CI 1.4-6.0) (among GWVs associated with "having seen killed or wounded victims"; "having been threatened with arms"; "having watched colleagues being seriously threatened or shot at"; water hygienic environment)	Age	Limitations: small study, self-reported soft outcomes and exposures

NOTE: BMI = body mass index; CDC = Centers for Disease Control and Prevention; CI = confidence interval; DU = depleted uranium; FSH = follicle-stimulating hormone; GW = Gulf War; GWV = Gulf War veterans; HFM = hemifacial microsomia; LH = luteinizing hormone; NDV = nondeployed veterans; NIFS = Nuclear Industry Family Study; OR = adjusted odds ratio; RR = adjusted risk ratio.

MULTISYMPTOM ILLNESSES

Since the mid-1990s, numerous studies have documented that deployment in the Gulf War entailed an increased risk of developing disabling complexes of self-reported symptoms among Gulf War veterans. Some reports suggest that as many as one quarter of US veterans who were deployed to the Persian Gulf in 1990-1991, about 175,000, are suffering from an array of symptoms that taken together has been called multisymptom illness, Gulf War illness, or Gulf War syndrome (RAC, 2008). However, veterans who were not deployed to the gulf also suffer from many of the same symptoms although the prevalence is not as great in this population. As summarized by Blanchard et al. (2005), these embraced a diversity of manifestations including "fatigue, musculoskeletal pain, sleep disturbances, cognitive dysfunction, moodiness and other symptoms." Following the earliest of these reports, investigators have considered the hypothesis that these symptoms reflect the presence of a novel and distinctive Gulf War disorder, that in turn is a consequence of exposure to one or more adverse environmental influences. Many approaches have been pursued in the effort to identify specific sets of symptoms and factors that uniquely distinguish this putative Gulf War complex. The Volume 4 committee took a slightly different approach to the issue of multisymptom illnesses compared with this committee. That committee looked at "unexplained illness" and the symptom reporting by the Gulf War deployed veterans and attempted to determine whether there appeared to be a unique illness that could be defined by the symptoms. The Update committee did not attempt to make such a determination, but rather accepted that multisymptom illness was a diagnostic entity and assessed the literature regarding the association between symptom reporting indicative of multisymptom illness and deployment to the Gulf War. Primary studies on multisymptom illness are summarized in Table 4-15.

The committee that wrote *Volume 6* of the *Gulf War and Health* series on the effects of deployment-related stress considered the long-term consequences of being in combat or deployed to a war zone. That committee concluded

> People deployed to a war zone may report more symptoms than people who are not deployed—the stress response results in a cascade of physiologic changes that can have profound effects on multiple organ systems. War-zone stressors might produce disruption in brain systems that mediate responses to stress and in central pain regulatory pathways that can result in greater reporting of physical and emotional symptoms. The continuation of altered physiologic states over months and years can contribute to the accumulation of a chronic stress burden that has adverse long-term health consequences. Much progress has been made in understanding the physiologic mechanisms of the stress response, particularly in animal models, but work remains to be done in human studies. Research on the effect of stressors on the endocrine, immune, cardiovascular, and gastrointestinal systems demonstrates the complexity of the interactions between those systems.

Factor Analyses and Surveys

As discussed in detail in *Volume 4*, two statistical techniques have been used by investigators to identify symptom clusters that could potentially be used to develop case definitions suggestive of a new syndrome: factor analysis and cluster analysis. Many of the studies reviewed by the committee use those techniques. The aims of the techniques are different: factor analysis seeks to identify groups of individuals' most prominent symptoms, whereas cluster analysis seeks to identify people who have similar symptoms. Factor analysis has been used far more frequently than cluster analysis in the major cohort studies. It seeks to identify a small number of groups of highly related variables among a much larger number of measured variables. In the context of Gulf War research, the measured variables are the symptoms that veterans report in surveys. Factor analysis aggregates veterans' symptoms into smaller groups to discern more fundamental, yet immeasurable, variables, which are referred to as factors.

Several factor analyses have been performed on Gulf War veterans (for example, Doebbling et al., 2000; Forbes et al., 2004) and were discussed in *Volume 4*. The update committee did not identify any new factor analysis studies of Gulf War veterans. In the initial such study, Haley and colleagues (1997) studied 249 Gulf War veterans and identified six factors that were suggested to constitute a Gulf War syndrome: syndrome 1—impaired cognition; syndrome 2—confusion-ataxia; syndrome 3—arthromyoneuropathy; syndrome 4—phobia-apraxia; syndrome 5—fever-adenopathy; and syndrome 6—weakness-incontinence. One potential limitation of this study was the relatively small cohort size and the absence of a nondeployed control group.

Another early factor analysis by Fukuda and colleagues at the CDC examined symptom sets in 3723 Air Force, Air Force Reserve, and Air National Guard veterans (1155 deployed and 2520 nondeployed). Two symptom complexes emerged as predominant: mood-cognition-fatigue and musculoskeletal. This group concluded that a chronic multisymptom illness (CMI) could be defined by the chronic presence (at least 6 months) of one or more symptoms from at least two of the following clusters: general fatigue, mood and cognitive abnormalities, and musculoskeletal pain (Fukuda et al., 1998). This syndrome was not completely specific to the Gulf War deployed veterans; the criteria were fulfilled by 39% of Gulf War veterans as compared to 14% of nondeployed veterans.

Nisenbaum et al. (2000) conducted a follow-up analysis of the cohort analyzed by Fukuda with the intention of defining a possible association between self-reported stressors in Gulf War deployment and the CMI. The authors surveyed 1002 (86.8%) cases including 58 (12.6%) and 401 (87.4%) classified as severe and mild to moderate. Participants were queried about potential stressors including type of primary duty, traumatic combat events, perception of a threat, preventive treatment for nerve gas exposure (pyridostigmine bromide), chemical hazards, adverse working conditions, family problems, and period of deployment. Multivariate analyses disclosed several self-reported factors that were associated with the higher likelihood of being a severe or mild-moderate case. Considering these two categories, the factors included (1) belief that biological or chemical weapons were used (OR 3.5, 95% CI 1.7-6.9, and OR 2.3, 95% CI 1.5-3.3, respectively), (2) pyridostigmine bromide use (OR 2.9, 95% CI 1.4-6.1, and OR 1.6, 95% CI 1.1-2.2, respectively), and (3) use of insect repellent (OR 2.4, 95% CI 1.3-4.5, and OR 1.7, 95% CI 1.2-2.3, respectively). Self-reported injuries were associated with severe illness (OR 2.1, 95% CI 1.1-4.3). The authors propose that "belief in a threat from biological or chemical weapons, suffering injuries that require medical attention, and use of insect repellent and pyridostigmine bromide, represent emotional, physical, and chemical stressors" that might lead to dysfunction of the hypothalamic-pituitary-adrenal and sympathetic-adrenal-medullary axes. In turn, this was thought potentially to cause "physiological and psychological changes" that might lead to chronic fatigue, mood-cognition, and musculoskeletal complaints.

In a population-based analysis, Ismail and associates (1999) identified three factors that accounted for 20% of the variance in UK Gulf War veterans: mood-cognition, respiratory symptoms, and peripheral nervous system symptoms. Comparison groups included cohorts of veterans who either served in Bosnia or were nondeployed. Many of the symptoms present in the Gulf War veterans were also present in Bosnian veterans.

Kang et al. (2002) performed another population-based factor analysis of 48 symptoms in larger cohorts of veterans either deployed (10,423 cases) or not deployed (8960) in the Gulf War. The study initially targeted 15,000 deployed veterans and 15,000 nondeployed veterans. One cluster of four symptoms was found to predominate (in mild or severe forms) in a subset of the Gulf War veterans (n = 277, 2.4%), who had also enhanced exposures to risk factors. A significantly higher prevalence of all 48 symptoms was observed among Gulf War deployed veterans compared to the nondeployed veterans (Kang et al., 2000). The four most frequently reported symptoms were runny nose, headache, unrefreshing sleep, and anxiety. Numerous chronic medical conditions—sinusitis, gastritis, and dermatitis—were reported more frequently by Gulf War veterans; many were reported about twice as often. The symptoms included blurred vision, loss of balance/dizziness, tremors/shaking, and speech difficulty. At least three of these four symptoms were present in 877 (7.7%) of the deployed veterans compared with 175 (1.8%) of the nondeployed veterans. The corresponding risk factors were consumption of contaminated food (for example, contaminated with oil or smoke), exposure to toxins (paint, solvents), and bathing in or drinking contaminated water. Kang and colleagues noted that a majority of cases (69%) with this set of four symptoms also met criteria for PTSD. Reciprocally, of cases meeting criteria for PTSD, about 11% experienced all four of these symptoms. Thus, these cases showed considerable overlap with PTSD. Also, when compared with the 6730 nondeployed veterans with none of the four symptoms, this group of 277 veterans had a higher incidence of other medical conditions, such as diarrhea, migraines, lumbago, hypertension, and tachycardia.

Ishoy et al. (1999a) conducted an epidemiological cross-sectional survey of 821 Danish veterans who had served as peacekeepers and in humanitarian relief in the Persian Gulf between April 1991 and January 1996, an interval that commenced after conclusion of the war. The veterans had a higher prevalence of neuropsychological, gastrointestinal, and skin symptoms when compared to controls. The neurological complaints included difficulty concentrating, sleep disturbance, fatigue, depression, headache, speech disturbances, and blurred vision. They also had more ICD-10 medical diagnoses compared with controls. Overall, the prevalence of these symptoms was about 20% greater, roughly comparable to the prevalence of such symptoms in US Gulf War veterans. Particularly striking was the development of these symptoms in a cohort whose tenure in the gulf began after conclusion of active war hostilities, implicating some common component of the experience that was, as the authors suggested, "independent of the actual war action."

Responses from the Iowa Persian Gulf Study were used by Doebbeling to explore whether there was a Persian Gulf War illness. The 1896 deployed veterans and 1799 nondeployed veterans were surveyed in 1995-1996 about the presence of 137 symptoms; the prevalence of symptoms was significantly increased in deployed (50%) compared with the nondeployed veterans (14%). Factor analyis identified three symptom clusters (somatic distress, psychological distress, and panic) in both the deployed and nondeployed veterans.

Whether there was a pattern to the multitude of symptoms reported by Australian male Gulf War veterans was studied by Forbes et al. (2004) also using factor analysis. The occurrence of 62 symptoms was assessed in 1322 deployed and 1459 nondeployed veterans. Three factors were identified—psycho-physiological distress, somatic distress, and arthroneuromuscular distress—in both deployed and nondeployed veterans. The authors report that the results did not suggest a unique pattern of self-reported symptoms in the deployed veterans.

To assess the persistence of multisymptom problems in Gulf War veterans, Blanchard (2006) performed a follow-up study of about 1061 deployed and 1128 nondeployed veterans who had participated in the initial studies of Gulf War CMI in the mid-1990s. Participants underwent examinations that included detailed medical and psychiatric histories, physical examinations (general and neurological), pulmonary function and nerve conduction tests, and both laboratory and neuropsychology studies. These investigators concluded that a decade after they were first studied, the Gulf War veterans showed a persistant prevalence of CMI (28.9%) compared with the nondeployed controls (15.8%). Moreover, the difference was exaggerated when only the most severely affected individuals were considered (7.0% vs 1.6%). In the deployed group, CMI correlated with higher combat exposure, while in the nondeployed group it correlated with full-time military service. CMI was associated with more fibromyalgia syndrome, chronic fatigue syndrome, arthralgias, dyspepsia, and metabolic syndrome in both the deployed and nondeployed cohorts. Among the deployed CMI cases, chronic fatigue syndrome was higher than in the nondeployed. In both groups (deployed and nondeployed), prewar non-PTSD anxiety disorders and depression were highly associated with CMI. The authors of this study conclude that "Ten years after the 1991 Gulf War, CMI is twice as prevalent in deployed veterans but still affects 15 percent of nondeployed veterans." They also note that at 10 years, the prevalence in the deployed group nonetheless seems to have decreased slowly over time; in the deployed group the 10-year prevalence (28.9%) is lower than it had been at 4 and 7 years (44.7% and 47%). Moreover, the authors argue that the critical predictor of CMI is stress. Blanchard and colleagues (2005) concluded with the caution that "Poor mental and physical functioning and metabolic syndrome in veterans with CMI portend a substantial future health-case burden."

Data from multiple factor studies of veterans in the United Kingdom and the United States were reanalyzed with a different statistical methodology involving dichtonous analysis of multiple lists of symptoms (Nisenbaum et al., 2004). This was undertaken to address the concern that biased findings may result when linear analysis of symptom sets is applied to data that are essentially binary (that is, a symptom is or is not present). The study's conclusions are broadly similar to those from other factor analyses: similar symptom categories are detected in Gulf War deployed and nondeployed veterans,

> except that the gastrointestinal factor in gulf veterans included other symptom types. Correlations among factors raise the question as to whether there is a general illness, even if not unique to gulf veterans, representing the common pathway underlying the identified factors.

Hospitalization Studies

Another approach to gauging the impact of Gulf War service is to assess the rates of hospitalizations of deployed versus nondeployed veterans in the years following deployment. Four studies have taken this approach. Gray et al. (1996) performed a retrospective multivariate, logistic regression analysis of the hospitalization rates of 547,076 deployed and 618,335 nondeployed veterans of the US Army, Navy, Marine Corps, and Air Force who remained on active duty through September 1993. In the 25-month period following the war (defined as August 1991 through September 1993), total hospitalizations of the deployed group were not increased as compared to the nondeployed group. In the deployed group, there was a small increase in admissions for testicular cancer and for genitourinary problems, ascribed in part to delayed care for problems that developed during the deployment itself. In the 25 months following the war, the deployed cohort had increased numbers of admissions for alcohol and drug abuse, and for adjustment reactions. The authors concluded that veterans of the Gulf War who remained on active duty through September 1993 were not at risk for unexplained disorders severe enough to merit hospitalization. They acknowledge that a potential limitation of this report is that it omits consideration of data both from those who left the military immediately after the war (before September 30, 1993) and from individuals whose symptoms developed after that date.

An extension of this study was subsequently provided by Knoke and colleagues (1998). These authors tested the hypothesis that the study by Gray et al. (1996) may have underestimated admissions for veterans with obscure, undiagnosed disorders, which might be missed by conventional ICD-9 coding. In this follow-up study, Knoke reviewed all admissions that entailed any "illness of unknown cause" as defined by 77 ICD-9 categories used by the CDC Emerging Infections Program to monitor death certificates for unexplained deaths. This study reviewed records for 552,111 deployed and 1,495,751 nondeployed veterans followed through March 1996. Briefly, after excluding a surge of admissions for evaluation of symptoms of unknown causes, this study found no excess of hospitalization for unexplained illnesses in deployed versus nondeployed veteran.

To encompass in this study those veterans who left service prior to September 1993 (for example, reservists and former veterans), Gray et al. (2000) also performed an analysis of all veterans admitted to three health-care systems in California, covering the deployment period 1991-1994. Because of limitations in acquiring data for discharged veterans, this study compared proportional morbidity ratios of discharge diagnoses between deployed and nondeployed veterans in each of the three systems, rather than hospitalization rates. Most major disease categories revealed no differences (for example, infectious diseases and cancer); in general, the deployed Gulf War veterans had overall proportions of hospitalizations that were similar to the nondeployed. The deployed cohort had a slight propensity for more hospitalizations for fractures, soft-tissue injuries, asthma, and other symptoms. The significance of these factors was difficult to assess.

Recently, Smith et al. (2006) have reexamined hospitalization rates using a longer follow-up period and including three comparative groups from three military theaters: Gulf War (lapsed time 10 years, 5 months, n = 445,465), post-Gulf War southwest Asia (9 years, 5 months, n = 249,047), and Bosnia (5 years, 1 month, n = 44,341). The central finding in this study is that individuals deployed to southwest Asia had slightly more hospitalizations that the Gulf War cohort, while the risk of hospitalization was slightly decreased for the Bosnian cohort. The authors conclude "It is unlikely that Gulf War veterans are at greater risk of hospitalization duc to specific exposure-related disease."

Other Reports

In a follow-up study to Kang et al. (2000, 2002), Kang et al. (2009) conducted a survey in 2005 to obtain health information from the 15,000 Gulf War deployed and 15,000 Gulf War era veterans originally surveyed in 1995. Responses to the postal questionnaire were received from 6111 deployed and 3859 era veterans. Unexplained multisymptom illness was assessed and defined as having several different symptoms that persisted for 6 months or longer and were not adequately explained by other diagnoses. Symptoms might include fatigue, muscle or joint pain, headaches, memory problems, digestive problems, respiratory problems, skin problems, or any other unexplained symptoms. Multisymptom illness was reported by 36.5% of the deployed and 11.7% of the era veterans for a risk ratio of 3.05 (95% CI 2.77-3.36), adjusted for age, sex, race, body mass index, current cigarette smoking, rank, branch of service, and unit component (active duty, National Guard, or reserve). This was the mostly widely reported medical condition for Gulf War veterans except for hepatitis. This study is limited in that only self-reports of symptoms were assessed.

To determine if framing the questions regarding health and symptoms might influence symptom reporting, Murphy et al. (2006) surveyed a group of 1647 UK active-duty military personnel about health problems 10 years after the Gulf War. Of those surveyed, 308 were subsequently identified as having served in the Gulf War while 1339 had not. Those deployed to the Gulf War were more likely than the control veterans to score above a cutoff on the 15-item symptom checklist (OR 1.84, 95% CI 1.17-2.91) and more likely to report the following individual symptoms, adjusted for age, sex, rank, and service branch: chest pain (OR 2.50, 95% CI 1.58-3.96); fatigue (OR 1.37, 95% CI 1.03-1.81); joint stiffness (OR 1.53, 95% CI 1.10-2.12); pain without swelling or redness in several joints (OR 1.60, 95% CI 1.07-2.39); feeling feverish (OR 2.66, 95% CI 1.05-6.73); feeling unrefreshed after sleep (OR 1.83, 95% CI 1.26-2.65); lump in throat (OR 3.21, 95% CI 1.39-7.41); diarrhea (OR 3.18, 95% CI 1.76-5.76); sore throat (OR 1.93, 95% CI 1.04-3.56); forgetfulness (OR 2.53, 95% CI 1.69-3.77); and ringing in ears (OR 1.82, 95% CI 1.08-3.10). The authors noted that among those surveyed, veterans who had served in the Gulf War were still in the military 10 years later whereas those who were not in the Gulf War may not have served that long, although the age distribution of the two cohorts was the same. The questionnaire did not ask any of the veterans about service in the Gulf War or other conflicts. This study is limited in that veterans who did not serve in the Gulf War may have served in other conflicts. Also, there was no assessment by a health-care professional (that is all symptoms were self-reports) and the study group was restricted to active-duty personnel, and therefore, veterans who may have served in the Gulf War or during the era and who had left the service were not included, perhaps leading to a healthy warrior bias.

Stimpson et al. (2006) surveyed UK veterans who had served only in the Gulf War (n = 2959), only in Bosnia (n = 2052), or both in the Gulf War and in Bosnia (n = 570), and a comparison era group of veterans who had not been deployed to either the Gulf War or Bosnia (n = 2614) for self-reports of CWP. A mailed questionnaire containing a pain manikin to ascertain the pattern and intensity of pain was sent to 12,592 male and female veterans in 1997; the response rate was 60-70%. Veterans were selected for each deployment group on the basis of stratified random sampling of all UK Gulf War veterans. Data from the shaded manikins were used to determine whether the pain pattern met the ACR definition of CWP. Compared with the era cohort, being deployed to the Gulf War increased the risk of reporting widespread pain (OR 1.82, 95% CI 1.51-2.20); being deployed to Bosnia did not increase the risk of reporting CWP (OR 1.06, 95% CI 0.83-1.36), but being deployed to both the Gulf War and Bosnia resulted in the most reporting of CWP (OR 2.04, 95% CI 1.52-2.73), even when adjusted for socioeconomic and demographic factors. The pattern of pain was similar in all the groups; the most common sites of pain were the back and knees. Veterans who reported pain in one limb were also 30 times more likely to report pain in the symmetrically opposite limb rather than a second limb on the same side of the body; the authors found this suggestive of "systemic pain" rather than pain from an injury. Although the sample was large, the study is limited by a lack of physical examination and a lack of indication as to whether the veterans had sustained injuries during deployment or were using pain medication at the time of the survey.

Using data from a self-report questionnaire, Proctor et al. (1998) compared health problems of 252 Gulf War deployed veterans from Fort Devens, Massachusetts, and New Orleans, Louisiana, with those of 48 era veterans who had been deployed to Germany. Among the musculoskeletal symptoms reported more frequently by the Fort Devens deployed veterans were joint pains (OR 2.6) and neck aches or stiffness (OR 2.7), and among the neurological symptoms with greater prevalence in both cohorts of deployed veterans were headaches (OR 4.2); all confidence intervals excluded 1.0. About 30% of the Gulf War veterans and 11% of the comparison group reported an inability to fall asleep (OR 3.4-3.6, 95% CI excludes 1.0).

Horn et al. (2006) compared the frequency of symptom reporting between deployed and era UK veterans of Gulf War and Iraq War. Iraq War veterans did not show the difference in symptom reporting between deployed (n = 3284) and nondeployed (n = 2408) male military personnel that had been seen for Gulf War veterans. The prevalence of each of the 15 most frequently reported symptoms for Gulf War veterans was significantly greater than for era veterans (ORs 1.9-3.9, all 95% CIs exclude 1.0). Compared with era veterans, more than 50% of the Gulf War deployed veterans reported feeling unrefreshed after sleep (OR 2.8, 95% CI 2.5-3.1), irritability or outbursts of anger (OR 3.5, 95% CI 3.2-4.0), headaches (OR 2.1, 95% CI 1.9-2.3), and fatigue (OR 2.7, 95% CI 2.4-3.0). Compared with era veterans, deployed veterans were three times more likely to be a fatigue case (based on a validated 13-item fatigue scale; OR 3.39, 95% CI 3.00-3.83) and twice as likely to report fair or poor general health (OR 2.00, 95% CI 1.70-2.35). UK Iraq war veterans showed no increase in fatigue or reports of poor or fair general health compared with their nondeployed counterparts.

Summary and Conclusions

There is increased reporting of multisymptom illness among those deployed in the Gulf War as seen in most of the studies conducted on Gulf War veterans. The phenomenon, which recurs in multiple studies from several countries, is predominantly subjective, without a consistent accompanying pattern of findings on physical examination or laboratory testing. The basis for this problem remains elusive but merits further analysis, along the lines of the investigations summarized in Chapter 5.

The committee concludes that there is sufficient evidence of association between deployment to Gulf War and chronic multisymptom illness.

Chronic Fatigue Syndrome

Chronic fatigue syndrome (CFS) is marked by severe and persistent fatigue with a cluster of other symptoms that have long been the focus of considerable controversy (Straus, 1991; Wessely, 1998). The study of unexplained fatiguing illnesses was greatly facilitated and legitimized in the last decade with the development of a case definition sponsored by the CDC (Box 4-1). CDC's case definition requires fatigue and related impairment in function, and the occurrence of four of eight other defining symptoms over at least 6 months (Fukuda et al., 1994;

Holmes et al., 1998). Of the eight symptoms, the most commonly reported are headaches, postexertional malaise, impaired cognition, and muscle pain (Buchwald and Garrity, 1994).

CFS is a diagnosis of exclusion. The CDC criteria require that three elements be completed as part of a comprehensive evaluation. The first element, determining whether the symptom criteria for CFS are present, requires that a person be queried specifically about length and severity of fatigue and about eight ancillary symptoms. The second element, determining whether other medical conditions are present, mandates a complete physical examination, a battery of specified laboratory tests, and a medical history. The third element, assessing exclusionary psychiatric conditions, requires an interview by a trained professional to obtain diagnostic information.

The etiology of CFS is unknown, and there are no widely accepted laboratory tests or pathologic physical signs (Epstein, 1995). Several biologic correlates of the syndrome have emerged, including dysregulation of the hypothalamic-pituitary-adrenal axis, immune activation, and other measures (Goshorn, 1998), but they might be present in only a minority of patients; and those findings are not specific to CFS. Although infectious agents may trigger some cases of CFS, a complex, multifactorial etiology that incorporates biologic, psychological, and social factors is likely (Wessely, 1998). The degree of disability associated with CFS is striking, with high rates of unemployment (Bombardier and Buchwald, 1996; Buchwald, 1996) and poor quality of life related to health (Hardt et al., 2001; Komaroff et al., 1996).

Thus, in this report, a primary study for CFS is one in which CFS has been diagnosed. A secondary study is one in which a CFS-like condition has been documented. Both primary and secondary studies needed to include a suitable control group so that findings could be interpreted. Other studies that estimated the prevalence of symptoms of "chronic fatigue" (Gray et al., 1999a; Unwin et al., 1999), or multisymptom illness (Fukuda et al., 1998), are not considered further in this section. Likewise, studies that used scalar measures of disability and poor quality of life related to health (Reid et al., 2001) as surrogates for the CDC criteria are not included. Finally, self-reports of CFS (Unwin et al., 1999) and self-reports of a physician diagnosis of CFS (Gray et al., 2002) were not included among the secondary studies because diagnostic data obtained that way are highly inaccurate. For example, in the Eisen et al. (2005) study, which the committee considered to be the only primary study, only two or three of 38 deployed and eight nondeployed veterans who self-reported CFS received a formal diagnosis after a comprehensive examination. Others, using a method of classifying a case of CFS based on cutoff scores on a fatigue scale and a functional status instrument, found that only 11% of veterans reporting a diagnosis of CFS met operational CFS study criteria.

Summary of *Volume 4*

Primary Studies

CFS was one of 12 primary health outcome measures studied by Eisen et al. (2005), who conducted medical evaluations in phase III of the nationally representative, population-based VA study. In the period 1999-2001, 1061 of 11,441 deployed and 1128 of 9476 nondeployed veterans selected were evaluated. Those veterans had participated in the phase I survey study conducted in 1995 (Kang et al., 2000). The veterans were randomly selected, and the researchers were blinded to their deployment status. The diagnosis of CFS was based on in-person interviews, examinations, and the strict application of the CDC criteria (Fukuda et al., 1994). The authors concluded that the population prevalence of CFS was higher in deployed than in nondeployed veterans: 1.6% vs 0.1% (OR 40.6, 95% CI 10.2-161.15). Study strengths are its

BOX 4-1
CDC Case Definition of Chronic Fatigue Syndrome

A diagnosis of chronic fatigue syndrome requires the presence of both the following:

- Clinically evaluated, unexplained, persistent or relapsing chronic fatigue that is of new or definite onset (that is, has not been lifelong), is not the result of ongoing exertion, is not substantially alleviated by rest, and results in substantial reduction in levels of occupational, educational, social, or personal activities. Clinical evaluation includes medical history, physical examination, laboratory studies, and psychiatric assessment.
- Concurrent occurrence of four or more of the following, which must have persisted or recurred during 6 or more consecutive months of illness and must not have predated the fatigue: self-reported impairment of short-term memory or concentration severe enough to cause substantial reduction in levels of occupational, educational, social, or personal activities; sore throat; tender cervical or axillary lymph nodes; muscle pain; multijoint pain without joint swelling or redness; headaches of a new type, pattern, or severity; unrefreshing sleep; and postexertional malaise lasting more than 24 hours.

SOURCE: Fukuda et al. (1994).

large, population-based design, stratified sampling method, analysis of participation bias, comprehensive examination, and use of computer-based algorithms by researchers who were blinded to deployment status. Study limitations include demographic differences between the deployed and nondeployed cohorts and the relatively low rate of participation in the study.

Secondary Studies

An earlier questionnaire study, conducted during phase I of the VA study, surveyed 11,441 deployed and 9476 nondeployed veterans (Kang et al., 2003). Several items in the 48-item symptom questionnaire served as the basis for meeting the case definition for CFS. After exclusion of veterans who self-reported medical conditions that could explain their fatigue, 4.9% of deployed and 1.2% of nondeployed veterans (OR 4.2, 95% CI 3.3-5.5) met the case definition. The investigators found that CFS was not related to the severity of combat stressors. The latter was assessed according to responses to questions on wearing chemical protective gear or hearing chemical alarms, being involved in direct combat duty, or witnessing any deaths. The study was limited by its reliance on solely self-reported symptoms without a physical or laboratory examination and on self-reported physician-diagnosed conditions. Thosc shortcomings resulted in a higher rate of CFS-like illness than was observed when the same cohorts were sampled and underwent more rigorous medical evaluations as in Eisen et al. (2005).

Proctor and colleagues (2001b) conducted in-person interviews of 180 Army veterans selected from the larger Fort Devens cohort to determine the prevalence of CFS. The deployed veterans were compared with 46 members of an air ambulance company deployed to Germany during the Gulf War. The prevalence was determined according to the symptom criteria specified by the CDC case definition (Fukuda et al., 1994). With that approach, the rate was higher in the Gulf War deployed than the Germany deployed group (7.5% vs 0%, $p = 0.02$). When additional information from self-reported medical or psychiatric conditions (such as substance abuse and bipolar disorder) and clinical psychiatric interviews was considered, the prevalence in Gulf War veterans decreased to 2%, which was no longer significant. The study demonstrated the importance of performing psychiatric assessments, but it was limited by the relatively small sample and the lack of medical or laboratory evaluations.

Canada deployed more than 4000 sea, land, and air troops to the gulf region; they participated in a naval blockade and were responsible for one-fourth of enemy interceptions in the gulf. A survey of the entire Canadian Gulf War force found that deployed veterans were at least five times as likely as nondeployed veterans to report symptoms of CFS (OR 5.27, 95% CI 3.95-7.03) (Goss Gilroy, 1998). Veterans were not interviewed or examined, and all data were obtained from self-reports. The CFS-like illness was based on responses to questions derived from the CDC criteria and a score above zero on the Chalder fatigue scale.[4] With only minor modifications, the items used in this study were the same as those used by the Iowa Persian Gulf Study Group (1997). The study was limited by the lack of in-person interviews and examinations and by the nontraditional assessment of CFS.

The Iowa Persian Gulf study (1997) surveyed 1896 deployed and 1799 nondeployed veterans who listed Iowa as their home state at the time of enlistment. The presence of a CFS-like condition was based on a combination of symptoms used in the CDC criteria (Fukuda et al., 1994) and scores on the Chalder fatigue scale. The investigators found that the prevalence differed by 1.4% (95% CI 0.9-2.0) after adjusting for age, sex, race, branch of military, and rank. Study limitations were the use of self-reports of symptoms on a questionnaire and the lack of medical evaluations. Although rigorously conducted and analyzed, the study suffers shortcomings similar to those of the Canadian study.

Updated and Supplemental Literature

The Update committee identified two new primary studies: Kelsall et al. (2006), who assessed health outcomes in Australian Gulf War veterans with chronic fatigue, and Ismail et al. (2008), who assessed UK Gulf War veterans for chronic fatigue and related disorders.

Between August 2000 and April 2002, Kelsall et al. (2006) conducted a cross-sectional study of chronic fatigue in male Australian Gulf War veterans. A total of 1456 deployed veterans participated (80.5% response rate of all who were deployed), and a comparison group consisted of 1588 individuals who served concurrently but were not deployed (56.8% response rate). Ascertainment was via a postal questionnaire plus a comprehensive medical evaluation that included neurologic and psychiatric tests, as well as the following laboratory tests: complete blood examination; erythrocyte sedimentation rate; urea; creatinine; electrolytes; serum calcium and phosphate; liver function tests; random plasma glucose; C-reactive protein; and serology tests (Epstein-Barr virus IgG, cytomegalovirus IgG, and hepatitis C core antibody). One percent of the Gulf War veterans and the comparison group had been diagnosed with CFS (adjusted OR 1.2, 95% CI 0.5-2.9). However, more Gulf War deployed veterans (7.9%) had prolonged fatigue lasting more than 6 months than did the comparison group (4.2%; aOR 1.9; 95% CI 1.4-2.7); and a similar increase was noted in the complaint of fatigue at all levels in the deployed group. In a small subset of controls who had been actively deployed elsewhere, the differences in complaints of chronic or prolonged fatigue were less apparent compared with the Gulf War deployed individuals and in fact failed to reach statistical significance; thus, there was an apparent active deployment effect. The odds of fatigue increased with reports of more PB tablets used, exposure to pesticides, belief in being near chemical weapons, and being in the gulf during air war. The strengths of this study are its relatively large size and national ascertainment. The weakness is

[4]The Chalder fatigue scale is widely used to measure physical and mental fatigue in CFS patients (Chalder et al., 1993).

that the exposure and symptom history was ascertained by self-report, raising a substantial possibility of biased recall.

Ismail et al. (2008) reported the prevalence of CFS and related disorders in UK veterans of the Gulf War. In this two-phase cohort study, randomly selected subsamples from a population-based cross-sectional postal survey of more than 10,000 military personnel were compared with control groups that included Bosnian peacekeepers and nondeployed military personnel. Comparisons were matched for total level of disability using a physical functioning scale. Gulf War veterans were more likely to be overweight, to be hypertensive, and to have elevated serum transaminase (AAT) levels. (It is possible that the AAT levels may reflect being overweight.) Among the disabled veterans, the adjusted OR for CFS was 7.8 (95% CI 2.5-24.5). CFS was present in 18% of disabled Gulf War veterans compared with only 3% of disabled nondeployed veterans. Remarkably, rates for other medically explainable conditions were not increased, indicating that the CFS symptoms were specifically increased in the Gulf War deployed population. Over half of veterans satisfying criteria for CFS had concomitant depression or anxiety disorder. The authors concluded that CFS was a medically unexplained condition associated with Gulf War service.

The Update committee identified one new secondary study. Lucas et al. (2007) administered a questionnaire about wartime exposures and symptoms experienced in 49 Gulf War veterans complaining of chronic fatigue matched to 44 healthy controls who were also deployed. For the purposes of the study, fatigue had to begin by July 1992. Fatigue was associated with exposure to oil fire, smoke, pesticides, contaminated food or water, Scud missiles, dead bodies, dead animals, and other environmental agents. There was also an association of fatigue with use of PB that increased 1.3% with every pill taken; there were also general trends toward worse health with PB exposure. This study was markedly limited by a very small sample size and a small number of individuals with PB intake data. There was also no adjustment made for multiple comparisons.

Summary and Conclusions

CFS and complaints of unexplained chronic fatigue appear to be increased in deployed Gulf War veterans compared to contemporaneous cohorts (either nondeployed or deployed elsewhere). This has been observed in several cross-sectional population-based studies that used self-reports to define CFS or chronic fatigue. However, the absolute prevalence of these symptoms has varied considerably from study to study. Associations between fatigue, subjective neurological symptoms, and exposures are also based entirely on retrospective self-reports.

Therefore, the committee concludes that there is a sufficient evidence for an association between deployment to the Gulf War and chronic fatigue syndrome. The underlying basis of the possible relationship is unclear, however, and further research is recommended.

TABLE 4-15 Multisymptom Illnesses

Reference	Design	Population	Outcomes	Results	Adjustments	Comments
Factor analyses and surveys						
Haley and Kurt, 1997 (Vol. 4)	Exploratory factor analysis of 52 symptoms	Active-duty and retired Navy GWVs (n = 249)	Factor-analysis derived syndromes	Impaired cognition Confusion-ataxia Arthromyoneuropathy Phobia-apraxia Fever-adenopathy Weakness-incontinence		Small cohort size, no nondeployed control group Accounted for 71% of observed variance
Fukuda et al., 1998 (Vol. 4)	Cross-sectional population survey; factor analysis (of 35 symptoms) to identify symptom categories in combination with clinical reasoning	3675 members of the air force, including National Guard, reserve, and active-duty components (1155 GWVs and 2520 NDVs) Factor analysis: n = 3255	Cases defined as having one or more symptoms from at least two of the three identified symptom categories: Fatigue Mood-cognition Musculoskeletal	GWV vs NDV: Mild-to-moderate cases (449 vs 354) OR 4.08 (95% CI 3.39-4.93) Severe cases (68 vs 18) OR 16.18 (95% CI 8.99-29.14)	Rank, sex, age, smoking status	Symptom categories accounted for 39% of common variance
Nisenbaum et al., 2000	Cross-sectional survey	1002 air force GWVs selected from the population described by Fukuda et al. (1998)	Association of self-reported exposures with mild-to-moderate and severe cases, as defined by Fukuda et al. (1998)	Belief that biological or chemical weapons were used, OR 3.5 (95% CI 1.7-6.9) and OR 2.3 (95% CI 1.5-3.3); PB, OR 2.9 (95% CI 1.4-6.1) and OR 1.6 (95% CI 1.1-2.2); Insect repellent, OR 2.4 (95% CI 1.3-4.5) and OR 1.7 (95% CI 1.2-2.3); Injuries requiring medical attention, severe cases only OR = 2.1 (95% CI 1.1-4.3)	Age, sex, smoking status, current rank	All exposures self-reported
Ismail et al., 1999 (Vol. 4)	Exploratory factor analysis of 52 symptoms (Based on survey conducted by	3214 male UK GWVs compared to 1770 Bosnia veterans and 2384 nondeployed era	Symptom categories	Mood-cognition Respiratory symptoms Peripheral nervous system symptoms Frequency of symptom reporting		Response rates: GWVs (76%), Bosnia veterans (42%), era veterans (56%) Factor categories

Reference	Design	Population	Outcomes	Results	Adjustments	Comments
	Unwin et al., 1999)	veterans		higher in GWVs compared to Bosnia and era cohorts, but similar correlations between symptoms for all cohorts		accounted for 20% of the common variance
Kang et al., 2002 (Vol. 4)	Exploratory factor analysis of 47 symptoms	GWVs (n = 10,423) compared to nondeployed era veterans (n = 8960)	Symptom clusters; association of symptom clusters with self-reported exposures	Five similar symptom clusters were found in both groups: Fatigue or depression Musculoskeletal/rheumatologic Gastrointestinal Pulmonary Upper respiratory Four symptoms comprised a neurologic cluster that appeared to be unique to GWVs: blurred vision, loss of balance/dizziness, tremors/shaking, and speech difficulty. 277 (2.4%) GWVs reported mild or severe problems with these symptoms, compared to 43 (0.45%) nondeployed. In addition, at least 3 out of 4 of these symptoms were observed in 877 (7.7%) GWVs vs 175 (1.8%) nondeployed veterans Exposures associated with four-symptom cases (n = 277) vs nonsymptomatic controls (n = 6730), $p < 0.0001$: Contaminated food (73% vs 21%); nerve gas (42% vs 5%); DU (29% vs 7%); toxic paint (51% vs 16%); bathed in or drank contaminated water (60% vs 19%); sexual assault (3.3% vs 0.4%); sexual harassment (15% vs 3%); Botulism vaccine (26% vs 9%)		69% response rate in GWVs and 60% in era controls 69% of the GWVs suffering all four symptoms also met criteria for PTSD

Reference	Design	Population	Outcomes	Results	Adjustments	Comments
Ishoy et al., 1999a (Vol. 4)	Cross-sectional	686 Danish peacekeepers deployed to gulf in 1990-1997 vs 231 age- and sex-matched armed forces nondeployed controls	Health examination by physician, including lung function and self-report questionnaire of symptoms	Deployed veterans reported higher prevalence ($p < 0.05$) of 17 out of 22 neuropsychological symptoms, 8 out of 14 gastrointestinal symptoms, and 8 out of 19 skin symptoms 81% of deployed veterans compared to 71% of controls had one or more ICD-10 diagnoses at examination ($p = 0.002$)		Participation rate: 83.6% deployed, 57.8% nondeployed
Blanchard et al., 2006 (Update)	Cross-sectional	1035 GWVs vs 1116 NDVs	CMI determined by medical examination in 1999-2001	Deployed vs nondeployed: CMI (all cases), 29% vs 16% (OR 2.16, 95% CI 1.61-2.90) Mild to moderate cases, 25% vs 15% (OR 1.92, 95% CI 1.41-2.63) Severe cases, 7% vs 1.6% (OR 4.65, 95% CI 2.27-9.52)	Age, sex, race, education, duty type, service branch, rank, income, combat exposure score, Khamisiyah exposure, psychiatric and other diagnoses prior to GW	Participation rate: 52% deployed, 39% nondeployed
Nisenbaum et al., 2004 (Vol. 4)	Dichotomous factor analysis (Reanalysis of survey results from Fukuda et al., 1998, and Ismail et al., 1999)	3454 male UK GWVs compared to 1979 Bosnia veterans and 2577 nondeployed era veterans 1163 deployed US Air Force veterans	Symptom clusters	UK cohort: Identified a cluster of gastrointestinal/urogenital symptoms that loaded to deployed veterans but not to either control group Confirmed factors identified by Ismail et al. (1999) were very similar across all three cohorts US Cohort: Gastrointestinal/respiratory Allergies Mood-cognition Musculoskeletal		No control group in US cohort

Reference	Design	Population	Outcomes	Results	Adjustments	Comments
Hospitalization studies						
Gray et al., 1996 (Update)	Retrospective cohort, hospitalizations from August 1991 through September 1993	547,076 active-duty GWVs, 618,335 NDVs	Hospital-discharge diagnoses of circulatory system disease in DoD hospital system (ICD-9 classification)	No increase in any-cause hospitalization among deployed GWVs	Prewar hospitalization, sex, age, race, service branch, marital status, rank, length of service, salary, occupation	Very short follow-up period; no outpatient data; restriction to DoD hospitals, and thus to persons remaining on active duty after the war; no adjustment for potential confounders such as smoking
Knoke et al., 1998 (Update)		552,111 deployed vs 1,479,751 nondeployed servicemembers in service during Gulf War and remaining there through 1996	Hospitalization records: DoD only, 1991-1996, ICD 799.9 (unexplained illness)	No excess in hospitalizations in this period when effect of CCEP was eliminated	Race, rank, salary, military branch, occupation, prewar hospitalization, sex	Active duty only, no assessment of outpatient treatment, respiratory findings removed after adjustment for VA screening-program attendance
Gray et al., 2000 (Update)	Retrospective cohort, hospitalizations from August 1991 through December 1994	652,979 GWVs, 652,922 randomly selected NDVs: 182,164 DoD hospitalizations; 16,030 VA hospitalizations; 5185 COSHPD hospitalizations	Hospital-discharge diagnoses in DoD, VA, and COSHPD hospital systems	Similar rates of hospitalization between deployed and nondeployed veterans	Age, sex, race (only for DoD PMR)	Able to assess only illnesses that resulted in hospitalization; possible undetected confounders PMR has lower sensitivity than a comparison of hospitalization rates would have
Smith et al., 2006 (Update)	Retrospective cohort study (cohort data from DMDC)	Active-duty personnel with a single deployment to: Gulf War theater (n = 455,465); southwest Asia, 1991-1998 (n = 249,047); Bosnia, 1995-1998 (n = 44,341)	Postdeployment hospitalization events (1991-2000)	Veterans of southwest Asia had slightly higher rate of hospitalization compared to deployed GWVs, while veterans of Bosnia had slightly lower rate of hospitalizations	Sex, age, marital status, pay grade, race/ethnicity, service branch, occupation, and predeployment hospitalization; time-dependent	Lower hazard ratio observed in veterans of Bosnia may be partially explained by shorter follow-up period Limitations: active-duty personnel only; hospitalizations at DoD facilities only

Reference	Design	Population	Outcomes	Results	Adjustments	Comments
					covariate to account for changing hospitalization methods, diagnostic criteria, and procedures	
Chronic fatigue syndrome (CFS)						
Eisen et al., 2005 (Vol. 4)	Population-based, cross-sectional, prevalence, in-person medical and psychiatric evaluations	1061 GWVs vs 1128 NDVs; selected from among those who had participated in 1995 National Health Survey of Gulf War Era Veterans and Their Families (mail and telephone survey) (Kang et al., 2000)	CFS based on in-person interviews according to CDC CFS criteria and exclusionary diagnoses from history, interviews, examinations, laboratory testing	OR 40.6, 95% CI 10.2-161.2	Age, sex, race, smoking, duty type, service branch, rank	Low participation rates (53% of deployed and 39% of nondeployed), but analysis of nonparticipants and participants reveals that participants, both deployed and nondeployed, are more likely to report symptoms of CFS
Kelsall et al., 2006 (Update)	Cross-sectional survey	1424 Australian male GWVs, 1548 male NDVs frequency matched by age and service type (Same population as Kelsall et al., 2004a,b, 2005)	Association of unexplained chronic fatigue and CFS determined in clinical assessment with self-reported exposure to various stressors	CFS in deployed veterans vs control groups OR 1.2 (95% CI 0.5-2.9) Chronic fatigue (≥ 6 months) OR 1.9 (95% CI 1.4-2.7) 91 (6.6%) GWVs had unexplained chronic fatigue vs 40 (2.9%) of controls (OR 2.3, 95% CI 1.6-3.4) Unexplained chronic fatigue in GWVs associated with PB (OR 2.8, 95% CI 1.3-6.1), oil smoke (OR 2.0, 95% CI 1.2-3.4), pesticides (OR 2.4, 95% CI 1.5-3.8), presence in chemical weapons area (OR 4.6, 95% CI	Age, service branch, rank; also education, marital status, smoking, and alcohol use for unexplained chronic fatigue.	Relatively large study with national ascertainment; response rate 80.5% for deployed, 56.8% for nondeployed Exposures self-reported; possible recall bias

Reference	Design	Population	Outcomes	Results	Adjustments	Comments
				2.7-7.8), and deployed during air war (OR 2.3, 95% CI 1.1-4.5)		
Ismail et al., 2008 (Update)	Two-phase cohort study; first phase population-based postal survey, second phase random sample of disabled phase 2 responders	111 deployed GWVs; 133 era veterans, including Bosnia peacekeepers; must have physical disability (less than 72.2 on SF-36 physical functioning scale from phase 1 survey) (Population derived from Unwin et al., 1999, and Ismail et al., 2002)	CFS determined through clinical assessment using CDC criteria	20 disabled GWVs (18%) and 4 disabled controls (3%), OR 7.8, 95% CI 2.5-24.5	Age, sex, rank, marital status, alcohol-disorders, selection bias via probability weights	Phase 1 response rate 70% for GWVs, 60% and 63% for Bosnia and era veterans, respectively. Phase 2 response rate 67% for GWVs, 55% and 43% for Bosnia and era veterans, respectively. 54% of GWVs with CFS had concomitant depression or anxiety disorder

NOTE: CCEP = Comprehensive Clinical Evaluation Program; CDC = Centers for Disease Control and Prevention; CFS = chronic fatigue syndrome; CI = confidence interval; CMI = chronic multisymptom illness; COSHPD = California Office of Statewide Health Planning and Development; CWP = chronic widespread pain; DMDC = Defense Manpower Data Center; DoD = Department of Defense; DU = depleted uranium; GWV = Gulf War veteran; NDV = nondeployed veteran; OR = odds ratio; PB = pyridostigmine bromide; PMR = personal medical record; VA = Department of Veterans Affairs.

EXTERNAL CAUSES OF MORTALITY

This section evaluates the findings on external causes of death among Gulf War veterans. Examples of major subgroups within this category include deaths due to accidents, such as motor vehicle accidents, and homicides and suicides. Studies of veterans of other wars, such as the Vietnam War, have found increased mortality from external causes, particularly in the years immediately following deployment (IOM, 2006). Primary studies on the mortality of Gulf War veterans are summarized in Table 4-16.

Summary of *Volume 4*

Primary Studies

For external causes of mortality, the Volume 4 committee identified four studies that met the criteria for primary studies (DASA, 2005; Kang and Bullman, 1996, 2001; Macfarlane et al., 2000).

In the first large mortality study of US Gulf War veterans, Kang and Bullman (1996) examined records from the VA BIRLS and deaths reported to the SSA for the period from 1991 to 1993.[5] The authors identified no excess all-cause mortality in deployed (n = 695,516) veterans compared with nondeployed veterans (n = 746,291), adjusted for age, race, marital status, branch of service, and type of unit. However, they did find higher mortality from motor vehicle accidents among deployed than among nondeployed veterans (RR 1.31, 95% CI 1.14-1.49), although the risk was lower than the expected rate based on overall US mortality (SMR 0.82, 95% CI 0.75-0.89) after adjustment for age, sex, race, and year of death. No increase in suicide or homicide among Gulf War veterans was found (Kang and Bullman, 1996). In a subsequent publication, Kang and Bullman (2001) found no excess mortality from motor vehicle accidents after 1993, a mortality pattern which is consistent with that following the Vietnam War (CDC, 1987; Thomas et al., 1991; Watanabe and Kang, 1995). Suicide rates were about equal through 1997 in deployed and nondeployed veterans (MRR 0.92, 95% CI 0.83-1.02). This later study again found no difference in all-cause mortality between deployed and nondeployed veterans, although it did find that the mortality rate in both cohorts was less than half of that expected for their civilian counterparts (Kang and Bullman, 2001).

Macfarlane et al. (2000) found no significant increase in mortality between UK Gulf War veterans (n = 53,462) and a control group of contemporaneous veterans (n = 53,450) matched by sex, age, branch of service, and level of fitness, the last factor included in an attempt to account for the healthy warrior effect. A small increase in accidental death was noted, but confidence intervals included 1.0 (MRR 1.18, 95% CI 0.98-1.42). The increase was primarily due to motor vehicle accidents (MRR 1.25, 95% CI 0.91-1.72). They did not did not address changes over time in excess external cause (or motor vehicle) mortality and did not find higher suicide or homicide rates in deployed compared to nondeployed veterans.

The UK Defence Analystical Service Agency (DASA, 2005) periodically publishes cumulative mortality figures for deployed veterans compared with Gulf War era controls. From April 1, 1991, to December 31, 2007, Gulf War veterans had no significant increase in mortality;

[5]The degree of completeness of these record systems was assessed with a validation study that used state vital-statistics data. Ascertainment was estimated at 89% of all deaths in the Gulf War cohort and comparison group.

however, DASA (2005) did observe small nonsignificant increases in transportation accident mortality (SMR 1.21, 95% CI 0.96-1.51), intentional self-harm (SMR 1.08, 95% CI 0.85-1.39), and other accidental mortality—including falls, drowning, and poisoning (SMR 1.07, 95% CI 0.74-1.54), but by 2007, these differences were not significant (DASA, 2009). When compared with earlier surveillance, these data show that any difference in the rate of external cause mortality in deployed veterans versus the era controls disappeared approximately 10 years after the war (DASA, 2005).

Secondary Studies

Two studies of external cause mortality in Gulf War veterans were identified as secondary studies by the Volume 4 committee. Writer et al. (1996) found an increased rate of noncombat mortality due to accidental injury in US active-duty troops stationed in the Gulf War compared to troops on active duty elsewhere between 1990 and 1991 (69% vs 41%, no indication of significance given). In a nested case-control study using the Gulf War-deployed and nondeployed cohorts assembled by Kang and colleagues (1996), Gackstetter et al. (2002) found that deployed veterans who died in motor vehicle accidents through 1995 (n = 1,343) were more likely to be male, younger, less educated, and never married than nondeployed controls (10 controls/case). They were also more likely to be enlisted, have combat occupations, and be in the National Guard or reserves and not in the Air Force.

Updated and Supplemental Literature

Primary Studies

The Update committee identified four new primary studies of external cause mortality: DASA (2009), Lincoln et al. (2006), Macfarlane et al. (2005), and Statistics Canada (2005).

Lincoln et al. (2006) conducted a nested case-control study to assess individual characteristics of Gulf War and other veterans associated with risk of fatal motor vehicle accidents. The authors used the same cohort and method of identifying fatal crashes as in the previous study of Kang and Bullman (1996), but additional, individual characteristics were assessed. They obtained demographic data from the DMDC and motor vehicle crash data from the Department of Transportation's Fatality Analysis Reporting System to identify 1318 motor vehicle crash fatalities between 1991 and 1995. They identified 765 motor vehicle deaths in deployed and 553 in era veterans (annual mortality rate 23.6, 95% CI 21.9-25.5) and found higher risk among those who were enlisted males, less educated, and did not use restraints. The deployed veterans may have been healthier initially, complicating the assessment of the full impact of deployment.

Macfarlane et al. (2005) conducted a cohort study of all UK Gulf War veterans (n = 51,753) and a matched cohort of 50,808 veterans not deployed to the Gulf. After 13 years of follow-up, they found little or no difference in overall mortality between those deployed and those not. A previously reported excess in non-disease-related mortality during the first 7 years of follow-up (MRR 1.31, 95% CI 1.06-1.63) was essentially absent in the later years (MRR 1.05, 95% CI 0.83-1.33). The strongest association was for transport accident deaths (MRR 1.44, 95% CI 1.13-1.84). Deployment was associated with little or no increased risk of intentional self-harm (MRR 1.04, 95% CI 0.80-1.36). Although the authors attempted to include all deployed UK veterans, the study is limited by the small size of the cohort.

Since publication of *Volume 4*, the Defence Analytical Services Agency (2009) has published updated summary statistics of mortality among deployed UK Gulf War veterans (n = 53,409) compared to a control group of era veterans (n = 54,143) from April 1, 1991, through December 31, 2007. The agency found no significant increase in the rate of all external cause mortality in UK Gulf War veterans versus era veterans (MRR 1.09, 95% CI 0.95-1.25), and in addition found no significant difference in the rate of mortality due to transportation accidents (MRR 1.17, 95% CI 0.94-1.45), other external cause injuries (MRR 1.04, 95% CI 0.74-1.45), or intentional self-harm and events of undetermined intent (MRR 1.12, 95% CI 0.89-1.40). The report also notes that the rate of mortality due to external causes has decreased from 1991 to 2007 for both deployed and nondeployed veterans, while the rate for a civilian cohort of similar size matched for age and sex has stayed relatively constant over the same time period.

A report from Statistics Canada (2005) used the cohort of Canadian veterans compiled by Goss Gilroy (1998) to compare mortality incidence between Gulf War deployed veterans (n = 5117) and a control group of era veterans (n = 6093), frequency matched for age, sex, and military duty status. Mortality data were obtained from the 1991-1999 Canadian Mortality Database. They found modest, but nonsignificant differences in mortality incidence among deployed veterans compared to nondeployed veterans due to all external causes (MRR 1.53, 95% CI 0.82-2.86), motor vehicle crashes (MRR 0.74, 95% CI 0.18-3.11), and suicide (MRR 1.17, 95% CI 0.46-2.95). The MRR for suicide was higher in the first 5 years of follow-up than in the second period. The overall risk of suicide was furthermore found to be comparable to (or lower than) the risk of suicide in the population (SMR 0.76, 95% CI 0.35-1.43). The report did find a significantly increased risk of mortality due to air and space crashes (MRR 5.50, 95% CI 1.16-26.0) in the deployed group, but the agency notes this might be explained by the fact that three times as many deployed veterans were in flight-related occupations (such as, pilots and navigators) as nondeployed veterans.

Bullman et al. (2005) examined the relationship between estimated exposure to chemical munitions destruction (sarin gas) at Khamisiyah in 1991 with cause-specific mortality of Gulf War veterans through December 31, 2000. Using the DoD's 2000 sarin plume exposure model (Rostker, 2000), 100,487 deployed military personnel were identified as potentially exposed and 224,980 were considered unexposed. The authors reported no increase in external-cause mortality risk among exposed veterans as compared to unexposed veterans (RR 1.01, 95% CI 0.92-1.10), and no increased risk of suicide (RR 1.05, 95% CI 0.88-1.25) or motor vehicle fatalities (RR 1.00, 95% CI 0.86-1.17). Similarly, no increased risk for any external-cause mortality, or suicide or motor vehicle fatality specifically, was observed when the authors divided the exposed group into persons exposed for either 1 or 2 days for comparison with the unexposed group.

Secondary Studies

Several additional secondary studies were identified. Gray and Kang (2006) published results of a review of the literature concerning health of Gulf War veterans. They particularly noted the excess mortality from motor vehicle accidents and the decline in this excess over time since the war. They noted and largely discounted the possibility that deployed veterans could have been healthier initially than their nondeployed counterparts, at least in the US mortality studies. Hooper et al. (2005) conducted a nested case-control study of risk factors for deaths from motor vehicle accidents among Gulf War era veterans, using largely the same underlying cohort and nearly identical case group, methods and subjects as Lincoln et al. (2006). Using a matched design and, after restrictions, 980 male cases and about 1300 controls, they identified younger age, lower education, and being unmarried as risk factors for fatal accidents among Gulf War veterans.

Summary and Conclusions

Since the last report, new studies have been published of external causes of death among Canadian and British veterans. These studies were small, reflecting the relatively small number of personnel deployed from these countries. In the British study, a previously reported increase in mortality from external causes had essentially disappeared with additional years of follow-up. In the Canadian study, there was an excess of deaths from air/space crashes among Gulf War veterans, but this may have been due to greater employment in the flight-related occupations. New studies concerning fatal motor vehicle accidents in US Gulf War era veterans focused on individual characteristics and found that younger age, lower education, and nonuse of restraints were risk factors for these fatal events. Perhaps the main limitation of all these new studies is shared with the older studies—deployed veterans may have been healthier initially, a difference which could tend to bias comparisons and obscure any effects of deployment to the gulf.

In conclusion, studies published to date have provided evidence of modestly higher mortality from transportation-related causes among Gulf War deployed veterans than other veterans. In US veterans, the excess is largely due to motor vehicle accidents, and has diminished and perhaps disappeared over time. A modestly higher mortality from airspace crashes that was noted in Canadian veterans may have been due to employment in flight-related occupations.

Therefore, the committee concludes that there is limited but suggestive evidence of an association between deployment to the Gulf War and an increase in mortality from external causes, primarily motor vehicle accidents, in the early years after deployment.

TABLE 4-16 External Causes of Mortality

Study	Design	Population	Outcomes	Results	Adjustments	Comments
Kang and Bullman, 1996, 2001 (Vol. 4)	Retrospective cohort, 2.4-year follow-up; Retrospective cohort, approximately 7-year follow-up	695,516 GWVs vs 746,291 NDVs	Mortality 1991-1997; Cox proportional hazards models	Increased deaths from motor vehicle accidents in Kang and Bullman, 1996 (RR 1.31, 95% CI 1.14-1.49) RRs became nonsignificant in Kang and Bullman, 2001 (RR 1.17, 95% CI 0.98-1.4) in 1994-1995; Increased HIV deaths in NDVs; no difference in potential nerve gas exposure; no homicide or suicide increase	Sex, age, race, marital status, branch of service, type of unit	Short duration of follow-up; healthy warrior effect may obscure difference
Macfarlane et al., 2000 (Vol. 4)	Cohort study	53,462 UK GWVs vs 53,450 UK NDVs	Mortality 1991-1999	Higher mortality in Gulf War veterans from external causes (MRR 1.18, 95% CI 0.98-1.42); no increase in homicide or suicide	Matching by sex, age, branch, fitness for service	
DASA, 2005 (Vol. 4)	Summary statistics of causes of death from April 1, 1991-June 30, 2005	53,409 UK GWVs vs 53,143 UK NDVs	Mortality 1991-June 2005	No increase in mortality except small and nonsignificant increase in “transport accidents” (SMR 1.21, 95% CI 0.96-1.51); “other external causes of accidental injury” (SMR 1.07, 95% CI 0.74-1.54); higher deaths from external causes disappeared about 10 years after Gulf War	Matching by sex, age, branch	
Lincoln et al., 2006 (Update)	Retrospective cohort and nested case-control; risk factors for motor vehicle crash	1318 cases of motor vehicle crash mortality (1991-1995) identified from	Annual motor vehicle mortality rate by risk factor	Higher motor vehicle annual mortality rate in deployed veterans: 23.56 (95% CI 21.9-25.3) for deployed vs 15.87 (95% CI 14.6-17.3) for		Deployed population possibly associated with greater risk-taking behavior (younger,

Study	Design	Population	Outcomes	Results	Adjustments	Comments
	fatality (Cohort derived from Kang and Bullman, 1996)	the VA's 1991 Gulf War cohort: 765 deployed GWVs, 553 era veterans; COD, demographic, and military records from DMDC and FARS		nondeployed per 100,000		less educated, not married)
Macfarlane et al., 2005 (Update)	Cohort; 13-year follow-up (Follow-up of Macfarlane et al., 2000)	51,753 UK GWVs and 50,808 NDVs, randomly selected, matched by age, sex, service branch, rank; also fitness for active service in the army and Royal Air Force	Mortality rates	All causes (MRR 1.03, 95% CI 0.92-1.15); external causes (MRR 1.19, 95% CI 1.02-1.39); transport accidents (MRR 1.44, 95% CI 1.13-1.84); intentional self-harm (MRR 1.04, 95% CI 0.80-1.36) No self-reported Gulf War theater exposure significantly associated with all cause, disease-related, or external mortality		Complete and long-term follow-up; cohort of moderate size; potentially other uncontrolled confounders
DASA, 2009 (Update)	Summary statistics of causes of death from April 1, 1991, to December 31, 2007	UK Gulf War veterans (n = 53,409) vs era veterans (n = 54,143)	Mortality data, causes of death classified based on ICD-10	All external cause mortality (MMR 1.09, 95% CI 0.95-1.25) No significant difference in mortality rate was found for any of the specific external causes of mortality included in the study	Single years of age structure of the gulf cohort at January 1, 1991	
Statistics Canada, 2005 (Update)	Retrospective cohort (Cohort based on Goss Gilroy, 1998)	5117 Canadian GWVs; 6093 Canadian NDVs, frequency matched for age,	Mortality and cancer incidences determined from the CMDB and CCDB, 1991-1999	All external causes (OR 1.53, 95% CI 0.82-2.86); motor vehicle crash (OR 0.74, 95% CI 0.18-3.11); air/space crash (OR 5.50, 95% CI 1.16-26.0);	Age, rank	

Study	Design	Population	Outcomes	Results	Adjustments	Comments
		sex, and military duty status		suicide (OR 1.17, 95% CI 0.46-2.95)		
Bullman et al., 2005 (Update)	Cohort mortality study; follow-up from March 1991 through 2000 (population from same source as Kang and Bullman, 1996, 2001)	100,487 US Army GWVs exposed to chemical warfare agents at Khamisiyah; 224,980 nonexposed army GWVs; exposure determined from the DoD plume model (Rostker, 2000)	Association of exposure to chemical warfare agents and mortality, determined through BIRLS, SSA; COD data from NDI	Exposed vs unexposed Any external cause: Relative risk 1.01 (95% CI 0.92-1.10) Suicide: RR 1.05 (95% CI 0.88-1.25) Motor vehicle fatalities: RR 1.00 (95% CI 0.86-1.17)	Age, race, sex, rank, unit component	Limitations: short latency, possible exposure misclassification

NOTE: BIRLS = Beneficiary Identification and Records Locator Subsystem (VA); CI = confidence interval; CMDB = Canadian MIS Data Base; COD = cause of death; DoD = Department of Defense; FARS = Fatality Analysis Reporting System (Department of Transportation); GWV = Gulf War veteran; HR = adjusted hazard ratio; MRR = mortality rate ratio; NDI = National Death Index; NDV = nondeployed veteran; OR = adjusted odds ratio; RR = adjusted risk ratio; SMR = standardized mortality ratio; SSA = Social Security Administration.

FEMALE VETERANS' HEALTH

Although women have always served in the military, primarily as nurses and clerks, the role of women in the military increased dramatically with the advent of an all volunteer military. During the Vietnam War, active-duty military women made up only 2.5% of the military forces. The Gulf War was among the first wars to see a sizable number of women in the military. During the Gulf War in 1990-1991, 33,000 to 37,000 military women were on the ground in the Persian Gulf, making up approximately 6.7% of the US military forces (Fricker et al., 2000).

Many of the studies discussed in this section were described in earlier sections in this chapter under specific health effects. This section pulls together the data on female veterans' health in an attempt to provide an overview of the deployment experiences of women who deployed to the Persian Gulf region, the health effects they experienced after their deployment, including mental health effects, and their hospitalization and mortality outcomes. Although men serving in the military may be subject to sexual assault and harassment, women in the military are far more likely to be subject to this behavior and this experience is also discussed.

Deployment Experiences

Women and men who deployed to the Gulf War theater in 1990-1991 experienced many of the same exposures and stressors. Although women were not allowed to serve in combat specialties, they were deployed as administrators, air-traffic controllers, logisticians, ammunition technicians, engineering-equipment mechanics, ordnance specialists, communicators, radio operators, drivers, law-enforcement specialists, and guards. Many female truck drivers hauled supplies and equipment into Kuwait. Some took enemy prisoners of war to holding facilities, and others flew helicopters and reconnaissance aircraft. Still others served on hospital, supply, oiler, and ammunition ships or served as public affairs officers and chaplains (DoD, 2004). As a result of their service in the Gulf War theater, female military personnel were exposed to many of the same environmental agents and other stressors as were males, that is, biological and chemical agents, oil-well fire smoke, heat, pesticides, solvents, fuels, burning rubbish, and combat-related exposures, such as Scud missiles, dead and wounded people, and difficult living conditions. Female military personnel were more likely to experience sexual harassment and assault than were male personnel (Wolfe et al., 1998).

Vogt et al. (2005) queried 317 Gulf War veterans (including 83 females) about combat and other deployment experiences such as handling human remains and dealing with prisoners of war, perceived threats, difficult living and working environments, concerns about family and relationship disruptions, lack of deployment social support, and sexual harassment. There were no male-female differences for most of the stressor measures. Women reported more exposure to interpersonal stressors, such as incidents of sexual harassment, and less postdeployment social support, whereas men reported more mission-related stressors, such as combat experiences. Wolfe et al. (1993) also found that men (n = 2136) and women (n = 208) reported similar Gulf War deployment experiences, with over 70% of men and women receiving chemical and biologic attack alerts and incoming fire from large arms, and about 50% of men and women had seen death or disfigurement of enemy troops. Men and women reported different deployment stressors when asked to rank their own experiences: almost half of the women reported combat exposure as their most significant stressor compared with 38% of men but about 25% of women and men reported a war-zone but noncombat event (such as a unit member's being injured or killed in nonmission activities or nearness to a prisoner-of-war riot) as their most significant stressor. Fewer than 10% of the women and men reported no stressful event during deployment.

The Iowa Persian Gulf War study was one of the few population-based US studies that investigated the health of women separately (Carney et al., 2003). Women were less likely to participate in combat than men, but 71% of women had at least one combat exposure. Women also reported similar prevalence of exposure to environmental agents, such as diesel fuel and smoke from oil-well fires. For men and women who were deployed to the Gulf War theater, the most frequently reported stressors for both sexes were seeing dead bodies or severely maimed or injured people, having a Scud missile explode within 1 mile, and having explosions other than Scuds within 1 mile; the men, however, reported significantly more exposure to combat. Overall, with the exception of combat exposure and sexual threat, women and men had similar deployment exposures.

In a study of US Navy health-care providers deployed to the Persian Gulf on a hospital ship days before the Gulf War, there was anticipation of large numbers of casualties and concerns for safety. Women were more likely to report having experienced depression; however, when training and experience were factored into the analysis with fear of injury and the stress of work demands, the sex difference for depression disappeared (Slusarcick et al., 2001).

Health Effects

For many of the studies discussed earlier in this chapter that assessed the prevalence of health effects in deployed and nondeployed Gulf War veterans, the numbers of women were so small that they were frequently not considered in the outcomes or were combined with the overwhelmingly male populations. However, there were a few studies that did distinguish between the female (deployed and nondeployed) and male veterans in the analyses concerning health outcomes. Most of the studies discussed here are also described in each health effect section where prevalence data by sex were also presented in the evidence table if available and therefore, are not repeated here.

Carney et al. (2003) observed that the patterns of health-care use by female veterans differed from that of male veterans: the former had significantly more outpatient, as well as inpatient, health care 5 years after the war. Women were also more likely than men to receive VA compensation (17% vs 7%), although their level of disability was similar.

Wolfe et al. (1998) found that among a cohort of Gulf War veterans from Fort Devens, Massachusetts, surveyed at 18-24 months after their return from the gulf, female veterans were about 6 times (ORs 5.6-6.4, 95% CIs 1.9-19.2) more likely to report having five or more health symptoms (compared with no health symptoms) than male veterans, whether or not they reported having been exposed to combat situations, poison gas or germ warfare, or had served in a transportation unit. Steele (2000) found that among Kansas Gulf War veterans, women were about 50% more likely to have Gulf War illness than men as of 1998 (OR 1.49, 95% CI 1.06-2.08) based on a telephone interview asking about physician-diagnosed or physician-treated medical conditions and chronic symptoms with onset after 1990.

Pierce (1997) assessed the health of 525 women who had been on active-duty or in the reserve or National Guard during the Gulf War, of whom 160 served in theater. The women were asked about their physical and emotional health 2 years after the war (time 1) and 4 years after the war (time 2). Compared to women deployed elsewhere, at time 1, women who had been deployed for more than 120 days reported more frequent skin rashes (1.17 vs 1.50, $p = 0.008$);

women deployed fewer than 120 days reported more depression as a general health measure (1.84 vs 2.22, p = 0.03) and more insomnia (1.92 vs 2.34, p = 0.04). There were more reports of unintentional weight loss in those deployed less than 120 days compared with those deployed elsewhere (p = 0.006) and a significant difference between those deployed less than 120 days and those deployed for more than 120 days (p = 0.006). Those who had left the military reported more frequent health problems. At time 2, skin rashes persisted in those who had served in theater less than 120 days, but differences in the other health conditions were no longer significant between the deployed and nondeployed women. Deployed women, however, regardless of the length of their service, reported more coughs, and those who were deployed for fewer than 120 days also reported more memory problems (p = 0.008). At time 2 only, women who had served in the gulf also were more likely to report lumps or cysts in the breast (p = 0.017), abnormal Pap test results (p = 0.036), and headaches (p = 0.0010), regardless of the length of their deployment. In a further study of female Air Force veterans 6 years after the war (Pierce, 2005), veterans who were deployed to the Persian Gulf area reported more frequently 29 of 48 symptoms compared with those deployed elsewhere, although the deployed women no longer reported more insomnia, unintentional weight loss, or memory problems than the nondeployed women. Women who had been deployed to the Gulf War were more likely (p < 0.001) to report the following symptoms than women who had not been deployed: skin rash; persistent cough; dizziness, faintness, or lightheadedness; forgetfulness, hoarseness, respiratory difficulties; tendency to bruise or bleed easily; itchy skin; and loss of energy. Reported health problems were not related to whether the woman was on active-duty, in the reserves, or a member of the National Guard.

In a similar study by Unwin et al. (2002), female UK veterans deployed to the Gulf War (n = 226) reported more frequently having 49 of the 50 medical conditions or symptoms assessed (the exception was asthma) than did female veterans deployed to Bosnia (n = 217) or era controls (n = 192). The most frequently reported symptoms in all three cohorts were headaches, fatigue, feeling unrefreshed after sleep, irritability and outbursts of anger, sleeping difficulties, and forgetfulness but the Gulf War veterans reported significantly more of each symptom compared with the other cohorts; ORs ranged from 1.5-3.7, all 95% CIs excluded 1.0 except for sleeping difficulties in deployed veterans versus nondeployed. The most frequently self-reported medical disorders for all three groups were premenstrual tension, back problems, and problems with periods, although the difference between the Gulf War veterans and the era veterans was not significant. The results for the symptom and medical condition reporting for female veterans were very similar to those for male UK Gulf War veterans (Unwin et al., 1999).

Frommelt et al. (2000) evaluated Pap smear results from a cohort of 6715 Air Force women who served on active duty between August 7, 1990, and March 1, 1991, and had routine Pap smears conducted in 1994. Pap smear test results were collected for 1446 female Gulf War veterans and 5269 female veterans who were not deployed to the Gulf. Overall, there were no observed differences in cervical pathology between the two groups. Among 26-30 years old veterans, a diagnosis of "other than within normal limits" occurred more frequently among Gulf War veterans (11.5%) compared with nondeployed veterans (6.6%, p – 0.013) in 1994, but no differences were detected among other age groups ranging from 20 and younger to over 50 years of age. The authors suggest there is no biologically plausible evidence to support an age-specific association between Gulf War service and abnormal cervical cytology.

Barth et al. (2009) assessed the long-term mortality for neurologic disorders in Gulf War veterans compared with nondeployed veterans between 1991 and the date of death or December

31, 2004, using a Cox proportional hazard model. Based on death certificates, among the 43,719 female Gulf War veterans, there was one death from ALS and none in the nondeployed female veterans; deployed male veterans also showed no increased risk for ALS. Ten female Gulf War veterans had died from brain cancer compared with 17 among the 99,027 nondeployed female veterans (rate ratio 1.50, 95% CI 0.68-3.30; adjusted for race, branch of service, type of unit, age, and marital status at entry to follow-up); men showed no increased risk for death from brain cancer. Being deployed did not increase the risk for MS or Parkinson's disease for deployed women compared with nondeployed women or men (deployed or nondeployed).

Being a woman slightly increased the likelihood of being diagnosed with chronic multisymptom illness 10 years after the Gulf War regardless of whether the female veteran was deployed (OR 1.41, 95% CI 0.94-2.13) or nondeployed (OR 1.29, 95% CI 0.81-2.04) although the increase was not significant (Blanchard et al., 2005).

Several studies have assessed the risk of adverse reproductive outcomes in female veterans who were deployed to the Gulf War. Kang et al. (2001) used data from the 1996 National Health Survey of Gulf War Era Veterans and Their Families of 30,000 veterans to estimate rates of spontaneous abortions, stillbirths, preterm births, birth defects, and infant mortality between deployed and era veterans, both men and women. There were 632 deployed female veterans compared with 691 female nondeployed veterans. Female veterans who were deployed reported more miscarriages and stillbirths compared with female nondeployed veterans but the differences were not different and there were no significant differences for preterm births or infant death. Deployed women also were more likely than nondeployed women to report giving birth to a child with a likely birth defect (OR 2.97, 95% CI 1.47-5.99), particularly one with a moderate to severe birth defect (OR 2.80, 95% CI 1.26-6.25). Deployed men also reported having more children with a likely birth defect (OR 1.94, 95% CI 1.37-2.74) and that the birth defect was moderate to severe (OR 1.78, 95% CI 1.19-2.66). Reported birth defects were categorized by study pediatricians as likely or unlikely based on the participants' descriptions of the infants' birth defect. In a 2005 follow-up study of the same Gulf War veterans, Kang et al. (2009) asked female veterans (1225 deployed and 851 nondeployed) about gynecological and reproductive outcomes. Compared with nondeployed veterans, the deployed female veterans reported more serious problems with premenstrual moods (OR 1.28, 95% CI 1.13-1.45) and more difficulty getting pregnant (OR 2.20, 95% CI 1.50-3.22). However, more deployed women had given birth in the 6 months prior to the survey (OR 2.11, 95% CI 0.89-5.04) and had experienced fewer miscarriages in the past 6 months (OR 0.42, 95% CI 0.15-1.17).

In a study of reproductive outcomes in Gulf War veterans conducted in 1996, Wells et al. (2006) found that female veterans were not at increased risk of reporting an adverse pregnancy outcome (OR 1.16, 95% CI 0.91-1.48), whether miscarriage, stillbirth, or ectopic pregnancy, compared with nondeployed female veterans. There was also no difference in the likelihood of having a low, normal, or high birth weight infant between deployed female veterans and nondeployed female veterans.

Mental Health Effects

Pierce (1997) found that 24% of 160 women deployed to the Gulf War theater met the criteria for PTSD based on the Mississippi scale for combat-related PTSD compared with 15% of the female veterans deployed elsewhere.

In a study of the prevalence and course of PTSD in a cohort of 2949 Gulf War veterans from Fort Devens, Massachusetts, that included 240 women, Wolfe et al. (1999a) found that

5 days after their return from deployment (time 1), 8% of the women and 3% of the men exceeded the cutoff point for PTSD on the Mississippi Scale for Combat-Related PTSD (OR 3.2, 95% CI 1.9-5.5). At 18-24 months after their return (time 2), however, this increased to 16% of the women and 7% of the men (OR 2.3, 95% CI 1.5-3.5) even after adjustment for combat exposure. Six percent of the women exceeded the cutoff point for PTSD at both time points, 2.2% exceeded it at time 1 only and 9% exceeded it at time 2 only, with 73% of the women who scored above the cutoff point at time 1 also scoring above the cutoff point at time 2.

Kang et al. (2005) used data collected in the National Health Survey of Gulf War Era Veterans and Their Families (Kang et al., 2000) to screen for PTSD among the respondents and to examine its association with sexual harassment and with sexual assault. Of the 11,441 Gulf War veterans surveyed 336 females (15.8%) and 1045 males (11.2%) met the screening criteria for PTSD. For women, sexual harassment while deployed was found to be associated with PTSD (OR 2.52, 95% CI 1.91-3.33), and sexual assault was even more strongly associated with PTSD (OR 5.41, 95% CI 3.19-9.17). When the intensity of combat was examined, a dose-response for the development of PTSD in women was found ranging from an OR of 1.47 from low combat to an OR of 4.03 (95% CI 1.97-8.23) for high combat exposure; men showed a similar trend.

In an assessment of deployment to the Gulf War as a risk factor for the development of mental disorders, Fielder et al. (2006) used a telephone interview with the Composite International Diagnostic Interview-Short Form/Diagnostic and Statistical Manual IV to diagnose any of 17 psychiatric disorders among deployed and nondeployed veterans. Compared with the 892 deployed male veterans, the 75 deployed female veterans had a higher 12-month prevalence of all disorders except for alcohol and drug dependence disorders. However, the 93 nondeployed female veterans also had a higher prevalence of the disorders than the 691 nondeployed male veterans, again with the exception of alcohol dependence.

Vogt et al. (2005) found that lack of social support in the Gulf War theater was a risk factor for the development of depression among women as were, to a lesser degree, concerns about family and relationship disruptions during deployment.

In a study of UK female veterans who had been deployed to the Gulf War, Rona et al. (2007) found that the 645 female veterans scored higher on the General Health Questionnaire-12 (GHQ-12; which measures psychological distress) (OR 1.49, 95% CI 1.02-2.17) and for fatigue (OR 1.48, 95% CI 1.03-2.31) than men. Differences in reports of PTSD, alcohol misuse, and general health perception were not significantly different between men and women. Comparing deployed female veterans with nondeployed female veterans, however, showed that the deployed female veterans had more symptoms of posttraumatic stress reaction (OR 13.80, 95% CI 3.13-60.78), higher scores on the GHQ-12 (OR 2.53, 95% CI 1.56-4.11), higher fatigue scores (OR 3.49, 95% CI 2.18-5.59), more physical symptoms (OR 21.70, 95% CI 5.05-93.19), and poorer general health perception (OR 2.57, 95% CI 1.23-5.40), only alcohol misuse was similar for the two groups.

Military Sexual Assault and Harassment

Sexual assault and harassment[6] are widely acknowledged stressors in the general population and are severe stressors when incurred in a war zone. In the military environment

---

[6]The US Army defines *sexual assault* as "intentional sexual contact, characterized by use of force, physical threat or abuse of authority or when the victim does not or cannot consent. Sexual assault includes rape, nonconsensual sodomy, indecent assault (unwanted, inappropriate sexual contact or fondling), or attempts to commit these acts."

with its overwhelmingly male population, sexual victimization is more likely to be experienced by women, regardless of their military occupation and background. The rate of reported sexual assault was about 70 per 100,000 uniformed servicemembers in 2002-2003 for all duty stations; 9% of the victims were men (DoD, 2004). Reported rates of sexual harassment of women in the military were about 46% and 24% in 1995 and 2002, respectively, compared to 8% and 3% for men for the same years. The female-to-male ratio for being a victim of sexual assault in the Gulf War was 16.5:1 and for sexual harassment 25:1 (Kang et al., 2005).

The 1995 National Health Survey of Gulf War Era Veterans and Their Families, conducted by the VA, found that of the 11,441 Gulf War veterans who responded (4202 women and 7239 men), 24% of the women reported having been subject to sexual harassment, and 3.3% reported sexual assault; only 0.6% of the men reported experiencing sexual harassment, and even fewer (0.2%) reported a sexual assault (Kang et al., 2005). Wolfe et al. (1998) interviewed 160 Army women on their return from the Gulf War and again 18-24 months later; the women reported rates of sexual assault of 7.3%, physical sexual harassment 33.1%, and verbal sexual harassment 66.2%—all of these rates are higher than those found in peacetime military and civilian populations. Goldzweig et al. (2006) reported rates of sexual harassment in studies of military personnel ranging from 55% to 79%, with sexual assault rates ranging from 4.2 to 7.3% in female active-duty personnel and 11 to 48% in female veterans.

Vogt et al. (2005) found that female veterans were more likely to report sexual harassment than men and that this harassment was a risk factor for the development of anxiety, but not for depression, even 10 years after deployment.

Hospitalization and Mortality

Several studies have looked at hospitalizations for Gulf War veterans in the years after deployment. Gray et al. (1996) reviewed discharge diagnoses at DoD hospitals between 1991-1993 for 1,165,411 Gulf War veterans (deployed and era) who remained on active duty after the war. Female veterans who had deployed were at greater risk than their nondeployed counterparts for hospitalizations for inflammatory disease of the ovary, fallopian tube, pelvic cellular tissue, and peritoneum (SMR 1.35, 95% CI 1.11-1.63), and for hospitalization for infertility (SMR 1.59, 95% CI 1.19-2.11). Hospitalizations for uterine leiomyoma, pain and other symptoms associated with the female genital organs, noninflammatory disorders of the cervix, and endometriosis were not significantly different between deployed and nondeployed female veterans. Knoke and Gray (1998) extended the time period of this study to 1996 and assessed postwar hospitalizations for active-duty veterans with at least one diagnosis of unexplained illnesses (ICD-9 code 799.9). Female veterans who had been deployed were at twice the risk of being hospitalized for an unexplained illness than were nondeployed female veterans (RR 2.11, 95% CI 2.04-2.18).

An evaluation of all-cause hospitalizations (excluding pregnancy-related causes) for Gulf War veterans who remained on active-duty between 1995-2004, found that female veterans, regardless of the armed service in which they served, were more likely to have been hospitalized in a DoD medical treatment facility than male veterans. Risk ratios ranged from 1.70 (95% CI 1.63-1.77) for Army veterans to 2.23 (95% CI 1.89-2.64) for female Marine Corps veterans (Hooper et al., 2008).

The Army defines *sexual harassment* as "a form of gender discrimination that involves unwelcome sexual advances, requests for sexual favors, and other verbal or physical conduct of a sexual nature" (US Army, 2005).

Between 1990 and 1997, being deployed to the Gulf War appears to have resulted in a slight increase in all-cause mortality for female veterans compared with female veterans who served in the military during the same time but were not deployed (OR 1.16, 95% CI 0.97-1.38). Deployed female veterans were at increased risk for death from external causes (OR 1.39, 95% CI 1.08-1.80), particularly motor vehicle accidents (OR 1.63, 95% CI 1.09-2.45). The vital status of 621,902 Gulf War veterans (7.0% women) was compared with that of 746,248 era controls (13.3% women) based on databases from the VA and the SSA and assessment of death certificates (Kang and Bullman, 2001).

Summary and Conclusions

Female Gulf War veterans experienced many of the exposures and stressors that male Gulf War veterans experienced while deployed to the Persian Gulf region in 1990-1991, including combat stressors such as seeing dead bodies and being near Scud missile explosions. In addition, female veterans were more likely to be subjected to sexual harassment and sexual assault than were male veterans.

The number of female military personnel who served in the Gulf War theater was much smaller (about 7%) than the number of males and this is reflected in the subsequent studies of the health effects of serving in the Gulf War. For this reason, few studies of Gulf War veterans include women, and most of these are unable to examine the health effects experienced by female veterans separately from male veterans because of small sample sizes. However, the few studies that did provide information on health effects seen in female Gulf War veterans who were deployed compared with female veterans who were in the military during the Gulf War but were not deployed, were reviewed by the Update committee. In general, the findings from the studies suggest that female Gulf War veterans suffer from many of the same health effects as do male Gulf War veterans but a larger proportion of them report more health symptoms, including Gulf War or multisymptom illness, than either male Gulf War veterans or nondeployed female veterans.

Although deployed female veterans report more adverse reproductive outcomes, these outcomes are often based on self-reports and there is no consistency in the type of adverse outcomes reported. For example, although more deployed female veterans reported giving birth to a child with a likely birth defect in 1996, by 2005, female veterans who had been deployed reported fewer miscarriages in the 6 months prior to the survey.

All of the studies of the mental health of female veterans indicate that the prevalence of mental health disorders was greater in deployed women compared to nondeployed women or to deployed men (even after adjustment for combat exposure). As with the deployed male veterans, increased exposure to combat stressors or sexual assault resulted in a greater risk for the development of PTSD. Female veterans were more likely to be the subject of sexual assault than male veterans, but male veterans were more likely to have mental health disorders as a result.

The committee concludes that female veterans who were deployed to the Gulf War have an increased prevalence of adverse health effects, including mental health disorders, compared with their nondeployed counterparts and with deployed male veterans.

REFERENCES

Abul, A. T., P. C. Nair, N. A. Behbehanei, and P. N. Sharma. 2001. Hospital admissions and death rates from asthma in Kuwait during pre- and post-Gulf War periods. *Annals of Allergy, Asthma, and Immunology* 86(4):465-468.

Al-Khalaf, B. 1998. Pilot study: The onset of asthma among the Kuwaiti population during the burning of oil wells after the Gulf War. *Environment International* 24(1-2):221-225.

Al-Turkait, F. A., and J. U. Ohaeri. 2008. Prevalence and correlates of posttraumatic stress disorder among Kuwaiti military men according to level of involvement in the first Gulf War. *Depression and Anxiety* 25(11):932-941.

ALS Association. 2008. *Who gets ALS.* http://www.alsa.org (accessed December 18, 2009).

Amato, A. A., A. McVey, C. Cha, E. C. Matthews, C. E. Jackson, R. Kleingunther, L. Worley, E. Cornman, and K. Kagan-Hallet. 1997. Evaluation of neuromuscular symptoms in veterans of the Persian Gulf War. *Neurology* 48(1):4-12.

American Psychiatric Association. 2000. *Diagnostic and Statistical Manual of Mental Disorders, Fourth Edition, Text Revision (DSM-IV-TR).* Washington, DC: American Psychiatric Publishing Association.

Ang, D. C., P. M. Peloso, R. F. Woolson, K. Kroenke, and B. N. Doebbeling. 2006. Predictors of incident chronic widespread pain among veterans following the first Gulf War. *Clinical Journal of Pain* 22(6):554-563.

Annegers, J. F., S. H. Appel, P. Perkins, and J. Lee. 1991. Amyotrophic lateral sclerosis mortality rates in Harris County, Texas. *Advances in Neurology* 56:239-243.

Araneta, M. R., C. A. Moore, R. S. Olney, L. D. Edmonds, J. A. Karcher, C. McDonough, K. M. Hiliopoulos, K. M. Schlangen, and G. C. Gray. 1997. Goldenhar syndrome among infants born in military hospitals to Gulf War veterans. *Teratology* 56(4):244-251.

Araneta, M. R. G., D. A. Destiche, K. M. Schlangen, R. D. Merz, M. B. Forrester, and G. C. Gray. 2000. Birth defects prevalence among infants of Persian Gulf War veterans born in Hawaii, 1989-1993. *Teratology* 62(4):195-204.

Araneta, M. R., K. M. Schlangen, L. D. Edmonds, D. A. Destiche, R. D. Merz, C. A. Hobbs, T. J. Flood, J. A. Harris, D. Krishnamurti, and G. C. Gray. 2003. Prevalence of birth defects among infants of Gulf War veterans in Arkansas, Arizona, California, Georgia, Hawaii, and Iowa, 1989-1993. *Birth Defects Research* 67(4):246-260.

Araneta, M. R., D. R. Kamens, A. C. Zau, V. M. Gastanaga, K. M. Schlangen, K. M. Hiliopoulos, and G. C. Gray. 2004. Conception and pregnancy during the Persian Gulf War: The risk to women veterans. *Annals of Epidemiology* 14(2):109-116.

Armon, C. 2003. An evidence-based medicine approach to the evaluation of the role of exogenous risk factors in sporadic amyotrophic lateral sclerosis. *Neuroepidemiology* 22(4):217-228.

Armon, C. 2004. Amyotrophic lateral sclerosis. In *Neuroepidemiology: From Principles to Practice*, edited by L. Nelson, C. Tanner, S. Van Den Eeden, and V. McGuire. New York: Oxford University Press. Pp. 162-187.

Armon, C., L. T. Kurland, J. R. Daube, and P. C. O'Brien. 1991. Epidemiologic correlates of sporadic amyotrophic lateral sclerosis. *Neurology* 41(7):1077-1084.

Armon, C., S. R. Brenner, R. Horner, and J. R. Feussner. 2004. Occurrence of amyotrophic lateral sclerosis among Gulf War veterans. *Neurology* 62(6):1027-1029.

Axelrod, B. N., and I. B. Milner. 1997. Neuropsychological findings in a sample of Operation Desert Storm veterans. *Journal of Neuropsychiatry and Clinical Neurosciences* 9(1):23-28.

Axelrod, S. R., C. A. Morgan, 3rd, and S. M. Southwick. 2005. Symptoms of posttraumatic stress disorder and borderline personality disorder in veterans of Operation Desert Storm. *American Journal of Psychiatry* 162(2):270-275.

Barbara, G., V. Stanghellini, R. De Giorgio, C. Cremon, G. S. Cottrell, D. Santini, G. Pasquinelli, A. M. Morselli-Labate, E. F. Grady, N. W. Bunnett, S. M. Collins, and R. Corinaldesi. 2004. Activated mast cells in proximity to colonic nerves correlate with abdominal pain in irritable bowel syndrome. *Gastroenterology* 126(3):693-702.

Barbara, G., V. Stanghellini, C. Cremon, R. De Giorgio, L. Gargano, R. Cogliandro, F. Pallotti, and R. Corinaldesi. 2008. Probiotics and irritable bowel syndrome: Rationale and clinical evidence for their use. *Journal of Clinical Gastroenterology* 42(Suppl 3):Pt 2.

Barrett, D. H., C. C. Doebbeling, D. A. Schwartz, M. D. Voelker, K. H. Falter, R. F. Woolson, and B. N. Doebbeling. 2002. Posttraumatic stress disorder and self-reported physical health status among U.S. military personnel serving during the Gulf War period: A population-based study. *Psychosomatics* 43(3):195-205.

Barth, S. K., H. K. Kang, T. A. Bullman, and M. T. Wallin. 2009. Neurological mortality among U.S. veterans of the Persian Gulf War: 13-year follow-up. *American Journal of Industrial Medicine* 52:663-670.

Black, D. W., C. P. Carney, V. L. Forman-Hoffman, E. Letuchy, P. Peloso, R. F. Woolson, and B. N. Doebbeling. 2004a. Depression in veterans of the first Gulf War and comparable military controls. *Annals of Clinical Psychiatry* 16(2):53-61.

Black, D. W., C. P. Carney, P. M. Peloso, R. F. Woolson, D. A. Schwartz, M. D. Voelker, D. H. Barrett, and B. N. Doebbeling. 2004b. Gulf War veterans with anxiety: Prevalence, comorbidity, and risk factors. *Epidemiology* 15(2):135-142.

Black, D. W., N. Blum, E. Letuchy, C. Carney Doebbeling, V. L. Forman-Hoffman, and B. N. Doebbeling. 2006. Borderline personality disorder and traits in veterans: Psychiatric comorbidity, healthcare utilization, and quality of life along a continuum of severity. *CNS Spectrums* 11(9):680-689.

Blanchard, M. 2006. The first author replies. *American Journal of Epidemiology* 164(7):709-710.

Blanchard, M. S., S. A. Eisen, R. Alpern, J. Karlinsky, R. Toomey, D. J. Reda, F. M. Murphy, L. W. Jackson, and H. K. Kang. 2005. Chronic multisymptom illness complex in Gulf War I veterans 10 years later. *American Journal of Epidemiology* 163(1):66-75.

Bombardier, C. H., and D. Buchwald. 1996. Chronic fatigue, chronic fatigue syndrome, and fibromyalgia: Disability and health-care use. *Medical Care* 34(9):924-930.

Bourdette, D. N., L. A. McCauley, A. Barkhuizen, W. Johnston, M. Wynn, S. K. Joos, D. Storzbach, T. Shuell, and D. Sticker. 2001. Symptom factor analysis, clinical findings, and functional status in a population-based case control study of Gulf War unexplained illness. *Journal of Occupational and Environmental Medicine* 43(12):1026-1040.

Brailey, K., J. J. Vasterling, and P. B. Sutker. 1998. Psychological aftermath of participation in the Persian Gulf War. In *The Environment and Mental Health: A Guide for Clinicians*, edited by A. Lundberg. London: Lawrence Erlbaum Associates. Pp. 83-101.

Buchwald, D. 1996. Fibromyalgia and chronic fatigue syndrome. Similarities and differences. *Rheumatic Disease Clinics of North America* 22(2):219-243.

Buchwald, D., and D. Garrity. 1994. Comparison of patients with chronic fatigue syndrome, fibromyalgia, and multiple chemical sensitivities. *Archives of Internal Medicine* 154(18):2049-2053.

Bullman, T. A., C. M. Mahan, H. K. Kang, and W. F. Page. 2005. Mortality in US Army Gulf War veterans exposed to 1991 Khamisiyah chemical munitions destruction. *American Journal of Public Health* 95(8):1382-1388.

Bunegin, L., H. C. Mitzel, C. S. Miller, J. F. Gelineau, and G. P. Tolstykh. 2001. Cognitive performance and cerebrohemodynamics associated with the Persian Gulf syndrome. *Toxicology and Industrial Health* 17(4):128-137.

California Birth Defects Monitoring Program. 2009. *Programs*. http://www.cdph.ca.gov/programs/CBDMP/Pages/default.aspx (accessed December 22, 2009).

Carney, C. P., T. R. Sampson, M. Voelker, R. Woolson, P. Thorne, and B. N. Doebbeling. 2003. Women in the gulf war: Combat experience, exposures, and subsequent health care use. *Military Medicine* 168(8):654-661.

CDC (Centers for Disease Control and Prevention). 1987. Postservice mortality among Vietnam veterans. The Centers for Disease Control Vietnam Experience Study. *JAMA* 257(6):790-795.

Cermelli, C., M. Vinceti, F. Beretti, V. Pietrini, G. Nacci, P. Pietrosemoli, A. Bartoletti, D. Guidetti, P. Sola, M. Bergomi, G. Vivoli, and M. Portolani. 2003. Risk of sporadic amyotrophic lateral sclerosis associated with seropositivity for herpesviruses and echovirus-7. *European Journal of Epidemiology* 18(2):123-127.

Chadwick, V. S., W. Chen, D. Shu, B. Paulus, P. Bethwaite, A. Tie, and I. Wilson. 2002. Activation of the mucosal immune system in irritable bowel syndrome. *Gastroenterology* 122(7):1778-1783.

Chalder, T., G. Berelowitz, T. Pawlikowska, L. Watts, S. Wessely, D. Wright, and E. P. Wallace. 1993. Development of a fatigue scale. *Journal of Psychosomatic Research* 37(2):147-153.

Cherry, N., F. Creed, A. Silman, G. Dunn, D. Baxter, J. Smedley, S. Taylor, and G. J. Macfarlane. 2001a. Health and exposures of United Kingdom Gulf War veterans. Part I: The pattern and extent of ill health. *Occupational and Environmental Medicine* 58(5):291-298.

Cherry, N., F. Creed, A. Silman, G. Dunn, D. Baxter, J. Smedley, S. Taylor, and G. J. Macfarlane. 2001b. Health and exposures of United Kingdom Gulf War veterans. Part II: The relation of health to exposure. *Occupational and Environmental Medicine* 58(5):299-306.

Chio, A., G. Benzi, M. Dossena, R. Mutani, and G. Mora. 2005. Severely increased risk of amyotrophic lateral sclerosis among Italian professional football players. *Brain* 128(3):472-476.

Coffman, C. J., R. D. Horner, S. C. Grambow, and J. Lindquist. 2005. Estimating the occurrence of amyotrophic lateral sclerosis among Gulf War (1990-1991) veterans using capture-recapture methods: An assessment of case ascertainment bias. *Neuroepidemiology* 24(3):141-150.

Cogliano, V. J., R. A. Baan, K. Straif, Y. Grosse, M. B. Secretan, F. El Ghissassi, and P. Kleihues. 2004. The science and practice of carcinogen identification and evaluation. *Environmental Health Perspectives* 112(13):1269-1274.

Compston, A. 2006. Making progress on the natural history of multiple sclerosis. *Brain* 129(3):561-563.

Coombe, M. D., and S. F. Drysdale. 1993. Assessment of the effects of atmospheric oil pollution in post war Kuwait. *Journal of the Royal Army Medical Corps* 139(3):95-97.

Cowan, D. N., R. F. DeFraites, G. C. Gray, M. B. Goldenbaum, and S. M. Wishik. 1997. The risk of birth defects among children of Persian Gulf War veterans. [comment]. *New England Journal of Medicine* 336(23):1650-1656.

Cowan, D. N., J. L. Lange, J. Heller, J. Kirkpatrick, and S. DeBakey. 2002. A case-control study of asthma among U.S. Army Gulf War veterans and modeled exposure to oil-well fire smoke. *Military Medicine* 167(9):777-782.

Creed, F., R. Levy, L. Bradley, C. Fransisconi, D. A. Drossman, B. Naliboff, and K. Olden. 2006. Psychosocial aspects of functional gastrointestinal disorders. In *Rome III: The Functional Gastrointestinal Disorders*, edited by D. A. Drossman, E. Corazziari, M. Delvaux, R. C. Spiller, N. J. Talley, W. G. Thompson, and W. E. Whitehead. McLean, VA: Degnon Associates. Pp. 295-368.

DASA (Defence Analytical Services Agency). 2005. *1990/1991 Gulf Conflict—UK Gulf Veterans Mortality Data: Causes of Death.* Newport, South Wales: National Statistics.

DASA. 2009. *1990/1991 Gulf Conflict—UK Gulf Veterans Mortality Data: Causes of Death, 31 Dec 2008.* Bath, UK: National Statistics. http://www.dasa.mod.uk/natstats/gulf/intro.html (accessed July 30, 2009).

David, A. S., L. Farrin, L. Hull, C. Unwin, S. Wessely, and T. Wykes. 2002. Cognitive functioning and disturbances of mood in UK veterans of the Persian Gulf War: A comparative study. *Psychological Medicine* 32(8):1357-1370.

Davis, L. E., S. A. Eisen, F. M. Murphy, R. Alpern, B. J. Parks, M. Blanchard, D. J. Reda, M. K. King, F. A. Mithen, and H. K. Kang. 2004. Clinical and laboratory assessment of distal peripheral nerves in Gulf War veterans and spouses. *Neurology* 63(6):1070-1077.

Dlugosz, L. J., W. J. Hocter, K. S. Kaiser, J. D. Knoke, J. M. Heller, N. A. Hamid, R. J. Reed, K. S. Kendler, and G. C. Gray. 1999. Risk factors for mental disorder hospitalization after the Persian Gulf War: U.S. Armed Forces, June 1, 1991-September 30, 1993. *Journal of Clinical Epidemiology* 52(12):1267-1278.

DoD (Department of Defense). 2004. *Task Force Report on Care for Victims of Sexual Assault.* Washington, DC.

Doebbeling, B. N., W. R. Clarke, D. Watson, J. C. Torner, R. F. Woolson, M. D. Voelker, D. H. Barrett, and D. A Schwartz. 2000. Is there a Persian Gulf War syndrome? Evidence from a large population-based survey of veterans and nondeployed controls. *American Journal of Medicine* 108(9):695-704.

Doyle, P., N. Maconochie, G. Davies, I. Maconochie, M. Pelerin, S. Prior, and S. Lewis. 2004. Miscarriage, stillbirth and congenital malformation in the offspring of UK veterans of the first Gulf War. *International Journal of Epidemiology* 33(1):74-86.

Drossman, D. A. 1998. Presidential address: Gastrointestinal illness and biopsychosocial model. *Psychosomatic Medicine* 60:258-267.

Drossman, D. A. 1999. Mind over matter in the postinfective irritable bowel. *Gut* 44(3):306-307.

Drossman, D. A. 2006. The Functional Gastrointestinal Disorders and the Rome III Process. In *Rome III: The Functional Gastrointestinal Disorders*, 3rd ed, edited by D. A. Drossman, E. Corazziari, M. Delvaux, R. Spiller, N. Talley, W. G. Thompson, and W. E. Whitehead. McLean, VA: Degnon Associates. Pp. 1-29.

Drossman, D., and Y. Ringel. 2004. Psychosocial factors in ulcerative colitis and Crohn's disease. In *Kirsner's Inflammatory Bowel Diseases,* 6th ed., edited by J. B. Kirsner and W. J. Sandborn. Elsevier Health Sciences.

Drossman, D. A., N. J. Talley, K. W. Olden, J. Leserman, and M. A. Barreiro. 1995. Sexual and physical abuse and gastrointestinal illness: Review and recommendations. *Annals of Internal Medicine* 123:782-794.

Drossman, D. A., M. Camilleri, E. A. Mayer, and W. E. Whitehead. 2002. AGA technical review on irritable bowel syndrome. *Gastroenterology* 123:2108-2131.

Drossman, D. A., E. Corazziari, M. Delvaux, R. C. Spiller, N. J. Talley, W. G. Thompson, and W. E. Whitehead. 2006. *Rome III: The Functional Gastrointestinal Disorders*. McLean, VA: Degnon Associates.

Dunlop, S. P., D. Jenkins, K. R. Neal, and R. C. Spiller. 2003. Relative importance of enterochromaffin cell hyperplasia, anxiety and depression in post-infectious IBS. *Gastroenterology* 125:1651-1659.

Dunphy, R. C., L. Bridgewater, D. D. Price, M. E. Robinson, C. J. I. Zeilman, and G. N. Verne. 2003. Visceral and cutaneous hypersensitivity in Persian Gulf War veterans with chronic gastrointestinal symptoms. *Pain* 102:79-85.

Eisen, S. A., H. K. Kang, F. M. Murphy, M. S. Blanchard, D. J. Reda, W. G. Henderson, R. Toomey, L. W. Jackson, R. Alpern, B. J. Parks, N. Klimas, C. Hall, H. S. Pak, J. Hunter, J. Karlinsky, M. J. Battistone, M. J. Lyons, and Gulf War Study Participating Investigators. 2005. Gulf War veterans' health: Medical evaluation of a U.S. cohort. *Annals of Internal Medicine* 142(11):881-890.

Elbaz, A., J. Clavel, P. J. Rathouz, F. Moisan, J.-P. Galanaud, B. Delemotte, A. Alpérovitch, and C. Tzourio. 2009. Professional exposure to pesticides and Parkinsons disease. *Annals of Neurology* 66(4):494-504.

Epstein, K. R. 1995. The chronically fatigued patient. *Medical Clinics of North America* 79(2):315-327.

Ezzati, M., and A. D. Lopez. 2003. Estimates of global mortality attributable to smoking in 2000. *Lancet* 362(9387):847-852.

Fiedler, N., G. Ozakinci, W. Hallman, D. Wartenberg, N. T. Brewer, D. H. Barrett, and H. M. Kipen. 2006. Military deployment to the Gulf War as a risk factor for psychiatric illness among US troops. *British Journal of Psychiatry* 188:453-459.

Forbes, A. B., D. P. McKenzie, A. J. Mackinnon, H. L. Kelsall, A. C. McFarlane, J. F. Ikin, D. C. Glass, and M. R. Sim. 2004. The health of Australian veterans of the 1991 Gulf War: factor analysis of self-reported symptoms. *Occupational and Enviornmental Medicine* 61:1014-1020.

Forman-Hoffman, V. L., P. M. Peloso, D. W. Black, R. F. Woolson, E. M. Letuchy, and B. N. Doebbeling. 2007. Chronic widespread pain in veterans of the first Gulf War: Impact of deployment status and associated health effects. *Journal of Pain* 8(12):954-961.

Franse, L. V., G. D. Valk, J. H. Dekker, R. J. Heine, and J. T. M. Van Eijk. 2000. "Numbness of the feet" is a poor indicator for polyneuropathy in type 2 diabetic patients. *Diabetic Medicine* 17(2):105-110.

Fricker, R. D., E. Reardon, D. M. Spektor, S. K. Cotton, J. Hawes-Dawson, J. E. Pace, and S. D. Hosek. 2000. *Pesticide Use During the Gulf War: A Survey of Gulf War Veterans*. Santa Monica, CA: RAND Corporation.

Frommelt, R. A., M. R. Peterson, and T. J. O'Leary. 2000. A comparison of cervical pathology between United States Air Force women who did and did not serve in the Persian Gulf War. *Annals of Epidemiology* 10(5):285-292.

Fukuda, K., S. E. Straus, I. Hickie, M. C. Sharpe, J. G. Dobbins, and A. Komaroff. 1994. The chronic fatigue syndrome: A comprehensive approach to its definition and study. *Annals of Internal Medicine* 121(12):953-959.

Fukuda, K., R. Nisenbaum, G. Stewart, W. W. Thompson, L. Robin, R. M. Washko, D. L. Noah, D. H. Barrett, B. Randall, B. L. Herwaldt, A. C. Mawle, and W. C. Reeves. 1998. Chronic multisymptom illness affecting Air Force veterans of the Gulf War. *JAMA* 280(11):981-988.

Fukudo, S., T. Normura, and M. Hongo. 1998. Impact of corticotropin-releasing hormone on gastrointestinal motility and adrenocorticotropic hormone in normal controls and patients with irritable bowel syndrome. *Gut* 42:845-849.

Gackstetter, G., S. DeBakey, D. Cowan, M. Paxton, R. Weaver, J. Lange, H. Kang, T. Bullman, A. Lincoln, and T. Hooper. 2002. Fatal motor vehicle crashes among veterans of the Gulf War era: A nested case-control study. *Annals of Epidemiology* 12(7):509.

Golan, D., E. Somer, S. Dishon, L. Cuzin-Disegni, and A. Miller. 2008. Impact of exposure to war stress on exacerbations of multiple sclerosis. *Annals of Neurology* 64:143-148.

Goldenberg, D. L., R. W. Simms, A. Geiger, and A. L. Komaroff. 1990. High frequency of fibromyalgia in patients with chronic fatigue seen in a primary care practice. *Arthritis and Rheumatism* 33(3):381-387.

Goldstein, G., S. R. Beers, L. A. Morrow, W. J. Shemansky, and S. R. Steinhauer. 1996. A preliminary neuropsychological study of Persian Gulf veterans. *Journal of the International Neuropsychological Society* 2(4):368-371.

Goldzweig, C. L., T. M. Balekian, C. Rolón, E. M. Yano, and P. G. Shekelle. 2006. The state of women veterans' health research: Results of a systematic literature review. *Journal of General Internal Medicine* 21(Suppl 3):S82-S92.

Goshorn, R. K. 1998. Chronic fatigue syndrome: A review for clinicians. *Seminars in Neurology* 18(2):237-242.

Goss Gilroy Inc. 1998. *Health Study of Canadian Forces Personnel Involved in the 1991 Conflict in the Persian Gulf.* Ottawa, Canada: Goss Gilroy Inc., and Department of National Defence.

Gray, G. C., and H. Kang. 2006. Healthcare utlization and mortality among veterans of the Gulf War. *Philisophical Transactions of the Royal Society B* 361:553-569.

Gray, G. C., B. D. Coate, C. M. Anderson, H. K. Kang, S. W. Berg, F. S. Wignall, J. D. Knoke, and E. Barrett-Connor. 1996. The postwar hospitalization experience of U.S. veterans of the Persian Gulf War. *New England Journal of Medicine* 335(20):1505-1513.

Gray, G. C., K. S. Kaiser, A. W. Hawksworth, F. W. Hall, and E. Barrett-Connor. 1999a. Increased postwar symptoms and psychological morbidity among U.S. Navy Gulf War veterans. *American Journal of Tropical Medicine and Hygiene* 60(5):758-766.

Gray, G. C., T. C. Smith, J. D. Knoke, and J. M. Heller. 1999b. The postwar hospitalization experience of Gulf War veterans possibly exposed to chemical munitions destruction at Khamisiyah, Iraq. *American Journal of Epidemiology* 150(5):532-540.

Gray, G. C., T. C. Smith, H. K. Kang, and J. D. Knoke. 2000. Are Gulf War veterans suffering war-related illnesses? Federal and civilian hospitalizations examined, June 1991 to December 1994. *American Journal of Epidemiology* 151(1):63-71.

Gray, G. C., R. J. Reed, K. S. Kaiser, T. C. Smith, and V. M. Gastanaga. 2002. Self-reported symptoms and medical conditions among 11,868 Gulf War-era veterans: The Seabee Health Study. *American Journal of Epidemiology* 155(11):1033-1044.

Grover, M., H. Herfarth, and D. A. Drossman. 2009. The functional-organic dichotomy: Post-infectious irritable bowel syndrome and inflammatory bowel disease-irritable bowel syndrome. *Clinical Gastroenterology and Hepatology* 7:48-53.

Gwee, K. A., Y. L. Leong, C. Graham, M. W. McKendrick, S. M. Collins, S. J. Walters, J. E. Underwood, and N. W. Read. 1999. The role of psychological and biological factors in postinfective gut dysfunction. *Gut* 44(3):400-406.

Haley, R. W. 2003. Excess incidence of ALS in young Gulf War veterans. *Neurology.* 61(6):750-756.

Haley, R. W., and T. L. Kurt. 1997. Self-reported exposure to neurotoxic chemical combinations in the Gulf War: A cross-sectional epidemiologic study. *Journal of the American Medical Association* 277(3):231-237.

Haley, R. W., S. Billecke, and B. N. La Du. 1999. Association of low PON1 type Q (type A) arylesterase activity with neurologic symptom complexes in Gulf War veterans. *Toxicology and Applied Pharmacology* 157(3):227-233.

Haley, R. W., J. L. Fleckenstein, W. W. Marshall, G. G. McDonald, G. L. Kramer, and F. Petty. 2000a. Effect of basal ganglia injury on central dopamine activity in Gulf War syndrome: Correlation of proton magnetic resonance spectroscopy and plasma homovanillic acid levels. *Archives of Neurology* 57(9):1280-1285.

Haley, R. W., W. W. Marshall, G. G. McDonald, M. A. Daugherty, F. Petty, and J. L. Fleckenstein. 2000b. Brain abnormalities in Gulf War syndrome: Evaluation with 1H MR spectroscopy. *Radiology* 215(3):807-817.

Haley, R. W., W. Vongpatanasin, G. I. Wolfe, W. W. Bryan, R. Armitage, R. F. Hoffmann, F. Petty, T. S. Callahan, E. Charuvastra, W. E. Shell, W. W. Marshall, and R. G. Victor. 2004. Blunted circadian variation in autonomic regulation of sinus node function in veterans with Gulf War syndrome. *American Journal of Medicine* 117(7):469-478.

Haley, R. W., J. S. Spence, P. S. Carmack, R. F. Gunst, W. R. Schucany, F. Petty, M. D. Devous, Sr., F. J. Bonte, and M. H. Trivedi. 2009. Abnormal brain response to cholinergic challenge in chronic encephalopathy from the 1991 Gulf War. *Psychiatry Research: Neuroimaging* 171(3):207-220.

Hardt, J., D., Buchwald, D., Wilks, M., Sharpe, W. A.,Nix, and U. T. Egle. 2001. Health-related quality of life in patients with chronic fatigue syndrome: An international study. *Journal of Psychosomatic Research* 51(2):431-434.

Higgins, E. M., K. Ismail, K. Kant, K. Harman, J. Mellerio, A. W. Du Vivier, and S. Wessely. 2002. Skin disease in Gulf War veterans. *QJM* 95(10):671-676.

Holmes, D. T., P. N. Tariot, and C. Cox. 1998. Preliminary evidence of psychological distress among reservists in the Persian Gulf War. *Journal of Nervous and Mental Disease* 186(3):166-173.

Hom, J., R. W. Haley, and T. L. Kurt. 1997. Neuropsychological correlates of Gulf War syndrome. *Archives of Clinical Neuropsychology* 12(6):531-544.

Hooper, T. I., S. F. DeBakey, A. Lincoln, H. K. Kang, D. N. Cowan, and G. D. Gackstetter. 2005. Leveraging existing databases to study vehicle crashes in a combat occupational cohort: Epidemiologic methods. *American Journal of Industrial Medicine* 48(2):118-127.

Hooper, T. I., S. F. Debakey, B. E. Nagaraj, K. S. Bellis, B. Smith, T. C. Smith, and G. D. Gackstetter. 2008. The long-term hospitalization experience following military service in the 1991 Gulf War among veterans remaining on active duty, 1994-2004. *BMC Public Health* 8:60.

Horn, O., L. Hull, M. Jones, D. Murphy, T. Browne, N. T. Fear, M. Hotopf, R. J. Rona, and S. Wessely. 2006. Is there an Iraq war syndrome? Comparison of the health of UK service personnel after the Gulf and Iraq wars. *Lancet* 367(9524):1742-1746.

Horner, R. D., K. G. Kamins, J. R. Feussner, S. C. Grambow, J. Hoff-Lindquist, Y. Harati, H. Mitsumoto, R. Pascuzzi, P. S. Spencer, R. Tim, D. Howard, T. C. Smith, M. A. Ryan, C. J. Coffman, and E. J. Kasarskis. 2003. Occurrence of amyotrophic lateral sclerosis among Gulf War veterans. *Neurology* 61(6):742-749.

Horner, R. D., S. C. Grambow, C. J. Coffman, J. H. Lindquist, E. Z. Oddone, K. D. Allen, and E. J. Kasarskis. 2008. Amyotrophic lateral sclerosis among 1991 Gulf War veterans: Evidence for a time-limited outbreak. *Neuroepidemiology* 31(1):28-32.

Hotopf, M., M. I. Mackness, V. Nikolaou, D. A. Collier, C. Curtis, A. David, P. Durrington, L. Hull, K. Ismail, M. Peakman, C. Unwin, S. Wessely, and B. Mackness. 2003. Paraoxonase in Persian Gulf War veterans. *Journal of Occupational and Environmental Medicine* 45(7):668-675.

Hyams, K. C., F. S. Wignall, and R. Roswell. 1996. War syndromes and their evaluation: From the U.S. Civil War to the Persian Gulf War. *Annals of Internal Medicine* 125(5):398-405.

Ikin, J. F., M. R. Sim, M. C. Creamer, A. B. Forbes, D. P. McKenzie, H. L. Kelsall, D. C. Glass, A. C. McFarlane, M. J. Abramson, P. Ittak, T. Dwyer, L. Blizzard, K. R. Delaney, K. W. A. Horsley, W. K. Harrex, and H. Schwarz. 2004. War-related psychological stressors and risk of psychological disorders in Australian veterans of the 1991 Gulf War. *British Journal of Psychiatry.* 185(2):116-126.

IOM (Institute of Medicine). 2006. *Amyotrophic Lateral Sclerosis in Veterans.* Washington, DC: The National Academies Press.

IOM. 2007. *Gulf War and Health, Volume 5: Infectious Diseases.* Washington, DC: The National Academies Press.

IOM. 2008. *Gulf War and Health: Updated Literature Review of Depleted Uranium.* Washington, DC: The National Academies Press.

Iowa Persian Gulf Study Group. 1997. Self-reported illness and health status among Gulf War veterans: A population-based study. *JAMA* 277(3):238-245.

Ishoy, T., P. Suadicani, B. Guldager, M. Appleyard, and F. Gyntelberg. 1999a. Risk factors for gastrointestinal symptoms. The Danish Gulf War Study. *Danish Medical Bulletin* 46(5):420-423.

Ishoy, T., P. Suadicani, B. Guldager, M. Appleyard, H. O. Hein, and F. Gyntelberg. 1999b. State of health after deployment in the Persian Gulf. The Danish Gulf War Study. *Danish Medical Bulletin* 46(5):416-419.

Ishoy, T., A. M. Andersson, P. Suadicani, B. Guldager, M. Appleyard, F. Gyntelberg, N. E. Skakkebaek, and S. Danish Gulf War. 2001a. Major reproductive health characteristics in male Gulf War veterans. The Danish Gulf War Study. *Danish Medical Bulletin* 48(1):29-32.

Ishoy, T., P. Suadicani, A.-M. Andersson, B. Guldager, M. Appleyard, N. Skakkebaek, and F. Gyntelberg. 2001b. Prevalence of male sexual problems in the Danish Gulf War Study. *Scandinavian Journal of Sexology* 4(1):43-55.

Ismail, K., B. Everitt, N. Blatchley, L. Hull, C. Unwin, A. David, and S. Wessely. 1999. Is there a Gulf War syndrome? *Lancet.* 353(9148):179-182.

Ismail, K., K. Kent, T. Brugha, M. Hotopf, L. Hull, P. Seed, I. Palmer, S. Reid, C. Unwin, A. S. David, and S. Wessely. 2002. The mental health of UK Gulf War veterans: Phase 2 of a two phase cohort study. *BMJ* 325(7364):576-582.

Ismail, K., K. Kent, R. Sherwood, L. Hull, P. Seed, A. S. David, and S. Wessely. 2008. Chronic fatigue syndrome and related disorders in UK veterans of the Gulf War 1990-1991: Results from a two-phase cohort study. *Psychological Medicine* 38(7):953-961.

Jones, M. P., J. B. Dilley, D. Drossman, and M. D. Crowell. 2006. Brain-gut connections in functional GI disorders: Anatomic and physiologic relationships. *Neurogastroenterology and Motility* 18(2):91-103.

Kamel, F., D. M. Umbach, T. L. Munsat, J. M. Shefner, H. Hu, and D. P. Sandler. 2002. Lead exposure and amyotrophic lateral sclerosis. *Epidemiology* 13(3):311-319.

Kamel, F., C. M. Tanner, D. M. Umbach, J. A. Hoppin, M. C. R. Alavanja, A. Blair, K. Comyns, S. M. Goldman, M. Korell, J. W. Langston, G. W. Ross, and D. P. Sandler. 2007. Pesticide exposure and self-reported Parkinson's disease in the agricultural health study. *American Journal of Epidemiology* 165(4):364-374.

Kang, H. K., and T. A. Bullman. 1996. Mortality among U.S. veterans of the Persian Gulf War. *New England Journal of Medicine* 335(20):1498-1504.

Kang, H. K., and T. A. Bullman. 2001. Mortality among US veterans of the Persian Gulf War: 7-year follow-up. *American Journal of Epidemiology* 154(5):399-405.

Kang, H. K., C. M. Mahan, K. Y. Lee, C. A. Magee, and F. M. Murphy. 2000. Illnesses among United States veterans of the Gulf War: A population-based survey of 30,000 veterans. *Journal of Occupational and Environmental Medicine* 42(5):491-501.

Kang, H., C. Magee, C. Mahan, K. Lee, F. Murphy, L. Jackson, and G. Matanoski. 2001. Pregnancy outcomes among U.S. Gulf War veterans: A population-based survey of 30,000 veterans. *Annals of Epidemiology* 11(7):504-511.

Kang, H. K., C. M. Mahan, K. Y. Lee, F. M. Murphy, S. J. Simmens, H. A. Young, and P. H. Levine. 2002. Evidence for a deployment-related Gulf War syndrome by factor analysis. *Archives of Environmental Health* 57(1):61-68.

Kang, H. K., B. H. Natelson, C. M. Mahan, K. Y. Lee, and F. M. Murphy. 2003. Post-traumatic stress disorder and chronic fatigue syndrome-like illness among Gulf War veterans: A population-based survey of 30,000 veterans. *American Journal of Epidemiology* 157(2):141-148.

Kang, H., N. Dalager, C. Mahan, and E. Ishii. 2005. The role of sexual assault on the risk of PTSD among Gulf War veterans. *Annals of Epidemiology* 15(3):191-195.

Kang, H. K., B. Li, C. M. Mahan, S. A. Eisen, and C. C. Engel. 2009. Health of US veterans of 1991 Gulf War: A follow-up survey in 10 years. *Journal of Occupational and Environmental Medicine* 51(4):401-410.

Karlinsky, J. B., M. Blanchard, R. Alpern, S. A. Eisen, H. Kang, F. M. Murphy, and D. J. Reda. 2004. Late prevalence of respiratory symptoms and pulmonary function abnormalities in Gulf War I veterans. *Archives of Internal Medicine* 164(22):2488-2491.

Kassinen, A., L. Krogius-Kurikka, H. Makivuokko, T. Rinttila, L. Paulin, J. Corander, E. Malinen, J. Apajalahti, and A. Palva. 2007. The fecal microbiota of irritable bowel syndrome patients differs significantly from that of healthy subjects. *Gastroenterology* 133:24-33.

Kellow, J. E., F. Azpiroz, M. Delvaux, G. F. Gebhart, H. Mertz, E. M. M. Quigley, and A. Smout. 2006a. Principles of applied neurogastroenterology: Physiology/motility-sensation. In *Rome III: The Functional Gastrointestinal Disorders*, 3rd ed, edited by D. A. Drossman, E. Corazziari, M. Delvaux, R. C. Spiller, N. J. Talley, W. G. Thompson, and W. E. Whitehead. McLean, VA: Degnon Associates. Pp. 89-160.

Kellow, J. E., F. Azpiroz, M. Delvaux, G. F. Gebhart, H. R. Mertz, E. M. M. Quigley, and A. Smout. 2006b. Principles of applied neurogastroenterology in the functional gastrointestinal disorders. *Gastroenterology* 130(5):1412-1420.

Kelsall, H. L., M. R. Sim, A. B. Forbes, D. C. Glass, D. P. McKenzie, J. F. Ikin, M. J. Abramson, L. Blizzard, and P. Ittak. 2004a. Symptoms and medical conditions in Australian veterans of the 1991 Gulf War: Relation to immunisations and other Gulf War exposures. *Occupational and Environmental Medicine* 61(12):1006-1013.

Kelsall, H. L., M. R. Sim, A. B. Forbes, D. P. McKenzie, D. C. Glass, J. F. Ikin, P. Ittak, and M. J. Abramson. 2004b. Respiratory health status of Australian veterans of the 1991 Gulf War and the effects of exposure to oil fire smoke and dust storms. *Thorax* 59(10):897-903.

Kelsall, H., R. Macdonell, M. Sim, A. Forbes, D. McKenzie, D. Glass, J. Ikin, and P. Ittak. 2005. Neurological status of Australian veterans of the 1991 Gulf War and the effect of medical and chemical exposures. *International Journal of Epidemiology* 34(4):810-819.

Kelsall, H., M. Sim, D. McKenzie, A. Forbes, K. Leder, D. Glass, J. Ikin, and A. McFarlane. 2006. Medically evaluated psychological and physical health of Australian Gulf War veterans with chronic fatigue. *Journal of Psychosomatic Research* 60(6):575-584.

Kelsall, H. L., M. R. Sim, J. F. Ikin, A. B. Forbes, D. P. McKenzie, D. C. Glass, and P. Ittak. 2007. Reproductive health of male Australian veterans of the 1991 Gulf War. *BMC Public Health* 7:79.

Kessler, R. C., A. Sonnega, E. Bromet., M. Hughes, and C.B. Nelson. 1995. Posttraumatic stress disorder in the National Comorbidity Survey. *Archives of General Psychiatry* 52(12):1048-1060.

Kessler, R. C., P. Berglund, O. Demler, R. Jin, K. R. Merikangas, and E. E. Walters. 2005a. Lifetime prevalence and age-of-onset distributions of DSM-IV disorders in the national comorbidity survey replication. *Archives of General Psychiatry* 62(6):593-602.

Kessler, R. C., T. C. Wai, O. Demler, and E. E. Walters. 2005b. Prevalence, severity, and comorbidity of 12-month DSM-IV disorders in the National Comorbidity Survey Replication. *Archives of General Psychiatry* 62(6):617-627.

Kieszak, S. M., W. D. Flanders, A. S. Kosinski, C. C. Shipp, and H. Karp. 1999. A comparison of the Charlson comorbidity index derived from medical record data and administrative billing data. *Journal of Clinical Epidemiology* 52(2):137-142.

Klooker, T. K., B. Braak, R. C. Painter, S. R. De Rooij, R. M. Van Elburg, R. M. Van Den Wijngaard, T. J. Roseboom, and G. E. Boeckxstaens. 2009. Exposure to severe wartime conditions in early life is associated with an increased risk of irritable bowel syndrome: A population-based cohort study. *American Journal of Gastroenterology* 104(9):2250-2256.

Knoke, J. D., and G. C. Gray. 1998. Hospitalizations for unexplained illnesses among U.S. veterans of the Persian Gulf War. [comment]. *Emerging Infectious Diseases* 4(2):211-219.

Knoke, J. D., G. C. Gray, and F. C. Garland. 1998. Testicular cancer and Persian Gulf War service. *Epidemiology* 9(6):648-653.

Knoke, J. D., T. C. Smith, G. C. Gray, K. S. Kaiser, and A. W. Hawksworth. 2000. Factor analysis of self-reported symptoms: Does it identify a Gulf War syndrome? *American Journal of Epidemiology* 152(4):379-388.

Komaroff, A. L., L. R. Fagioli, T. H. Doolittle, B. Gandek, M. A. Gleit, R. T. Guerriero, R. J. Kornish II, N. C. Ware, J. E. Ware Jr, and D. W. Bates. 1996. Health status in patients with chronic fatigue syndrome and in general population and disease comparison groups. *American Journal of Medicine* 101(3):281-290.

Kroenke, K., P. Koslowe, and M. Roy. 1998. Symptoms in 18,495 Persian Gulf War veterans. Latency of onset and lack of association with self-reported exposures. *Journal of Occupational & Environmental Medicine* 40(6):520-528.

Kuzma, J. M., and D. W. Black. 2006. Chronic widespread pain and psychiatric disorders in veterans of the first Gulf War. *Current Pain and Headache Reports* 10(2):85-89.

Lakatta, E. G. 2002. Cardiovascular ageing in health sets the stage for cardiovascular disease. *Heart Lung and Circulation* 11(2):76-91.

Lang, K. A., and J. Saylor. 1995. Gastrointestinal symptoms and the Gulf War syndrome. *Gastroenterology* 108(4):A23.

Lange, G., L. A. Tiersky, J. B. Scharer, T. Policastro, N. Fiedler, T. E. Morgan, and B. H. Natelson. 2001. Cognitive functioning in Gulf War illness. *Journal of Clinical and Experimental Neuropsychology* 23(2):240-249.

Lange, J. L., D. A. Schwartz, B. N. Doebbeling, J. M. Heller, and P. S. Thorne. 2002. Exposures to the Kuwait oil fires and their association with asthma and bronchitis among gulf war veterans. *Environmental Health Perspectives* 110(11):1141-1146.

Levine, P. H., H. A. Young, S. J. Simmens, D. Rentz, V. E. Kofie, C. M. Mahan, and H. K. Kang. 2005. Is testicular cancer related to Gulf War deployment? Evidence from a pilot population-based study of Gulf War era veterans and cancer registries. *Military Medicine* 170(2):149-153.

Levy, R. L., W. E. Whitehead, M. R. Von Korff, and A. D. Feld. 2000. Intergenerational transmission of gastrointestinal illness behavior. *American Journal of Gastroenterology* 95(2):451-456.

Levy, R. L., K. W. Olden, B. D. Naliboff, L. A. Bradley, C. F. Francisconi, D. A. Drossman, and F. Creed. 2006. Psychosocial aspects of the functional gastrointestinal disorder. *Gastroenterology* 130:1447-1458.

Lincoln, A. E., T. I. Hooper, H. K. Kang, S. F. Debakey, D. N. Cowan, and G. D. Gackstetter. 2006. Motor vehicle fatalities among Gulf War era veterans: Characteristics, mechanisms, and circumstances. *Traffic Injury Prevention* 7(1):31-37.

Lindem, K., T. Heeren, R. F. White, S. P. Proctor, M. Krengel, J. Vasterling, P. B. Sutker, J. Wolfe, and T. M. Keane. 2003a. Neuropsychological performance in Gulf War era veterans: Traumatic stress symptomatology and exposure to chemical-biological warfare agents. *Journal of Psychopathology and Behavioral Assessment.* 25(2):105-119.

Lindem, K., S. P. Proctor, T. Heeren, M. Krengel, J. Vasterling, P. B. Sutker, J. Wolfe, T. M. Keane, and R. F. White. 2003b. Neuropsychological performance in Gulf War era veterans: Neuropsychological symptom reporting. *Journal of Psychopathology and Behavioral Assessment.*(2):121-127.

Lindem, K., R. F. White, T. Heeren, S. P. Proctor, M. Krengel, J. Vasterling, J. Wolfe, P. B. Sutker, S. Kirkley, and T. M. Keane. 2003c. Neuropsychological performance in Gulf War era veterans: Motivational factors and effort. *Journal of Psychopathology and Behavioral Assessment.* 25(2):129-138.

Longstreth, G. F. 2006. Functional dyspepsia—Managing the conundrum. *New England Journal of Medicine* 354(8):791-793.

Longstreth, G. F., W. G. Thompson, W. D. Chey, L. A. Houghton, F. Mearin, and R. C. Spiller. 2006. Functional bowel disorders. *Gastroenterology* 130(5):1480-1491.

Lucas, K. E., P. C. Rowe, and H. K. Armenian. 2007. Latency and exposure-health associations in Gulf War veterans with early fatigue onsets: A case-control study. *Annals of Epidemiology* 17(10):799-806.

Macfarlane, G. J., E. Thomas, and N. Cherry. 2000. Mortality among UK Gulf War veterans. *Lancet* 356(9223):17-21.

Macfarlane, G. J., A.-M. Biggs, N. Maconochie, M. Hotopf, P. Doyle, and M. Lunt. 2003. Incidence of cancer among UK Gulf War veterans: Cohort study. *British Medical Journal* 327(7428):1373-1375.

Macfarlane, G. J., M. Hotopf, N. Maconochie, N. Blatchley, A. Richards, and M. Lunt. 2005. Long-term mortality amongst Gulf War Veterans: Is there a relationship with experiences during deployment and subsequent morbidity? *International Journal of Epidemiology* 34(6):1403-1408.

Mackness, B., M. I. Mackness, S. Arrol, W. Turkie, and P. N. Durrington. 1997. Effect of the molecular polymorphisms of human paraoxonase (PON1) on the rate of hydrolysis of paraoxon. *British Journal of Pharmacology* 122(2):265-268.

Maconochie, N., P. Doyle, E. Roman, G. Davies, P. G. Smith, and V. Beral. 1999. The nuclear industry family study: Linkage of occupational exposures to reproduction and child health. *British Medical Journal* 318(7196):1453-1454.

Maconochie, N., P. Doyle, and C. Carson. 2004. Infertility among male UK veterans of the 1990-1 Gulf war: Reproductive cohort study. *British Medical Journal* 329(7459):196-201.

Magruder, K. M., B. C. Frueh, R. G. Knapp, L. Davis, M. B. Hamner, R. H. Martin, P. B. Gold, and G. W. Arana. 2005. Prevalence of posttraumatic stress disorder in Veterans Affairs primary care clinics. *General Hospital Psychiatry* 27(3):169-179.

McCauley, L. A., M. Lasarev, D. Sticker, D. G. Rischitelli, and P. S. Spencer. 2002. Illness experience of Gulf War veterans possibly exposed to chemical warfare agents. *American Journal of Preventive Medicine* 23(3):200-206.

McDiarmid, M. A., J. P. Keogh, F. J. Hooper, K. McPhaul, K. Squibb, R. Kane, R. Dipino, M. Kabat, B. Kaup, L. Anderson, D. Hoover, L. Brown, M. Hamilton, D. Jacobson-Kram, B. Burrows, and M. Walsh. 2000. Health effects of depleted uranium on exposed Gulf War veterans. *Environmental Research* 82(2):168-180.

McDiarmid, M. A., K. Squibb, S. Engelhardt, M. Oliver, P. Gucer, P. D. Wilson, R. Kane, M. Kabat, B. Kaup, L. Anderson, D. Hoover, L. Brown, and D. Jacobson-Kram. 2001. Surveillance of depleted uranium exposed Gulf War veterans: Health effects observed in an enlarged "friendly fire" cohort. *Journal of Occupational and Environmental Medicine* 43(12):991-1000.

McDiarmid, M. A., S. Engelhardt, M. Oliver, P. Gucer, P. D. Wilson, R. Kane, M. Kabat, B. Kaup, L. Anderson, D. Hoover, L. Brown, B. Handwerger, R. J. Albertini, D. Jacobson-Kram, C. D. Thorne, and K. S. Squibb. 2004. Health effects of depleted uranium on exposed Gulf War veterans: A 10-year follow-up. *Journal of Toxicology and Environmental Health—Part A* 67(4):277-296.

McDiarmid, M. A., S. M. Engelhardt, M. Oliver, P. Gucer, P. D. Wilson, R. Kane, M. Kabat, B. Kaup, L. Anderson, D. Hoover, L. Brown, R. J. Albertini, R. Gudi, D. Jacobson-Kram, C. D. Thorne, and K. S. Squibb. 2006. Biological monitoring and surveillance results of Gulf War I veterans exposed to depleted uranium. *International Archives of Occupational and Environmental Health* 79(1):11-21.

McDiarmid, M. A., S. M. Engelhardt, M. Oliver, P. Gucer, P. D. Wilson, R. Kane, A. Cernich, B. Kaup, L. Anderson, D. Hoover, L. Brown, R. Albertini, R. Gudi, D. Jacobson-Kram, and K. S. Squibb. 2007a. Health surveillance of Gulf War I veterans exposed to depleted uranium: Updating the cohort. *Health Physics* 93(1):60-73.

McDiarmid, M. A., K. Squibb, S. Engelhardt, P. Gucer, and M. Oliver. 2007b. Surveillance of Gulf War I veterans exposed to depleted uranium: 15 years of follow-up. *European Journal of Oncology* 12(4):235-242.

McDiarmid, M. A., S. M. Engelhardt, C. D. Dorsey, M. Oliver, P. Gucer, P. D. Wilson, R. Kane, A. Cernich, B. Kaup, L. Anderson, D. Hoover, L. Brown, R. Albertini, R. Gudi, and K. S. Squibb. 2009. Surveillance results of depleted uranium-exposed Gulf War I veterans: Sixteen years of follow-up. *Journal of Toxicology and Environmental Health Part A* 72(1):14-29.

McDonald, W.I., A. Compston, G. Edan, D. Goodkin, H.P. Hartung, F.D. Lublin, H.F. McFarland, D.W. Paty, C.H. Polman, S.C. Reingold, M. Sandberg-Wollheim, W. Sibley, A. Thompson, S. van den Noort, B.Y. Weinshenker, J.S. Wolinsky.. 2001. Recommended diagnostic criteria for multiple sclerosis: Guidelines from the International Panel on the diagnosis of multiple sclerosis. *Annals of Neurology* 50(1):121-127.

McGuire, V., W. T. J. Longstreth, T. D. Koepsell, and G. van Belle. 1996. Incidence of amyotrophic lateral sclerosis in three counties in western Washington state. *Neurology* 47(2):571-573.

McGuire, V., W. T. Longstreth Jr, L. M. Nelson, T. D. Koepsell, H. Checkoway, M. S. Morgan, and G. Van Belle. 1997. Occupational exposures and amyotrophic lateral sclerosis: A population-based case-control study. *American Journal of Epidemiology* 145(12):1076-1088.

McKenzie, D. P., J. F. Ikin, A. C. McFarlane, M. Creamer, A. B. Forbes, H. L. Kelsall, D. C. Glass, P. Ittak, and M. R. Sim. 2004. Psychological health of Australian veterans of the 1991 Gulf War: An assessment using the SF-12, GHQ-12 and PCL-S. *Psychological Medicine* 34(8):1419-1430.

McKeown, E. S., S. D. Parry, R. Stansfield, J. R. Barton, and M. R. Welfare. 2006. Postinfectious irritable bowel syndrome may occur after non-gastrointestinal and intestinal infection. *Neurogastroenterology and Motility* 18(9):839-843.

Murphy, D., R. Hooper, C. French, M. Jones, R. Rona, and S. Wessely. 2006. Is the increased reporting of symptomatic ill health in Gulf War veterans related to how one asks the question? *Journal of Psychosomatic Research* 61(2):181-186.

Murphy, F. M., H. Kang, N. A. Dalager, K. Y. Lee, R. E. Allen, S. H. Mather, and K. W. Kizer. 1999. The health status of Gulf War veterans: Lessons learned from the Department of Veterans Affairs Health Registry. *Military Medicine* 164(5):327-331.

Murray, C. D., J. Flynn, L. Ratcliffe, M. R. Jacyna, M. A. Kamm, and A. V. Emmanuel. 2004. Effect of acute physical and psychological stress on gut autonomic innervation in irritable bowel syndrome. *Gastroenterology* 127:1695-1703.

National Institute of Neurological Disorders and Stroke. 2006. Conference Report: NIH Peripheral Neuropathy Conference, October 22-24, 2006, Bethesda, MD.

National Institute of Neurological Disorders and Stroke. 2009. *Amyotrophic Lateral Sclerosis Fact Sheet.* http://www.ninds.nih.gov/disorders/amyotrophiclateralsclerosis/detail_amyotrophiclateralsclerosis.htm (accessed December 4, 2009).

Nelson, L. M., V. McGuire, W. T. Longstreth, and C. Matkin. 2000. Population-based case-control study of amyotrophic lateral sclerosis in western Washington State. I. Cigarette smoking and alcohol consumption. *American Journal of Epidemiology* 151(2):156-163.

Nicolson, G. L., M. Y. Nasralla, J. Haier, and J. Pomfret. 2002. High frequency of systemic mycoplasmal infections in Gulf War veterans and civilians with amyotrophic lateral sclerosis (ALS). *Journal of Clinical Neuroscience* 9(5):525-529.

Nimnuan, C., S. Rabe-Hesketh, S. Wessely, and M. Hotopf. 2001. How many functional somatic syndromes? *Journal of Psychosomatic Research* 51(4):549-557.

Nisenbaum, R., D. H. Barrett, M. Reyes, and W. C. Reeves. 2000. Deployment stressors and a chronic multisymptom illness among Gulf War veterans. *Journal of Nervous and Mental Disease* 188(5):259-266.

Nisenbaum, R., K. Ismail, S. Wessely, C. Unwin, L. Hull, and W. C. Reeves. 2004. Dichotomous factor analysis of symptoms reported by UK and US veterans of the 1991 Gulf War. *Population Health Metrics* 2(1):8.

O'Toole, B. I., R. P. Marshall, D. A. Grayson, R. J. Schureck, M. Dobson, M. French, B. Pulvertaft, L. Meldrum, J. Bolton, and J. Vennard. 1996. The Australian Vietnam Veterans Health Study: III. Psychological health of Australian Vietnam veterans and its relationship to combat. *International Journal of Epidemiology* 25(2):331-340.

Page, W. F., C. M. Mahan, T. A. Bullman, and H. K. Kang. 2005. Health effects in Army Gulf War veterans possibly exposed to chemical munitions destruction at Khamisiyah, Iraq: Part I. Morbidity associated with potential exposure. *Military Medicine* 170(11):935-944.

Pasquina, P. F., T. K. Joseph, and L. Foster. 2004. Decreased prevalence of peripheral nerve pathology by electrodiagnostic testing in Gulf War veterans. *Military Medicine* 169(11):868-871.

Pearce, J. M. S. 2004. Myofascial pain, fibromyalgia or fibrositis? *European Neurology* 52(2):67-72.

Penman, A. D., R. S. Tarver, and M. M. Currier. 1996. No evidence of increase in birth defects and health problems among children born to Persian Gulf War veterans in Mississippi. *Military Medicine* 161(1):1-6.

Petruccelli, B. P., M. Goldenbaum, B. Scott, R. Lachiver, D. Kanjarpane, E. Elliott, M. Francis, M. A. McDiarmid, and D. Deeter. 1999. Health effects of the 1991 Kuwait oil fires: A survey of US Army troops. *Journal of Occupational and Environmental Medicine* 41(6):433-439.

Pierce, P. F. 1997. Physical and emotional health of Gulf War veteran women. *Aviation Space and Environmental Medicine* 68(4):317-321.

Pierce, P. F. 2005. Monitoring the health of Persian Gulf War veteran women. *Military Medicine* 170(5):349-354.

Pizarro, J., R. C. Silver, and J. Prause. 2006. Physical and mental health costs of traumatic war experiences among Civil War veterans. *Archives of General Psychiatry* 63(2):193-200.

Proctor, S. P., T. Heeren, R. F. White, J. Wolfe, M. S. Borgos, J. D. Davis, L. Pepper, R. Clapp, P. B. Sutker, J. J. Vasterling, and D. Ozonoff. 1998. Health status of Persian Gulf War veterans: Self-reported symptoms, environmental exposures and the effect of stress. *International Journal of Epidemiology* 27(6):1000-1010.

Proctor, S. P., R. Harley, J. Wolfe, T. Heeren, and R. F. White. 2001a. Health-related quality of life in Persian Gulf War veterans. *Military Medicine* 166(6):510-519.

Proctor, S. P., K. J. Heaton, R. F. White, and J. Wolfe. 2001b. Chemical sensitivity and chronic fatigue in Gulf War veterans: A brief report. *Journal of Occupational and Environmental Medicine* 43(3):259-264.

Proctor, S. P., R. F. White, T. Heeren, F. Debes, B. Gloerfelt-Tarp, M. Appleyard, T. Ishoy, B. Guldager, P. Suadicani, F. Gyntelberg, and D. M. Ozonoff. 2003. Neuropsychological functioning in Danish Gulf War veterans. *Journal of Psychopathology and Behavioral Assessment* 25(2):85-93.

Proctor, S. P., K. J. Heaton, T. Heeren, and R. F. White. 2006. Effects of sarin and cyclosarin exposure during the 1991 Gulf War on neurobehavioral functioning in US Army veterans. *Neurotoxicology* 27(6):931-939.

Pulling, M. C., M. Orsborn, B. J. Olson, S. Hunt, and D. J. Kearney. 2008. 181 striking prevalence of irritable bowel syndrome in former prisoners of war: Analysis of risk factors. *Gastroenterology* 134(4 Suppl 1):A-31.

RAC (Research Advisory Committee on Gulf War Veterans' Illnesses). 2008. *Gulf War Illness and the Health of Gulf War Veterans: Scientific Findings and Recommendations.* Washington, DC: US Government Printing Office.

Reid, S., M. Hotopf, L. Hull, K. Ismail, C. Unwin, and S. Wessely. 2001. Multiple chemical sensitivity and chronic fatigue syndrome in British Gulf War veterans. *American Journal of Epidemiology* 153(6):604-609.

Riddle, M., R. Gormley, D. Tribble, B. Cash, and C. Porter. 2009. Post-infectious functional gastrointestinal disorders in the U.S. Military. *American Journal of Gastroenterology* 104(Suppl):S484-S500.

Ritz, B. R., A. D. Manthripragada, S. Costello, S. J. Lincoln, M. J. Farrer, M. Cockburn, and J. Bronstein. 2009. Dopamine transporter genetic variants and pesticides in Parkinson's disease. *Environmental Health Perspectives* 117(6):964-969.

Rivera-Zayas, J., M. Arroyo, and E. Mejias. 2001. Evaluation of Persian Gulf veterans with symptoms of peripheral neuropathy. *Military Medicine* 166(5):449-451.

Roland, P. S., R. W. Haley, W. Yellin, K. Owens, and A. G. Shoup. 2000. Vestibular dysfunction in Gulf War syndrome. *Otolaryngology - Head and Neck Surgery* 122(3):319-329.

Rona, R. J., N. T. Fear, L. Hull, and S. Wessely. 2007. Women in novel occupational roles: Mental health trends in the UK Armed Forces. *International Journal of Epidemiology* 36(2):319-326.

Rose, M. R., M. K. Sharief, J. Priddin, V. Nikolaou, L. Hull, C. Unwin, R. Ajmal-Ali, R. A. Sherwood, A. Spellman, A. David, and S. Wessely. 2004. Evaluation of neuromuscular symptoms in UK Gulf War veterans: A controlled study. *Neurology* 63(9):1681-1687.

Rostker, B. 2000. *Case Narrative: US Demolition Operations at Khamisiyah.* Department of Defense. http://www.gulflink.osd.mil/khamisiyah_ii/ (accessed December 3, 2009).

Rowland, L. 2000. Hereditary and acquired motor neuron diseases. In *Merritt's Neurology*. 10th ed, edited by L. Rowland. Philadelphia, PA: Lippincott Williams and Wilkins. Pp. 708-714.

Roy-Byrne, P., L. Arguelles, M. E. Vitek, J. Goldberg, T. M. Keane, W. R. True, and R. K. Pitman. 2004. Persistence and change of PTSD symptomatology—A longitudinal co-twin control analysis of the Vietnam Era Twin Registry. *Social Psychiatry and Psychiatric Epidemiology* 39(9):681-685.

Sharief, M. K., J. Priddin, R. S. Delamont, C. Unwin, M. R. Rose, A. David, and S. Wessely. 2002. Neurophysiologic analysis of neuromuscular symptoms in UK Gulf War veterans: A controlled study. *Neurology* 59(10):1518-1525.

Sherer, T. B., R. Betarbet, and J. T. Greenamyre. 2001. Pathogenesis of Parkinson's disease. *Current Opinion in Investigational Drugs* 2(5):657-662.

Shih, R. A., H. Hu, M. G. Weisskopf, and B. S. Schwartz. 2007. Cumulative lead dose and cognitive function in adults: A review of studies that measured both blood lead and bone lead. *Environmental Health Perspectives* 115(3):483-492.

Siddique, N., R. Sufit, and T. Siddique. 1999. Degenerative motor, sensory, and autonomic disorders. In *Textbook of Clinical Neurology*, 1st ed, edited by C. Goetz and E. Pappert. Philadelphia, PA: W.B. Saunders Company. Pp. 695-717.

Sillanpaa, M. C., L. M. Agar, I. B. Milner, E. C. Podany, B. N. Axelrod, and G. G. Brown. 1997. Gulf War veterans: A neuropsychological examination. *Journal of Clinical and Experimental Neuropsychology* 19(2):211-219.

Sim, M., M. Abramson, P. A. Forbes, D. Glass, J. Ikin, P. Ittak, H. Kelsall, K. Leder, D. McKenzie, and J. McNeil. 2003. *Australian Gulf War Veterans' Health Study.* Canberra, Australia: Department of Veterans' Affairs. http://www.dva.gov.au/aboutDVA/publications/health_research/aus_gulf_war_vets/Pages/pdf%20table%20of%20contents.aspx (accessed October 5, 2009).

Simmons, R., N. Maconochie, and P. Doyle. 2004. Self-reported ill health in male UK Gulf War veterans: A retrospective cohort study. *BMC Public Health* 4(1):27.

Slusarcick, A. L., R. J. Ursano, M. P. Dinneen, and C. S. Fullerton. 2001. Factors associated with depression on a hospital ship deployed during the Persian Gulf War. *Military Medicine* 166(3):248-252.

Smith, B., T. C. Smith, M. A. K. Ryan, and G. C. Gray. 2006. A comparison of the postdeployment hospitalization experience of U.S. military personnel following service in the 1991 Gulf War, Southwest Asia after the Gulf War, and Bosnia. *Journal of Occupational and Environmental Hygiene* 3(12):660-670.

Smith, T. C., G. C. Gray, and J. D. Knoke. 2000. Is systemic lupus erythematosus, amyotrophic lateral sclerosis, or fibromyalgia associated with Persian Gulf War service? An examination of Department of Defense hospitalization data. *American Journal of Epidemiology* 151(11):1053-1059.

Smith, T. C., J. M. Heller, T. I. Hooper, G. D. Gackstetter, and G. C. Gray. 2002. Are Gulf War veterans experiencing illness due to exposure to smoke from Kuwaiti oil well fires? Examination of Department of Defense hospitalization data. *American Journal of Epidemiology* 155(10):908-917.

Smith, T. C., G. C. Gray, J. C. Weir, J. M. Heller, and M. A. Ryan. 2003. Gulf War veterans and Iraqi nerve agents at Khamisiyah: Postwar hospitalization data revisited. *American Journal of Epidemiology* 158(5):457-467.

Sostek, M. B., S. Jackson, J. K. Linevsky, E. M. Schimmel, and B. G. Fincke. 1996. High prevalence of chronic gastrointestinal symptoms in a National Guard Unit of Persian Gulf veterans. *American Journal of Gastroenterology* 91(12):2494-2497.

Spiller, R., and E. Campbell. 2006. Post-infectious irritable bowel syndrome. *Current Opinion in Gastroenterology* 22:13-17.

Squibb, K. S., and M. A. McDiarmid. 2006. Depleted uranium exposure and health effects in Gulf War veterans. *Philosophical Transactions of the Royal Society of London - Series B: Biological Sciences* 361(1468):639-648.

Statistics Canada. 2005. *The Canadian Persian Gulf Cohort Study: Detailed Report.* http://www.dnd.ca/health-sante/pub/rpt/PDF/GW-GG-Rep-Rap-eng.pdf (accessed July 13, 2009).

Steele, L. 2000. Prevalence and patterns of Gulf War illness in Kansas veterans: Association of symptoms with characteristics of person, place, and time of military service. *American Journal of Epidemiology* 152(10):992-1002.

Stimpson, N. J., C. Unwin, L. Hull, T. David, S. Wessely, and G. Lewis. 2006. Prevalence of reported pain, widespread pain, and pain symmetry in veterans of the Persian Gulf War (1990-1991): The use of pain manikins in Persian Gulf War health research. *Military Medicine* 171(12):1181-1186.

Storzbach, D., D. S. Rohlman, W. K. Anger, L. M. Binder, and K. A. Campbell. 2001. Neurobehavioral deficits in Persian Gulf veterans: Additional evidence from a population-based study. *Environmental Research* 85(1):1-13.

Straus, S. E. 1991. History of chronic fatigue syndrome. *Reviews of Infectious Diseases* 13 (Suppl 1).

Stretch, R. H., P. D. Bliese, D. H. Marlowe, K. M. Wright, K. H. Knudson, and C. H. Hoover. 1995. Physical health symptomatology of Gulf War-era service personnel from the states of Pennsylvania and Hawaii. *Military Medicine* 160(3):131-136.

Stretch, R. H., P. D. Bliese, D. H. Marlowe, K. M. Wright, K. H. Knudson, and C. H. Hoover. 1996a. Psychological health of Gulf War-era military personnel. *Military Medicine* 161(5):257-261.

Stretch, R. H., D. H. Marlowe, K. M. Wright, P. D. Bliese, K. H. Knudson, and C. H. Hoover. 1996b. Post-traumatic stress disorder symptoms among Gulf War veterans. *Military Medicine* 161(7):407-410.

Susser, E., and P. E. Shrout. 2009. Two plus two equals three? Do we need to rethink lifetime prevalence? *Psychological Medicine* (E-published ahead of print):1-3.

Sutker, P. B., J. M. Davis, M. Uddo, and S. R. Ditta. 1995. War zone stress, personal resources, and PTSD in Persian Gulf War returnees. *Journal of Abnormal Psychology* 104(3):444-452.

Thomas, H. V., N. J. Stimpson, A. Weightman, F. Dunstan, and G. Lewis. 2006. Pain in veterans of the Gulf War of 1991: A systematic review. *BMC Musculoskeletal Disorders* 7:74.

Thomas, T. L., H. K. Kang, and N. A. Dalager. 1991. Mortality among women Vietnam veterans, 1973-1987. *American Journal of Epidemiology* 134(9):973-980.

Toomey, R., H. K. Kang, J. Karlinsky, D. G. Baker, J. J. Vasterling, R. Alpern, D. J. Reda, W. G. Henderson, F. M. Murphy, and S. A. Eisen. 2007. Mental health of US Gulf War veterans 10 years after the war. *British Journal of Psychiatry* 190:385-393.

Toomey, R., R. Alpern, J. J. Vasterling, D. G. Baker, D. J. Reda, M. J. Lyons, W. G. Henderson, H. K. Kang, S. A. Eisen, and F. M. Murphy. 2009. Neuropsychological functioning of U.S. Gulf War veterans 10 years after the war. *Journal of the International Neuropsychological Society* 15(5):717-729.

Tuteja, A. K., K. G. Tolman, N. J. Talley, M. Samore, G. J. Stoddard, S. Batt, and G. N. Verner. 2008. Bowel disorders in Gulf War veterans. *Gastroenterology* 134(4):A-31.

Unwin, C., N. Blatchley, W. Coker, S. Ferry, M. Hotopf, L. Hull, K. Ismail, I. Palmer, A. David, and S. Wessely. 1999. Health of UK servicemen who served in Persian Gulf War. *Lancet* 353(9148):169-178.

U.S. Army. 2005. *U.S. Army Sexual Assault and Prevention Program.* http://www.sexualassault.army.mil/content/faqs.cfm (accessed July 18, 2007).

Valenti, M., F. E. Pontieri, F. Conti, E. Altobelli, T. Manzoni, and L. Frati. 2005. Amyotrophic lateral sclerosis and sports: A case-control study. *European Journal of Neurology* 12(3):223-225.

Van Den Heuvel, C., E. Thornton, and R. Vink. 2007. Traumatic brain injury and Alzheimer's disease: a review. *Progress in Brain Research* 161:303-316.

Vasterling, J. J., K. Brailey, H. Tomlin, J. Rice, and P. B. Sutker. 2003. Olfactory functioning in Gulf War-era veterans: Relationships to war-zone duty, self-reported hazards exposures, and psychological distress. *Journal of the International Neuropsychological Society* 9(3):407-418.

Verret, C., M. A. Jutand, C. De Vigan, M. Begassat, L. Bensefa-Colas, P. Brochard, and R. Salamon. 2008. Reproductive health and pregnancy outcomes among French Gulf War veterans. *BMC Public Health* 8(141).

Vogt, D. S., A. P. Pless, L. A. King, and D. W. King. 2005. Deployment stressors, gender, and mental health outcomes among Gulf War I veterans. *Journal of Traumatic Stress* 18(3):272-284.

Watanabe, K. K., and H. K. Kang. 1995. Military service in Vietnam and the risk of death from trauma and selected cancers. *Annals of Epidemiology* 5(5):407-412.

Weisskopf, M. G., E. J. O'Reilly, M. L. McCullough, E. E. Calle, M. J. Thun, M. Cudkowicz, and A. Ascherio. 2005. Prospective study of military service and mortality from ALS. *Neurology* 64(1):32-37.

Wells, T. S., L. Z. Wang, C. N. Spooner, T. C. Smith, K. M. Hiliopoulos, D. R. Kamens, G. C. Gray, and P. A. Sato. 2006. Self-reported reproductive outcomes among male and female 1991 Gulf War era US military veterans. *Maternal and Child Health Journal* 10(6):501-510.

Werler, M. M., J. E. Sheehan, and A. A. Mitchell. 2005. Gulf War veterans and hemifacial microsomia. *Birth Defects Research* 73(1):50-52.

Wessely, S. 1998. The epidemiology of chronic fatigue syndrome. *Epidemiologia e Psichiatria Sociale* 7(1):10-24.

Wessely, S. 2005. Risk, psychiatry and the military. *British Journal of Psychiatry* 186:459-466.

White, R. F., S. P. Proctor, T. Heeren, J. Wolfe, M. Krengel, J. Vasterling, K. Lindem, K. J. Heaton, P. Sutker, and D. M. Ozonoff. 2001. Neuropsychological function in Gulf War veterans: Relationships to self-reported toxicant exposures. *American Journal of Industrial Medicine* 40(1):42-54.

Wilcox, A. J., C. R. Weinberg, J. F. O'Connor, D. D. Baird, J. P. Schlatterer, R. E. Canfield, E. G. Armstrong, and B. C. Nisula. 1988. Incidence of early loss of pregnancy. *New England Journal of Medicine* 319(28):189-194.

Winkenwerder, W., Jr. 2002. *Case Narrative: US Demolition Operations at Khamisiyah, Final Report.* US Department of Defense. http://www.gulflink.osd.mil/khamisiyah_iii/ (accessed December 3, 2009).

Wolfe, F., H. A. Smythe, M. B. Yunus, R. M. Bennett, C. Bombardier, D. L. Goldenberg, P. Tugwell, S. M. Campbell, M. Abeles, P. Clark, A. G. Fam, S. J. Farber, J. J. Fiechtner, C. M. Franklin, R. A. Gatter, D. Hamaty, J. Lessard, A. S. Lichtbroun, A. T. Masi, G. A. Mccain, W. J. Reynolds, T. J. Romano, I. J. Russell, and R. P. Sheon. 1990. The American College of Rheumatology 1990 criteria for the classification of fibromyalgia. *Arthritis and Rheumatism* 33(2):160-172.

Wolfe, J., P. J. Brown, and J. M. Kelley. 1993. Reassessing war stress: Exposure and the Persian Gulf War. *Journal of Social Issues* 49(4):15-31.

Wolfe, J., F., K. Ross, J. Anderson, I. J. Russell, and L. Hebert. 1995. The prevalence and characteristics of fibromyalgia in the general population. *Arthritis and Rheumatism* 38(1):19-28.

Wolfe, F., J. Anderson, D. Harkness, R. M. Bennett, X. J. Caro, D. L. Goldenberg, I. J. Russell, and M. B. Yunus. 1997. Health status and disease severity in fibromyalgia: Results of a six-center longitudinal study. *Arthritis and Rheumatism* 40(9):1571-1579.

Wolfe, J., S. P. Proctor, J. D. Davis, M. S. Borgos, and M. J. Friedman. 1998. Health symptoms reported by Persian Gulf War veterans two years after return. *American Journal of Industrial Medicine* 33(2):104-113.

Wolfe, J., D. J. Erickson, E. J. Sharkansky, D. W. King, and L. A. King. 1999a. Course and predictors of posttraumatic stress disorder among Gulf War veterans: A prospective analysis. *Journal of Consulting & Clinical Psychology* 67(4):520-528.

Wolfe, J., S. P. Proctor, D. J. Erickson, T. Heeren, M. J. Friedman, M. T. Huang, P. B. Sutker, J. J. Vasterling, and R. F. White. 1999b. Relationship of psychiatric status to Gulf War veterans' health problems. *Psychosomatic Medicine* 61(4):532-540.

Writer, J., R. DeFraites, and J. Brundage. 1996. Comparative mortality among US military personnel in the Persian Gulf and worldwide during Operations Desert Shield and Desert Storm. *Journal of the American Medical Association* 275(2):118-121.

Wurzelmann, D., R. Pena, L. Cortes, P. Valladares, P. Heidt, and D. R. Morgan. 2008. Positive association between traumatic war experiences in the Sandinista Revolution and subsequent IBS: A population-based study in Nicaragua. *Gastroenterology* 134(1):A-112.

5

CONCLUSIONS AND RECOMMENDATIONS

The Update committee was asked to review, evaluate, and summarize the literature on the health outcomes identified in *Gulf War and Health, Volume 4: Health Effects of Serving in the Gulf War* (IOM, 2006), with an emphasis on those outcomes that appeared to occur at higher incidence or prevalence in veterans deployed to the Gulf War, in particular: cancer, amyotrophic lateral sclerosis (ALS) and other neurologic diseases, birth defects and other adverse pregnancy outcomes, and postdeployment psychiatric conditions. The committee also was asked to review studies on cause-specific mortality in Gulf War veterans as recommended in the 2006 report and to identify any emerging health outcomes seen in Gulf War veterans. In preparing this report, the Update committee modified the health outcomes that were reviewed in *Volume 4*. For example, the Update committee included genitourinary outcomes, considered multisymptom illness as a separate entity rather than using the ICD category of "symptoms, signs, and abnormal clinical and laboratory findings," and did not include multiple chemical sensitivity or chronic fatigue syndrome as separate outcomes, but rather considered them as multisymptom illnesses. Furthermore, the Update committee included the diseases and disorders identified in the several hospitalization and mortality studies in the discussion of each relevant health outcome, rather than as a separate outcome.

The approaches used by the Volume 4 committee and the Update committee for reviewing the literature differed and are reflected in the separate conclusions reached by the two committees. Because the task of the Volume 4 committee was to catalog the health outcomes that appeared to have greater prevalence in veterans who had been deployed to the Gulf War compared with veterans who served in the military at the same time but were not deployed to the Persian Gulf area, the Volume 4 committee did not specifically evaluate the strength of association between deployment to the Gulf War and individual health outcomes. Rather it categorized studies on whether the health outcomes seen in veterans were based on self-reports (including self-reports of physician diagnoses) or on objective measures such as a physical examination by a health-care provider and/or laboratory tests. Using that approach, the Volume 4 committee found that deployed veterans more frequently reported symptoms indicative of multisymptom illness (although the symptoms did not appear to constitute a unique syndrome, illness, or symptom complex), psychiatric disorders such as posttraumatic stress disorder (PTSD), gastrointestinal disorders, skin disorders, joint pain, and respiratory disorders. However, when objective measures were used to diagnose the health outcomes seen in deployed and nondeployed veterans, the results were different. Deployed veterans were more likely to experience injury or death from motor vehicle accidents in the years immediately after the war, to possibly be at increased risk of ALS, and one study showed more birth defects in offspring of deployed veterans. Objective measures failed to show an increased prevalence of hospitalizations among active-duty Gulf War veterans, cancer (results for testicular cancer were inconsistent), peripheral neuropathy, cardiovascular disease, diabetes, or pulmonary function. The committee noted the few studies that attempted to link specific exposures, such as oil-well fire smoke and possible nerve agents released at Khamisiyah, to health outcomes. Only self-reports of exposure to oil-well fires were linked to an increase in self-reported respiratory symptoms that were suggestive of asthma and bronchitis.

As described in Chapter 4, the Update committee used a different approach for reviewing the literature. It considered studies that used only self-reports by Gulf War veterans to be secondary studies for most health outcomes; the major exception to this rule was multisymptom illness. However, some health outcomes, such as fibromyalgia or irritable bowel syndrome, lack objective diagnostic tests and are diagnosed based on symptom reporting that meet accepted criteria (for example, the Centers for Disease Control and Prevention criteria for chronic fatigue syndrome and the Rome criteria for irritable bowel syndrome). When the symptom reporting was sufficiently descriptive to meet the diagnostic criteria for that outcome, those studies were considered to be primary if the other evaluation criteria for a primary study (described in Chapter 4) were met. Studies that used objective measures to diagnose a health outcome were also considered to be primary if they met the other evaluation criteria.

The conclusions reached by the committee regarding the strength of the association between deployment to the Gulf War and each health outcome are summarized below. The committee notes that the majority of studies that it reviewed were conducted on both men and women, but for most studies, results for women were not presented separately as the number of women was relatively small. Results specific for women were presented in Chapter 4.

Sufficient Evidence of a Causal Relationship

Evidence is sufficient to conclude that a causal relationship exists between being deployed to the Gulf War and a health outcome. The evidence fulfills the criteria for sufficient evidence of a causal association in which chance, bias, and confounding can be ruled out with reasonable confidence, and is supported by several of the other considerations used to assess causality: strength of association, dose-response relationship, consistency of association, temporal relationship, specificity of association, and biological plausibility.

- PTSD.

Sufficient Evidence of an Association

Evidence suggests an association, in that a positive association has been observed between deployment to the Gulf War and a health outcome in humans; however, there is some doubt as to chance, bias, and confounding.

- Other psychiatric disorders, including generalized anxiety disorder, depression, and substance abuse, particularly alcohol abuse. Furthermore these psychiatric disorders persist for at least 10 years after deployment.
- Gastrointestinal symptoms consistent with functional gastrointestinal disorders such as irritable bowel syndrome and functional dyspepsia.
- Multisymptom illness.
- Chronic fatigue syndrome.

Limited/Suggestive Evidence of an Association

Some evidence of an association between deployment to the Gulf War and a health outcome in humans exists, but this is limited in that substantial doubt exists regarding chance, bias, and confounding.

- ALS.
- Fibromyalgia and chronic widespread pain.
- Self-reported sexual difficulties.
- Mortality from external causes, primarily motor vehicle accidents, in the early years after deployment.

Inadequate/Insufficient Evidence to Determine Whether an Association Exists

The available studies are of insufficient quality, validity, consistency, or statistical power to permit a conclusion regarding the presence or absence of an association between deployment to the Gulf War and a health outcome in humans.

- Any cancers.
- Disorders of the blood and blood forming organs.
- Endocrine, nutritional, and metabolic diseases.
- Neurocognitive and neurobehavioral performance.
- Multiple sclerosis.
- Other neurologic outcomes, such as Parkinson's disease, dementia, and Alzheimer's disease.
- Cardiovascular disorders.
- Respiratory diseases.
- Structural gastrointestinal diseases.
- Skin diseases.
- Musculoskeletal disorders.
- Other specific conditions of the genitourinary system.
- Specific birth defects.
- Adverse pregnancy outcomes such as miscarriage, stillbirth, preterm birth, and low birth weight.
- Fertility problems.

Limited/Suggestive Evidence of No Association

There are several adequate studies, covering the full range of levels of exposure that humans are known to encounter, that are mutually consistent in not showing an association between exposure to a specific agent and a health outcome at any level of exposure. A conclusion of no association is inevitably limited to the conditions, levels of exposure, and length of observation covered by the available studies. In addition, the possibility of a very small elevation in risk at the levels of exposure studied can never be excluded.

- Peripheral neuropathy.
- Mortality from cardiovascular disease in the first 10 years after the war.

- Decreased lung function in the first 10 years after the war.
- Hospitalization for genitourinary diseases.

QUALITY OF THE STUDIES

Virtually all the reports in the Gulf War and Health series have called for improved studies of Gulf War and other veterans. This committee reiterates that need but notes that at almost 20 years after the war, it is difficult, if not impossible, to reconstruct the exposures to which the veterans were subjected in theater. It is similarly difficult after so many years to establish the predeployment physical and mental health status of these veterans for comparison purposes. Nevertheless,

- To date, while many studies have been conducted on Gulf War veterans, their quality is varied and many of them have substantial methodological limitations. As a result uncertainty remains concerning the relationship between deployment to the Gulf War and health outcomes. These limitations include:
    - Lack of representativeness of the Gulf War population in some studies, affecting external validity such that what we have learned from the samples studied cannot be easily extrapolated to all Gulf War veterans.
    - Low participation rates and, indeed, differential participation rates in many studies, affecting internal validity due to selection bias. For example, the significantly higher response rate among deployed veterans compared with nondeployed control groups observed in many studies may result from greater participation of deployed troops because they were already experiencing health problems.
    - Studies that may have been too narrow in their assessment of health status (for example, self-reported outcomes such as hypertension, diabetes, or cardiovascular disease), or use of data collection instruments that might have been too insensitive (or invalid) to detect abnormalities in deployed veterans (for example, death certificates or hospital-discharge diagnoses).
    - There is a particular problem with self-reported exposures, especially when respondents are aware of media reports linking outcomes with putative exposures.
    - Timing of the investigation relative to the latent period for some health outcomes (for example, cancer, and some neurologic outcomes, such as MS, ALS, or Parkinson's disease, for which there might be a long time between exposure and disease onset).
    - Use of cross-sectional studies that limit assessment of temporality, symptom duration and chronicity, latency of onset, severity, and prognosis.
- Future studies of Gulf War veterans, and indeed any veteran population, need to be adequately designed in order to:
    - Provide sufficient statistical power (precision).
    - Ensure validity, including the avoidance of bias, such as recall and response bias, meaning that efforts should be made to encourage equal participation among deployed and nondeployed individuals with the goal of avoiding participation rates linked to general health and symptom presence, and to ensure comparable assessment of the severity and frequency of reported symptoms.

- Improve disease measurement to avoid misclassification; for example, including information collected from non-DoD hospitals in studies of hospitalization, obtaining cancer incidence data from existing cancer registries, validating self-reports of health outcomes, and using the least error-prone measures of these outcomes.
- Better characterize deployment and potentially related adverse environmental influences; for example, collect information on the length and location of deployment or job and task descriptions.
- Measure and adjust for possible confounding factors; for example, lifestyle factors (such as smoking and risk-taking behaviors) or predeployment physical and psychological health status.

POSSIBLE CAUSES OF MULTISYMPTOM ILLNESS IN VETERANS

During its deliberations, the Update committee held two public sessions at which it heard from numerous interested parties including representatives of veterans' service organizations and individual Gulf War veterans. The committee was also asked by VA secretary Gen. Shinseki to invite representatives of the VA Research Advisory Committee on Gulf War Veterans' Illnesses (RAC) to make presentations to the committee on the findings and conclusions in its report, *Gulf War Illness and the Health of Gulf War Veterans*, released in November 2008, to "ensure that the basis for any differences between these reports can be efficiently and accurately communicated and considered by the latest IOM committee."

The Update committee concluded, based on a comprehensive review of the human epidemiologic literature, that there is sufficient evidence of an association between deployment to the Gulf War and multisymptom illness (see Chapter 4). The RAC, however, had concluded that the constellation of symptoms called Gulf War illness was caused by exposure to pyridostigmine bromide (PB) and to pesticides during the Gulf War, and that other exposures might also be implicated in Gulf War illness. The Update committee felt it was important to consider this major RAC conclusion regarding the cause of Gulf War illness and the evidence used to support that conclusion in order to respond to Gen. Shinseki's request. A comprehensive assessment of all the evidence on PB and pesticides exposures in the Gulf War was beyond the Update committee's formal scope of work. The committee, therefore, limited its assessment to those studies used by the RAC to support its conclusion on the cause of Gulf War illness. The committee believed that its assessment of those RAC studies was best presented in an appendix.

Although the Update committee did not assess the biological plausibility of the link between PB and pesticides and Gulf War illness, in keeping with its charge to examine the strength of association between deployment to the Gulf War and various human health outcomes, the committee critically examined the human exposure studies cited by the RAC as evidence that PB and pesticides are causally associated with Gulf War illness (see Appendix A). However, in contrast to the RAC report, the Update committee found that human epidemiologic evidence was not sufficient to establish a causative relationship between any specific drug, toxin, plume, or other agent, either alone or in combination, and Gulf War illness. Given this important issue, the Update committee also undertook an assessment of the key experimental research studies that were cited in the RAC report as supporting the plausibility of this association. This focused assessment of the experimental literature, summarized in Appendix A, did not meet, in the committee's opinion, a threshold that would lead to the conclusion that any Gulf War illness-related problems could reasonably be expected to result from these putative exposures. Indeed, the committee concludes that many key questions remain unanswered. This is true both with respect to the underlying cause or causes of the multisystem illness complex experienced by so many of the Gulf War soldiers, and also with respect to the adequacy of the experimental studies that have addressed the potential contribution of any external agent to the development, course, or persistence of this perplexing disorder. The committee concludes that it is essential to keep in mind that other etiologic factors may also play a role, and research into this matter must continue. The committee also concludes that it is possible that the specific cause(s) of the many and diverse symptoms reported by the veterans may never be determined given the limitations of the available data. To not acknowledge the uncertainty of what we know and the real possibility of not being able to identify a cause of the veterans' illnesses would be a disservice to medical science and more importantly to the men and women who served so courageously in this battleground.

There are other areas of research that might be conducted on the etiology of Gulf War illness. The constellation of unexplained symptoms associated with the Gulf War illness complex could result from interplay between both biological and psychological factors. However, it is important to remember that there are a number of different causes for a disease, but due to the paucity of data it will be difficult to disentangle these for Gulf War illness. The symptoms of Gulf War illness could have a single cause, different causes in different individuals, or require multiple factors operating in combination.

Studies that lead to a better understanding of how biological and psychological factors give rise to variety of symptoms are needed as they may be the key to understanding and treating the Gulf War illness complex. For example, certain exposures may lead to alterations in blood–brain barrier permeability, neural pathways or transmitters, or neuroendocrine systems. It is also important to consider the effects of chronic stress, and, given the physical environment in the Persian Gulf, thermal dysregulation, an area that has received little attention to date.

THE PATH FORWARD

After almost two decades of research on Gulf War veterans, important questions remain unanswered. What are the causes of the multisymptom illness experienced by veterans? How does predeployment health status influence the risk of developing Gulf War illness? Why do some veterans suffer a constellation of many symptoms whereas others experience isolated symptoms or only some components of the illness, and still others who served in the same battleground seemingly with similar exposures remain entirely without symptoms? Why do some veterans who were not on the ground in the Persian Gulf area (for example, Australian troops at sea), or others who arrived after the conclusion of the battle (for example, Danish forces), also experience symptoms of Gulf War illness? How severe and disabling are residual Gulf War symptoms? What are the most effective treatments for veterans who do suffer from multisymptom illness, and should the treatments vary depending on specific symptoms? Beyond the perplexing problem of Gulf War illness, what are the overall long-term physical and mental health consequences of serving in the Gulf War?

The committee believes that the path forward for veterans has two branches. The first is continued surveillance of Gulf War veterans. Such surveillance might include the following:

- Although further investigations based solely on self-reports are not likely to contribute significantly to increased understanding of Gulf War illness, well-designed follow-up studies of mortality, cancer, and neurologic and psychiatric outcomes will continue to be valuable. Well-designed, adequately powered studies of MS and ALS incidence following deployment are also needed.
- Methodologically robust cohorts need to be assembled now and followed carefully to track the development of ALS, MS, brain cancer, and psychiatric conditions, as well as the appearance of additional health issues that occur at a later age, such as other cancers, cardiovascular disease, and neurodegenerative diseases. Several well-characterized cohorts have already been established that could form the basis of future studies. For example, the US cohort studied by the VA; the two UK cohorts; and the Canadian, Danish, and Australian cohorts. Relatively small cohorts, such as the Canadian or Australian veterans, might not be useful for outcomes with low incidence (for example, ALS or brain cancer), but they might be very useful for tracking frequently seen health outcomes such as Gulf War illness, cardiovascular and respiratory diseases, other cancer types, neurodegenerative conditions such as dementia, and some psychiatric disorders.
- With regard to functional gastrointestinal disorders (irritable bowel syndrome and functional dyspepsia), recent evidence supports the need for two types of studies: one type will determine the role of prior acute gastroenteritis among deployed soldiers in the development of these disorders, and the second type will use symptom-specific criteria (for example, Rome criteria) to clarify the association of medical and psychosocial comorbidities with functional gastrointestinal disorders and their severity.
- Uncommon genetic variants or rare environmental events may not be recognized as associated with an outcome of interest unless very large numbers of individuals are studied or sophisticated capture methods are used to explore specific hypotheses. It is possible, for example, that new and objective information related to exposures might become available in the future that could improve our ability to estimate individual exposures and to assess health effects in groups of Gulf War veterans according to specific exposures.

In addition to epidemiologic studies, the committee believes that a second branch of inquiry is important. This consists of a renewed research effort with substantial commitment to well-organized efforts to better identify and treat multisymptom illness in Gulf War veterans. Given the high reported prevalence of persistent symptoms, plus the steady advances in understanding genetics, molecular diagnostics, and imaging, it is possible now to plan and carry out adequately powered studies to identify inherited genetic variants, molecular profiles of gene expression, other epigenetic markers (such as modifications of DNA structure related to environmental exposures), specific viral exposures, signatures of immune activation, or brain changes identified by sensitive imaging measures—all these are traits that distinguish Gulf War veterans with persistent medical symptoms from healthy deployed or nondeployed veterans. The committee is optimistic that a rigorous, adequately powered analysis would identify useful biomarkers that might not only be helpful for symptomatic veterans of the Gulf War but also for nondeployed veterans and for civilians with a range of medically unexplained symptoms including chronic fatigue, muscle and joint pains, sleep disturbances, difficulty with concentration, and depression.

As with many other disorders, it is likely that Gulf War illness results from an interplay of genetic and environmental factors; genetics may play a larger role for some affected individuals, whereas the environment is predominant for others. In general, the more complex and heterogeneous a disorder, the larger the number of subjects needed to unravel its etiology. The value of identifying even minor genetic contributors to an unknown disease cannot be overstated, as such discoveries can reveal previously unknown causative pathways that can also clarify potential environmental agents as well as potential therapeutic targets.

Subsequent investigations should also explore the biology of Gulf War illness in the context of identifying targets for therapies. These studies might include, but are not limited to, the following goals:

- Determine whether inflammation is associated with Gulf War illness.
- Evaluate the status of genetic variation in genes that respond to environmental toxicants, such as paraoxonase 1 (PON1). Variants of these genes could be present differentially in sufferers of Gulf War illness.
- Improve understanding of the basic symptom complex of Gulf War illness. For example, what is the nature of specific complaints, their severity, and the resulting disability?
- Enhance understanding of the objective correlates of Gulf War illness. For example, can sleep disturbances or potential dysfunction of the autonomic nervous system be better understood?
- Validate reported biomarkers of Gulf War illness, including anatomic and functional imaging findings and published immune associations.
- There is a dearth of organized clinical trials to examine potential treatments for the observed symptoms experienced by Gulf War veterans. Aligned with the effort to improve care pathways for Gulf War illness sufferers, there should be a focused effort to consider the development of clinical trials informed by the best biological data related to the cause of Gulf War illness.

Answers to these questions will help to address the issue of possible causes of Gulf War illness and, more importantly, are essential for the development of effective treatments.

Detailed planning with access to the very best expertise in medicine, epidemiology, toxicology, imaging, molecular biology, and clinical trials will maximize the chances of success. Careful clinical ascertainment and development of unbiased assembled samples of adequate size are additional prerequisites. For example, given the likely small effect size of any genetic variant that might contribute to multisymptom illness, DNA samples from a cohort of 10,000 affected and an equal number of unaffected individuals might be required for a genome-wide exploration of susceptibility for modifier genes contributing to multisymptom illness. Patient cohorts of this size are now routinely collected for modern investigations of complex illnesses. Given current estimates that more than 250,000 US Gulf War veterans have persistent unexplained medical symptoms, it is feasible to collect two such cohorts for genetic analysis (the first for identification of associated variants and the second for replication). The funding needs to support a study of this magnitude would be substantial but could also present a new opportunity to promote cooperation among different funding sources and provide high-level coordination for an important health problem. A new consortium among the VA, DoD, and National Institutes for Health (NIH) could be established for this purpose, perhaps with participation by the private sector for drug development and clinical trials. The participation and perhaps leadership of the Clinical Translational Sciences Consortium at the NIH would also be worth exploration. The overall goal would be to provide a centrally coordinated but facile organization capable of creating an adequately powered dataset and then encouraging practical and innovative science aimed at understanding the basis of unexplained symptoms in Gulf War veterans and developing effective treatments in order to alleviate their suffering as rapidly and completely as possible.

APPENDIX A

CHOLINESTERASE INHIBITORS AND MULITSYMPTOM ILLNESSES

Numerous studies of Gulf War veterans have identified an association between self-reported multisymptom illness and self-reported exposures to several cholinesterase-inhibiting agents, including the drug pyridostigmine bromide (PB), cholinesterase- and noncholinesterase-inhibiting pesticides, and the cholinesterase-inhibiting nerve gases, sarin and cyclosarin. This appendix reviews some of the known health effects that can result from these potential exposures and addresses the evidence potentially linking those exposures to multisymptom illness, including what is often called Gulf War illness. This appendix discusses how Gulf War veterans might have been exposed to cholinesterase inhibitors, the physiologic and toxicologic actions of these chemicals, and reviews some of the studies that have attempted to link various chemical agents to symptoms indicative of cholinesterase inhibition of veterans.

When a person chooses to move a body part such as a finger, the brain sends a signal first down through the spinal cord, then from the spinal cord out the nerves of the arm and into the hand. The nerves carry an impulse down their length somewhat like an electrical current is conducted down a wire. This impulse reaches the muscles of the finger and the muscle contracts in response and the finger moves. These nerves, which carry the signal, are long nerves called motor neurons. Despite the analogy, the conduction of the impulse differs from electricity moving through a wire in several respects. First, the impulse moves along the nerve as a result of the nerve cell changing its internal charge from negative to positive along its length in a wave like fashion. Second, when a nerve connects with the muscle it does not transmit the electrical signal directly, like electricity crossing a wired junction, but instead the end of the nerve fiber releases a chemical (called a neurotransmitter). This chemical moves across a narrow space (called a synapse) between the nerve and the muscle and binds to molecules on the surface of the muscle that are concentrated around the synapse. When the neurotransmitter binds to these molecules, the molecules cause a change in the membrane of the muscle cell, which causes the muscle to contract. This same phenomenon of nerve impulse and chemical transmitter crossing a synapse occurs when nerves connect to other nerves, and when nerves connect to glands, such as the salivary glands. In these situations, the neurotransmitter crossing the synapse results in the continuation of the nerve impulse or the secretion of the gland.

There are several neurotransmitters in the body, with acetylcholine being one of the most common. Neurons that use acetylcholine as a neurotransmitter are referred to as cholinergic. The enzyme cholinesterase plays an essential role in terminating the chemical signal between a cholinergic neuron and the nerve, muscle, or gland that is being stimulated. Acetylcholinesterase (AChE) acts to quickly metabolize acetylcholine into choline and acetic acid, rendering it inactive. It is critical for the normal function of the nervous system. When AChE is inhibited, acetylcholine can accumulate causing overstimulation of the cholinergic junctions and organs controlled by cholinergic neurons. Tissues innervated by cholinergic neurons include muscles (both smooth and voluntary); glands such as salivary, pancreas, and lachrymal; and certain parts of the brain. Thus inhibition of cholinesterase can cause overactivity of a wide variety of bodily functions. This overactivity is characteristic of poisoning by cholinesterase inhibitors (Bardin et al., 1994).

EXPOSURES TO CHOLINESTERASE INHIBITORS AND OTHER PESTICIDES DURING THE GULF WAR

Pesticides

Pesticides are defined by the federal Fungicide Insecticide Fumigant Rodenticide Act as any substance that kills, repels, or mitigates a pest. Under this definition, insect repellents such as diethyltoluamide (DEET) would be considered pesticides. Several types of pesticides were used in the Gulf War theater, among the most common were organophosphates, carbamates, and pyrethroids.

Organophosphate pesticides are chemicals in wide use as insecticides in agricultural and nonagricultural applications. They were initially developed by German scientists prior to World War II. They range in toxicity from very mildly toxic to extremely toxic and are toxic by mouth, inhalation, or dermal absorption. Most organophosphate pesticides require activation by an enzyme system known as the cytochrome P450 system. This system oxidizes a portion of the molecule making it much more toxic than the parent compound. It is this active molecule that binds to the cholinesterase molecule, blocking the action of the enzyme and leading to the accumulation of the neurotransmitter acetylcholine. This accumulation of acetylcholine and the overstimulation of the nerves, glands, and muscles that are innervated by cholinergic neurons, lead to the signs and symptoms seen in organophosphate poisonings. The organophosphate binds to the active site and slowly forms a covalent bond with the enzyme, thus irreversibly inhibiting the cholinesterase enzyme. The enzyme is replaced by the body over time.

Carbamates are a group of chemicals that, like organophosphates, are commonly used as insecticides. They also inhibit cholinesterase. The inhibition they cause tends to be less long lasting than inhibition with organophosphates, because unlike organophosphates, they do not go through a permanent bonding (covalent bonding) with the cholinesterase molecule. They are short acting, and the enzyme reactivates when the concentration of the carbamate in the system is reduced.

Permethrin is a low to moderate toxicity pesticide in the class of pesticides known as pyrethroids. This class is derived from natural pesticides, which are found in chrysanthemums. Permethrin alters the function of nerve ion gates by destabilizing the neuronal ion balance. This instability results in neurons firing more easily and in uncoordinated neuronal discharges. These uncoordinated discharges are largely responsible for the insecticidal effect of the chemical.

The most serious consequence of overexposure to pyrethroids is seizure activity. This however, is rare in humans as the toxicity of pyrethroids is far less for warm-blooded animals than for cold-blooded ones. Acute exposure in humans is generally characterized by burning or irritating sensations in the fingers and lips.

DEET is a liquid insect repellent that can be applied to the skin or clothing. Despite the wide use of the chemical, there have been relatively few reports of systemic toxicity. Children appear to be most at risk for DEET toxicity, particularly when it is used excessively.

Illnesses associated with DEET include contact dermatitis and eye irritation. DEET is efficiently absorbed across the gut and skin. High blood levels can lead to encephalopathy, which can have severe long-term consequences including flaccid paralysis and areflexia. Fatal poisonings have been reported. No studies of chronic low-level exposure to DEET in humans were identified by the Update committee.

Illness Associated with Cholinesterase Inhibitors and Pesticides

Acute illness due to cholinesterase inhibition from chemicals such as organophosphates, carbamates, PB, or sarin manifests with symptoms and signs resulting from toxic effects on the central and peripheral nervous system. Central nervous system (CNS) symptoms and signs include confusion, headache, loss of consciousness, and, in severe overexposures, death due to respiratory center depression. Peripheral symptoms and signs include salivation, lacrimation, blurry vision, excessive bronchial secretions, sweating, weakness, muscle fasciculations, diarrhea, and loss of bladder control. Severe cholinesterase inhibition can result in death primarily because of respiratory failure. This failure results from a combination of bronchial secretions, bronchial constriction, weakened respiratory muscle function, and inhibited respiratory drive.

Symptoms and signs resulting from chronic low-level exposure to cholinesterase inhibitors are less well defined and some physiological accommodation can occur, leading to the amelioration of some symptoms. Persistent signs and symptoms after a severe acute poisoning have been more frequently studied. Several studies have identified persistent neurobehavioral changes lasting years after recovery from severe organophosphate pesticide poisoning (Delgado et al., 2004; London et al., 1998; Rosenstock et al., 1991; Savage et al., 1988; Steenland et al., 1994; Wesseling et al., 2002).

In addition to acute toxic reactions, two other syndromes have been identified with overexposure to organophosphate pesticides: intermediate syndrome and organophosphate-induced delayed polyneuropathy (OPIDP). Intermediate syndrome occurs after an acute severe organophosphate intoxication and manifests as severe weakness, generally showing up 48 hours after the acute illness begins. This weakness can lead to respiratory failure if there is no intervention to support respiration (De Bleecker et al., 1993). OPIDP results from exposure to a select group of organophosphate chemicals that are capable of binding to and inhibiting a neuronal enzyme known as neuropathy target esterase. This syndrome usually appears about 2 weeks after the poisoning. It is characterized by weakness in the extremities and is understood to be due to a degenerative neuropathy of long motor neurons (Lotti and Morreto, 2005).

While in the Gulf War theater, servicemembers might have had exposure to three distinct groups of cholinesterase inhibitors: sarin or cyclosarin nerve gas, PB, and organophosphate and/or carbamate pesticides. Other common pesticide exposures were to insect repellents containing DEET and permethrin. Pesticides were used to control fleas, flies, and other insects. PB was used as a prophylactic antidote for exposure to nerve gas, which was known to have been previously used by Iraqi forces.

The most complete documentation of the use of pesticides, cholinesterase inhibitors, and PB pills by Gulf War veterans was conducted by the RAND Corporation for the Department of Defense (DoD). The RAND report *Pesticide Use During the Gulf War: A Survey of Gulf War*

Veterans (Fricker et al., 2000) collected information by phone survey in 1999 from 2005 randomly sampled veterans from the estimated 469,047 Gulf War veterans who were believed to be on the ground in theater during Operations Desert Shield and Desert Storm in 1990-1991. Fricker et al. found that about 66% of respondents reported use of pesticides in some form. Veterans reported using pesticides during the Gulf War in a variety of ways, including personal use—for example, application of lotions, sprays, and personal use of flea collars, and field use—for example, broadcast applications in eating areas or use of pest strips in eating areas or toilet facilities. The survey focused on the form of pesticide used because most respondents were unable to provide the names of the pesticides they used or saw others use.

Fricker et al. (2000) imputed the active ingredients from the form of the pesticide reportedly used and other information provided by the respondents. It was necessary to impute the ingredients because most of the respondents could not recall the name, color, or smell of the pesticides they used or saw used. The investigators estimated that 50% of veterans applied DEET in some form, 6% used permethrin, and 3% used a sulfur pesticide. A small percentage of veterans, an estimated 13,000, used tick or flea collars and were able to correctly identify those products. The survey investigators were able to identify the active ingredients in pesticides used in field use of pesticides with even less certainty than pesticides used in personal use applications. They imputed that possible active ingredients in aerosols were alethrin, permethrin, resmethrin, phenothrin (all pyrethroids), chlorpyrifos and malathion (both organophosphates), propoxure (a carbamate), and DEET (a hydrocarbon repellent).

Pyridostigmine Bromide

PB is a pharmaceutical cholinesterase inhibitor used widely in the treatment of myasthenia gravis, an autoimmune neuromuscular condition, and a vascular condition known as orthostatic hypotension. In both cases, the mechanism of the drug is to reversibly inhibit the enzyme cholinesterase, which allows the accumulation of acetylcholine leading to overstimulation of the acetylcholine receptors. In the case of myasthenia gravis, these receptors are voluntary muscle receptors, which due to the disease are decreased in concentration. In the case of orthostatic hypotension, the increase in acetylcholine stimulates receptors that increase venous blood return and increase blood pressure. It is provided as a small white tablet, taken orally.

Symptoms of Toxicity from PB Overexposure.

Pyridostigmine bromide when taken in excess produces symptoms similar to those produced by overexposure to organophosphate or carbamate pesticides. These symptoms are due to the excess of acetylcholine in the body. Excess secretions such as saliva, bronchial secretions, sweating, and tearing may be seen. Muscles may fibrillate and become weak. Diarrhea, nausea, frequent or uncontrolled urination, as well as confusion or irritability may occur. Other symptoms include blurred vision and pupillary constriction, bronchospasm, and, in severe cases, pulmonary edema (Medline Plus, 2008). In terms of long-term effects of PB, the Food and Drug Administration has summarized the existing knowledge and concluded that despite a long history of PB being used in the treatment of myasthenia gravis no evidence of long-term health effects has emerged to date (FDA, 2009).

PB tablets were provided by the DoD to military personnel in the Gulf War theater as a prophylactic against cholinesterase-inhibiting nerve gas. The theory behind the use of PB for such prophylaxis is that by reversibly inhibiting a portion of the acetylcholine receptors in the body, a sufficient percentage of the receptors will be protected and will reactivate so as to permit survival in the case of a nerve gas exposure. The RAND survey reported that about 50% of the Gulf War deployed personnel in the Army and Marine Corps/Navy used PB pills. Of those who used the pills, 95% of whom reported taking 3 or fewer pills per day for fewer than 30 days out of the month. The median use was 20 pills per 30-day period. It was also noted that those self-reporting the most PB use also tended to self-report more frequent use of pesticides.

Nerve Gas

The nerve gases sarin and cyclosarin are extremely potent cholinesterase-inhibiting chemicals. Sarin, also known as GB for German B, and cyclosarin, also known as GF, were first developed by German scientists near the start of World War II.

Sarin and cyclosarin have a potency far exceeding that of pesticidal cholinesterase inhibitors. The acute effects are effectively those of overexposure to organophosphate or carbamate pesticides. Long-term effects in humans have been identified among survivors of the sarin attacks in Japan. Chronic symptoms such as forgetfulness, depressed mood, and loss of interest or apathy were more common in victims of sarin toxicity than controls up to 10 years after their acute illness (Yanagisawa et al., 2006). Some neuropsychological performance measures were also seen to be worse among sarin victims compared with controls 3 years after acute exposure (Nishiwaki et al., 2001), and PTSD symptoms were common in a very small sample of previously poisoned victims (Ohtani et al., 2004). There are very few events that permit study of the long-term effects of sarin exposure, and no human studies exclusively of cyclosarin were found in the literature. However, the persistent abnormalities seen in sarin victims that last long after the acute toxicity has resolved appear to be similar to the long-term neurobehavioral effects seen after acute intoxication from organophosphate pesticides (Delgado et al., 2004; London et al., 1998; Rosenstock et al., 1991; Savage et al., 1988; Steenland et al., 1994; Wesseling et al., 2002).

Khamisiyah was a munitions storage site that was destroyed by US forces during Operation Desert Storm in March 1991. Servicemembers involved in the demolition were unaware that the bunker also contained the sarin and cyclosarin. A plume of nerve gas was released from the demolition that drifted in a decreasing concentration gradient away from the site on the prevailing winds (see *Volume 4*, Chapter 2, for a more detailed discussion of the Khamisiyah plume modeling).

The DoD attempted to determine the number and identity of the troops potentially exposed to nerve gas from the Khamisiyah demolition. The DoD modeled potential exposures in 1997 and 2000. The approaches used by the DoD on each occasion have come under strong criticism by a variety of critics, including the General Accounting Office, which conducted an independent investigation of the Khamisiyah modeling efforts by the DoD (GAO, 2004). Although the number of people exposed in each model did not differ significantly, the location of those troops did.

The time during which nerve gas may have been released from Khamisiyah is uncertain because there were aerial attacks as well as ground detonations of explosives at this site. No reports of acute symptoms among potentially exposed military personnel have been linked to the nerve gas relesases from the Khamisiyah demolition. However, very low-level exposure to sarin or cyclosarin may cause symptoms indistinguishable from systemic viral illnesses or mild bacterial illnesses and thus the symptoms might be confused with other illnesses commonly seen in an unhygienic theater of war. Only one peer-reviewed study was identified that used symptom reports from 5555 Gulf War army veterans. The symptom reports were obtained by a mailed survey prior to the DoD's release of information about possible nerve gas exposure from the Khamisiyah demolition (Page et al., 2005a). This study found that the 1898 veterans who were potentially exposed to the Khamisiyah plume did not have higher rates of 48 symptoms queried compared with 3336 nonexposed veterans. Of the 31 medical conditions about which respondents were asked, the potentially exposed veterans reported slightly higher rates of only two: enteritis (risk ratio [RR] 1.19, 95% confidence interval [CI] 1.0-1.43) and colitis (RR 1.39, 95% CI 1.14-1.70) in the preceding 12 months. The analysis adjusted for age, sex, race, rank, marital status, and unit component; potential exposure was based on the 2000 DoD plume modeling (Page et al., 2005b).

LONG-TERM EFFECTS OF LOW DOSES OF CHOLINESTERASE INHIBITORS

Whether long-term, low-dose (nonintoxicating) exposures to cholinesterase inhibitors results in CNS illness has not been determined (Keifer and Firestone, 2007). Organophosphate-exposed workers in California who showed reduced cholinesterase levels during routine monitoring had no decrease in neuropsychological function on 27 neurological and neuropsychological tests compared with controls (Ames et al., 1995). Neurological and neuropsychological tests of South African workers exposed to organophosphate pesticides also found no association between history of chronic organophosphate exposure and test performance; however, previous organophosphate poisoning was predictive of lowered test performance (London et al., 1998). Chronic neurologic effects have been studied in another group of organophosphate-exposed workers: sheep dippers. The most highly exposed sheep dippers showed an increase in neurological symptoms and decreases in neuropsychological test performance and peripheral sensory function (Pilkington et al., 2001; Stephens et al., 1995, 1996).

The US Agricultural Health Study, the largest cohort study of pesticide-exposed workers to date, found self-reported retinal degeneration to be associated with fungicide exposure (Kamel et al., 2007). Bessler et al. (2006), studying the same cohort, a history of an acute exposure to a high concentration of pesticide was significantly associated with self-reported, doctor-diagnosed depression in men and women. The self-reported, doctor-diagnosed depression was also associated with the highest level of self-reported lifetime, cumulative pesticide exposure in men but not in women (Besseler et al., 2008). This study is unique in identifying an association between chronic high levels of nonintoxicating exposure and depression. However, the study did not find a dose-response effect across the three levels of lifetime cumulative exposure and considered cumulative exposure to all pesticides in its exposure classification, not just those that inhibited cholinesterase. The Agricultural Health Study also found increased self-reports of Parkinson's disease to be associated with increased use of pesticides (Kamel et al., 2007). This finding reinforced other studies that found an increased risk of Parkinsonism among rural residents, farm residents, and pesticide-exposed populations. Costello et al. (2009) recently found a strong association between subjects objectively assessed for the presence of Parkinsonism and exposure to pesticides as indicated by historically confirmed residence in proximity to sprayed agricultural land in California (Costello et al., 2009).

STUDIES IN GULF WAR POPULATIONS

Several studies of Gulf War veterans have found an association between self-reported multisystem illness and self-reported exposure to pesticides, nerve gas, or PB, or some combination of them. Haley and Kurt first reported this association in 1997. Some 249 veterans of a naval construction battalion (Seabees) responded to a mailed questionnaire about health symptoms and exposure including pesticide and PB tablet use and nerve gas-related events. Principal component analysis was used to reduce symptoms to three syndromes: syndrome 1 "impaired cognition," syndrome 2 "confusion-ataxia," and syndrome 3 "arthromyoneuropathy." Work in security during the war was significantly associated with the risk of syndrome 1 (RR 5.4, 95% CI 1.8-16). Syndrome 2 was associated with reports of experiencing a nerve gas attack (RR 8.0, 95% CI 2.3-25.9) or being in sector 7 during a specified period, an area and time of potential exposure to nerve gas drift. Risk of syndrome 2 also increased with the scale of adverse effects to PB. Syndrome 3 was found to be associated with the amount of insect repellent that veterans reported using on their skin and with the scale of symptoms they reported in response to taking PB tablets. The risk for syndromes 2 or 3 was not associated with the amount of PB tablets consumed.

Ishoy et al. (1999a,b) conducted a cross-sectional interview and examination-based study of 686 (83.6%) of Danish personnel who were deployed to the Gulf on a peacekeeping mission after the end of hostilities. A sex-, age-, and profession-matched control group of 231 individuals (57.8% of 400 potential participants) who could have been but were not deployed to the Gulf were included for comparison. There was no adjustment for potential confounders in the analysis, and Gulf War veterans were significantly older, taller, heavier, more likely male, and had higher diastolic blood pressure than the nondeployed counterparts. Since their deployment to the gulf, the Danish peacekeepers were significantly more likely to have a wide variety of symptoms including headaches, blurry vision, numbness or tingling of hands of feet, balance difficulties, depression and concentration problems, fatigue, sleep difficulty, nightmares, nervousness and agitation, and difficulty pronouncing words correctly. A significant difference was found between the two groups for undiagnosed skin problems as well. Only minor differences were found between the groups for hematological parameters (Ishoy et al., 1999a). Focusing on gastrointestinal difficulties in the same cohort, Ishoy et al. (1999b) found that using a bivariate analysis, 15 of 24 exposures were associated with one or more gastrointestinal symptoms, including diarrhea and rumbling of the stomach. In logistic regression analysis, three factors remained significant, including burning waste/manure, use of insecticides against cockroaches, and low physical activity. Two other factors approached significance: tooth brushing with water contaminated with chemicals, and bathing or drinking contaminated water (fumes, oil, chemicals). As the number of these self-reported exposures increased, the risk for ongoing multisymptom illness increased (trend test not reported). The authors pointed out that in reviewing the Hill criteria for causation, the associations they found to be strongest were biologically plausible and were consistent with general medical knowledge, specifically the association between exposure to waste and infection-related gastrointestinal symptoms and inadequate vector control (cockroaches), resulting in microbial contamination and infectious gastrointestinal illnesses. It is important to point out that, except for a few people, the Danish study participants were not present in the gulf during combat operations and served primarily as support personnel and peacekeeping forces.

In a further analysis of the Danish cohort, Suadicani et al. (1999) examined the association between self-reported exposures and neuropsychological symptoms. While most self-reported exposures were significantly associated with neuropsychological symptoms on bivariate analysis, in multiple linear regression models only a few remained significant. The authors found that threats such as "observing colleagues or friends being threatened with arms or shot at" remained the only psychosocial exposure predictive of neuropsychological symptoms after controlling for demographics and potential confounders. Job demand factors such as "occasional or frequent demand of high degrees of concentration, dissatisfaction with the physical work environmental, and unwillingness from immediate superiors to listen to one's problems were significant predictors of neuropsychological symptoms in a multivariable model." Among self-reported physical factors that remained significantly associated with neuropsychological factors after adjusting for confounders in a logistic model were "bathing in or drinking contaminated water, exposure to depleted uranium, contact with dead animals, and burning of waste or manure." An analysis of the prevalence of clusters of neuropsychological symptoms showed that physicochemical factors interacted with psychological factors in predicting symptoms; however, the physicochemical factor alone was not predictive of symptoms. Insecticides and use of lotions or sprays, which were significant in bivariate analysis, were no longer significant in the multivariate modeling. No information was provided on PB, presumably because it was not used by peacekeepers after the conflict. The authors demonstrated that the number of psychosocial factors reported by the participants increased so did the likelihood that the participant suffered from three to five neuropsychological symptoms.

Nisenbaum et al. (2000) provided a self-administered questionnaire on symptoms and Gulf War deployment stressors to four Air Force units on base in January-March of 1995. Using the Centers for Disease Control and Prevention (CDC) definition of chronic multisymptom illness (Fukuda et al., 1998), the authors classified cases as mild to severe depending on the severity of the case-defining symptoms. They conducted logistic regression analyses for possible risk factors to compare severe disease with no disease and mild-moderate disease with no disease. The response rate was not clearly defined in the report, although unit participation rates were provided in the Fukuda paper. Of those 1163 Gulf War veterans who participated, 1002 had complete data and remained in the final analysis. Several self-reported deployment stressor (exposures) were found to be significantly associated with severe illness, including belief that biological or chemical weapons were used, PB use, and regular insect repellent use. Having sustained injuries that required medical attention was associated only with severe illness, and an interaction term of PB use and insect repellent use was not significant.

Spencer et al. (2001) conducted a nested case-control study based on responses to a mailed survey of a random sample of 2343 of 8603 Washington and Oregon Gulf War veterans. The response rate of locatable veterans was 55% overall. Cases were defined as having reported at least one of three symptom types (fatigue, cognitive/psychological, or musculoskeletal). Controls had none of the three symptom types or had symptoms that were explained by existing medical conditions. Cases and controls were examined with a history, screening physical, a neurological examination, a 4-hour neurobehavioral battery, and laboratory tests. The results were reviewed by a clinical determination committee composed of appropriate medical specialists. Exposures were assessed by a self-reported 142-item list that was reduced by elimination of redundant factors and cluster analysis to 9 factors representing a total of 42 exposure variables. The authors found that on the basis of multivariate modeling, the greatest risks for unexplained illness were sun-related exposure, the presence of a medical condition that the individual sought medical care for while in theater, and conditions of combat. No association was found for self-reported PB and/or insect repellent use. Exposure to oil-well fires was also not significantly associated with being a case.

Cherry et al. (2001) conducted a cross-sectional study of self-reported symptoms and exposures among 7971 UK Gulf War veterans. They had good participation with an 85.5% response rate. Principal component analysis of 94 symptoms resulted in seven factors: psychological, neurological, peripheral, respiratory, gastrointestinal, concentration, and appetite. These factors were developed using data from about half the cohort and were tested on the other half of the cohort for validation. Severity scores were derived using a Likert-like scale, and a manikin drawing was used to identify the extent of symptoms, such as tingling and pain. Using multilinear regression with adjustment for potential confounders, symptom severity scores were associated with the number of inoculations, days handling pesticides, and days exposed to burning oil wells. Regression of exposure against the seven factors found a statistically significant association between the "peripheral" factor (thought to be related to peripheral neuropathy) and the number of inoculations and the number of days handling pesticides. Days handling pesticides also associated with the "neurological" factor. Reported number of days of use of insect repellents was associated with peripheral, respiratory, and appetite factors.

Information derived from the manikins included numbness and tingling (possibly related to peripheral neuropathy) and widespread pain (thought to possibly be functional). Handling of pesticides and use of insect repellent were associated with numbness and tingling, and use of insect repellent, seeking medical care while in the gulf, and reporting side effects from PB were significantly associated with widespread pain. The authors discuss potential bias in detail and conclude, on the basis of their data, that pesticides or inoculations cannot be shown to be responsible for peripheral neuropathy in these veterans. They do suggest that objective measures for ill health are available and should be applied to this cohort (Cherry et al., 2001).

Gray et al. (2002) reported on a cross-sectional mail survey of 17,599 US deployed and nondeployed Seabees. Response rates were 64% overall with 56% of Gulf War deployed, 30% of other deployed, and 15% of nondeployed veterans responding. Significantly more self-reported multisymptom diseases and also more isolated symptoms were reported by Gulf War deployed veterans compared with nondeployed and other deployed veterans. Gulf War deployed Seabees were significantly more likely to report having more of all 33 symptoms and conditions asked when compared with the other two groups on the basis of logistic regression analyses that controlled for age, sex, race/ethnicity, and duty status. Deployed Seabees were also significantly more likely to report suffering from a wide variety of disorders than either nondeployed or other deployed, including digestive disorders, chronic fatigue syndrome (CFS), posttraumatic stress disorder (PTSD), multiple chemical sensitivity, irritable bowel syndrome, and skin rash. Deployed Seabees also reported more depression and were more likely to report being in fair or poor health than the other two groups. This study explored associations between meeting the definition for Gulf War illness and self-reported exposures. Depending on the multivariate analytic approach, there were weak associations between Gulf War illness and the following:

- being exposed to fumes from munitions,
- pesticide exposure,
- drinking contaminated water,
- being exposed to sandstorms,
- seeing someone killed,

- contact with dead animals,
- having food poisoning in one's unit,
- use of PB,
- use of ciprofloxacin,
- use of gas masks,
- drinking from a desert bag,
- receiving botulism toxin,
- being single,
- being female, and
- service type.

On the basis of multilinear analysis, no association was found between Gulf War illness and receipt of several other vaccines, being exposed to oil-well fire smoke or jet fuel use in tents, wearing a flea collar, wearing insect repellent-treated uniforms, seeing dead bodies, eating local food or suffering food poisoning, or having direct combat exposure.

Wolfe et al. (2002) surveyed 2949 US Army soldiers from Fort Devens, Massachusetts, who had been deployed to the Persian Gulf; 1290 responded with self-reports of symptoms and exposures. A respondent was classified as having met the CDC criteria for multisymptom illness if they had at least one symptom in two of three symptom clusters: fatigue, mood and cognition, and musculoskeletal. Approximately 60% of respondents met the criteria for multisymptom illness. The authors found that after controlling for demographic factors, exposure to oil-well fires, the smell of chemicals in the air, having a heater in one's tent, using a clinic while in the gulf, receiving an anthrax shot, and consuming PB pills showed a relationship with self-reported multisymptom illness (Wolfe et al., 2002).

Mahan et al. (2005) analyzed the responses of 5555 army veterans to the National Health Survey of Gulf War Era Veterans (Kang et al., 2000). This survey was collected on a sample of 15,000 troops deployed to the gulf and 15,000 troops who were not deployed there. The survey was mailed before some of the Gulf War veterans received notification of possible nerve gas exposure from the Khamisiyah detonation. Some 11,441 veterans responded to the questionnaire. Respondents were classified as either exposed or unexposed to the plume based on their unit locations and the 2000 DoD modeling of the drift plume. The authors controlled for age, sex, unit composition, when comparing the prevalence of 47 self-reported symptoms in the two groups of veterans. No significant differences in symptom prevalence were found except for severe wheezing and joint swelling, both of which were more common among the unexposed respondents. Among the 31 self-reported illnesses, colitis and enteritis were reported by a greater percentage of exposed veterans compared with unexposed veterans. There was no significant difference in measures of impairment such as being limited in work by one's health, and no differences in self-ratings of health status. Exposed and unexposed veterans reported similar numbers of medical office visits and hospitalizations. The investigators found no difference in the self-reports of symptom-based conditions such as PTSD and CFS between the two groups. The results remained the same regardless of whether exposure was based on the 1995 plume model or the 2000 plume model (Mahan et al., 2005).

ANIMAL STUDIES

The Update committee has also evaluated selected studies of the effects of potential Gulf War intoxicants on animals. While this was not within its original charge, and a comprehensive examination of all of the pertinent literature was beyond its expertise, the committee nonetheless felt that this effort has merit, both for defining potential health hazards of Gulf War service and in designing potential future investigations. Accordingly, members of the committee reviewed the animal studies listed in Table 6 of the VA Research Advisory Committee's report (RAC, 2008), focusing on two questions. First, do data from those animal studies demonstrate that stress can amplify the effects of intoxicants or drugs such as PB, in either the peripheral or the CNS? Second, do these animal studies document long-term adverse effects from short-term exposures to these agents?

With respect to the first question, perhaps the two most salient observations are studies by Friedman et al. (1996) and Abdel-Rahman et al. (2002). Friedman's group examined the inhibition of brain AChE levels in FVB/N mice without and with stress (induced by forced swimming). They reported that the forced swimming stress paradigm was associated with enhanced inhibition of brain AChE by intraperitoneal pyridostigmine (0.1 mg/kg), concurrently with diminished integrity of the blood-brain barrier (measured by enhanced entry of Evans Blue dye and plasmid DNA). Independently of stress, intraperitoneal pyridostigmine also increased the level of RNA encoding brain c-fos and AChE. In hippocampal slice cultures, pyridostigmine enhanced expression of c-fos (but not synaptophysin) and produced a concomitant increase in evoked CA1 electrical activity. These investigators proposed that by altering the permeation properties of the blood–brain barrier, stress can amplify the CNS effects of peripherally delivered pyridostigmine, a compound with a quarternary amine thought to not normally enter the CNS. This model might explain how doses of pyridostigmine that do not normally produce CNS symptoms—such as nervousness, headaches, drowsiness, attention deficits, subnormal cognition—can trigger such symptom complexes. Aspects of the Friedman study are reinforced by the finding of Abdel-Rahman et al. (2002) that in rats stress imposed by restricting movement enhances neural effects of three simultaneously administered toxins: pyridostigmine (1.3 mg/kg/d), DEET (40 mg/kg/d), and permethrin (0.13 mg/kg/d). When superimposed on a stress paradigm, these compounds reduced the integrity of the blood-brain barrier in several regions (cingulate cortex, dentate gyrus of the hippocampus, lateral dorsal nucleus of the thalamus, and the dorsomedial nucleus of the hypothalamus); in each region, there was evidence of neuronal death and astrogliosis.

The model developed in the Friedman report has obvious relevance to understanding how brief exposures to low doses of intoxicants might have unexpected adverse effects on the CNS in Gulf War veterans. It is of interest, therefore, that Lallement et al. (1998, 2001) who also investigated the impact of stress on brain permeation by pyridostigmine, reached somewhat different conclusions. In the Lallement studies, stress was induced by heat rather than exercise in guinea pigs. Using two methods to significantly increase core temperatures, no evidence of loss of integrity of the blood-brain barrier was found. The authors urged caution in translating the results of the Friedman report to Gulf War phenomena in humans (Lallement et al., 1998). In a follow-up study of pyridostigmine administered subcutaneously to guinea pigs over 6 days, only rare and focal evidence of disruption of the blood-brain barrier was found (Lallement, 2001). In studies of CD-1 and FVB/N mice, Grauer et al. (2000) were not able to demonstrate brain permeation by pyridostigmine (0.4 mg/kg, intramuscular or intraperitoneal), using two paradigms of stress (swimming and cold), a result that directly contradicts the conclusions of the Friedman report. While Grauer et al. did not explicitly evaluate properties of the blood-brain barrier, they inferred that it must have remained intact in the absence of any effect of peripheral pyridostigmine on brain AChE levels. This view is in alignment with a report from Telang et al. (1999) that radiolabeled pyridostigmine failed to permeate the brains of FVB/N mice, even after swim-induced stress.

A second important question that animal studies might help answer is whether short-term exposures to intoxicants can lead to long-term consequences for the CNS. Of interest in this context is the report by van Helden that a 5-hour exposure to sarin induces changes in the power spectrum of electroencephalograms (EEGs; plots of the intensity of EEG activity as a function of EEG frequency) that can be detected 1 year after exposure. Moreover, the change in the EEG occurs at a much lower dose than the appearance of miosis, which is among the most subtle clinical manifestations of sarin exposure (van Helden et al., 2004).

These findings are broadly consistent with earlier reports from Burchfiel and Duffy (1982) who found long-term changes in the EEGs of rhesus monkeys after a single high dose of sarin. High doses of sarin have been shown to result in derangements of the EEG, visual-evoked potentials, and event-related potentials as seen in human following the sarin incidents in Japan (Yanagisawa et al., 2006). What is less clear is whether the severity and intensity of putative sarin exposures of Gulf War veterans approaches those of the Japanese cases or the animal studies.

The Update committee finds that these animal studies address but do not resolve the questions about whether in the context of stress, low-level intoxicants that are otherwise well tolerated may exert adverse effects on the CNS; and whether brief exposures to some intoxicants can exert long-lasting (albeit subtle) neurotoxic effects on the brain. Because the animal data on these points are inconsistent or contradictory, the greatest need is for further investigation of these issues in the context of the symptoms of some Gulf War veterans. Specifically, investigations can focus on whether there are factors that confer heightened sensitivity to stress and intoxicants on some veterans such that they experience an increased adverse response to the brief exposures? Are there clinical tools that help define objective findings that correlate with peripheral and central Gulf War symptom complexes? Will subtle but quantitative measures of cortical function, brain oscillators, or central autonomic parameters—using techniques such as functional MRI, polysomnography, event-evoked potentials—reveal persistent abnormalities that have thus far eluded definition? In the committee's view, these questions are among the set of issues that merit further analysis in the effort to understand and treat Gulf War illness.

GENETIC SUSCEPTIBILITY TO CHOLINESTERASE INHIBITORS

Multisymptom illness is striking for the lack of uniformity of symptoms among deployed veterans and that only a minority of the deployed cohort is symptomatic. To the extent that multisymptom illness in Gulf War veterans might be a consequence of exposure to toxins such as cholinesterase inhibitors, a potential explanation for this nonuniformity is the high degree of polymorphism in the proteins that detoxify a wide range of intoxicants. Foremost among these are the paroxonases, three esterases that metabolize oxidized lipids (PON1, 2, and 3). PON1 also metabolizes the highly toxic oxon forms of organophosphate insecticides, such as chlorpyrifos and diazinon (Aldridge, 1953; Furlong et al., 1989). Naturally occurring genetic variations in the genes encoding the paroxonases determine the expression levels and functions of the PON proteins. For example, polymorphisms in the PON1 gene include the coding variants L55M and Q192R, as well as regulatory polymorphisms C-108T and A-162G (Brophy et al., 2001; Costa et al., 2005; Davies et al., 1996). There are also functionally significant polymorphisms in the butyrylcholinesterase (BuChE) gene that reduce BuChE levels and activity (Jensen et al., 1995). Variants in these genes have been implicated as determinants of normal aging and in various disorders, such as neurodegenerative and cardiovascular diseases (Benmoyal-Segal et al., 2005). Several studies have incriminated PON1 polymorphisms in ALS (reviewed by Wills et al., 2009).

Golomb (2008) reviewed studies found through a search of the National Library of Medicine's PubMed database, using the key words "Gulf War," "epidemiology," and "acetylcholinesterase inhibitors." She concluded that these studies—combined with veterans' self-reports of exposures in the Gulf War theatre (including those cited earlier in this report), and studies of people occupationally exposed to cholinesterase inhibitors—supported, through "triangular evidence," a causative association between exposure to cholinesterase inhibitors during deployment in the Gulf War and Gulf War illness. However, after a review of the primary sources cited by Golomb, the Update committee believes that more study is needed before any clear association can be inferred between Gulf War illness (multisymptom illness) and any inherited variability in PON1 or BChE genes.

An initial association between rare PON1 genotypes and multisymptom illness was first suggested by Haley et al. (1999) in a study of 25 symptomatic US Gulf War veterans, but the finding failed to reach statistical significance ($p = 0.08$ before correction for multiple comparisons). The authors also reported that the rare genotypes had reduced functional activity (Haley et al., 1999). In contrast to Haley et al., Mackness et al. (2000), in a larger study of 152 UK veterans with multisymptom illness, could find no association between genotype status and multisymptom illness and, furthermore, no function-genotype association for PON1 could be identified either in veterans with multisymptom illness or in controls. Although Mackness et al. (2000) did initially report an association of symptoms of Gulf War illness with reduced PON1 activity, in a follow-up study apparently with a different UK veteran cohort, Hotopf et al. (2003) concluded that reduced PON1 activity was found in deployed veterans regardless of whether they had symptoms of multisymptom illness. Because reduced PON1 activity may accompany states of chronic inflammation, the author postulated that inflammation might explain the reduced activity in deployed soldiers.

Golomb (2008) cites a US Army report (Lockridge, 1999) that states that rare genetic variants of BChE are present at a statistically increased frequency in Gulf War veterans with multisymptom sufferers. A second Department of Defense study (Sastre and Cook, 2004) found no evidence of any genotype-function correlations with BChE but, like the Lockridge study, did find an association between multisymptom illness symptoms and carriers of rare BChE genotypes who also self-reported PB exposure. However, the numbers of carriers of rare genotypes were small in both these studies—11 out of 226 veterans in Lockridge (1999) and 28 out of 304 veterans in Sastre and Cook (2004).

Thus, the Update committee concludes that current evidence raises the possibility of an association between multisymptom illness and genotypes of both BChE and PON1, but no definitive conclusions can be drawn. These data may represent an extremely important clue to the etiology of chronic symptoms seen both in the Gulf War veterans and in some civilian populations. The committee strongly recommends that well-designed studies be undertaken and replicated to more robustly test the hypothesis that naturally occurring variants in detoxifying enzymes for AChE inhibitors may be susceptibility factors for the development of myltisumptom illness.

Human studies of Gulf War veterans have consistently shown increased symptom reports among a portion of the deployed veterans compared with nondeployed veterans (see Chapter 4). Unfortunately, objective exposure information is generally lacking, and most studies have depended upon self-reports of both exposure and illness and symptoms. No consistent relationship is apparent between specific exposures and symptoms across these studies. Studies of genetic differences in metabolizing or buffering toxins and their relationship to multisymptom illness may hold promise for understanding multisymptom illness given that genes represent an unbiased measure of susceptibility.

THE ROLE OF CHOLINESTERASE INHIBITORS AND PESTICIDES IN MULTISYMPTOM ILLNESS

While pesticide and PB use appear to have been widespread during the Gulf War, there is no evidence that Gulf War veterans suffered acute toxicity from either nerve gas or pesticides on a wide scale during and after the conflict. Except for an association with Parkinsonism, there remains substantial doubt as to whether long-term illness results from low-level chronic exposure to pesticides, including cholinesterase inhibitors. The Agricultural Health Study, the largest study of a pesticide-exposed cohort to date, has confirmed what had been reported from smaller studies of acute pesticide exposures, that is, CNS disorders may persist after acute exposures cease. Two groups of people with chronic, nonintoxicating pesticide exposures have been studied. Studies of UK sheep dippers with organophosphate exposures and one study of pesticide applicators in Iowa and North Carolina have found persistent long-term CNS effects from chronic exposure to high levels of pesticides (Beseler et al., 2008). In the latter study, no dose-response relationship was seen, and pesticides were not restricted to cholinesterase inhibitors. Low-level chronic pesticide exposure has been implicated in Parkinsonism in multiple studies and a causal association with a specific mixture of pesticides (herbicides and fungicides, neither of which are cholinesterase inhibitors) during a vulnerable period of life may explain why stronger associations with pesticide use were not found earlier and more frequently (Costello et al., 2009).

Animal studies have provided mixed results in terms of central and persistent effects of exposure to cholinesterase inhibitors and pesticides, and many questions remain. These questions include: whether the blood-brain barrier can be breached by PB during stress and whether persistent changes in peripheral or CNS function can be induced by exposure to cholinesterase inhibitors at levels comparable to those experienced by Gulf War veterans.

Studies of Gulf War veterans have not used uniform descriptions of possible exposures in theater and the exposures assessments are based almost exclusively on self-reports by veterans, often years after deployment, making it difficult to compare studies. The same is true for symptom reporting by the veterans. The terminology used by the researchers for the veterans' symptoms can differ markedly as is evident from the factor analysis studies described in the section on "Multisymptom Illnesses" in Chapter 4.

There have been several studies that have found associations between self-reported exposures to pesticides, nerve gas, PB, and mixtures thereof, and self-reported symptoms and multisymptom illness. However, several well-designed studies have concluded that no association exists for such exposures, and other stress-related and environmental factors appear to be more important. Due to the publicity surrounding multisymptom illness and its possible associations with environmental exposures stimulated by early studies of Gulf War veterans, obtaining unbiased results through studies using self-reports of symptoms and exposures seems unlikely at this point. Studies of genetic differences, such as polymorphisms in genes responsible for metabolic inactivation of toxins (PON1 variants) or buffering of toxic load (BChE levels), may hold promise given the objective nature of these potential modifying factors and their likely effect on biologically active doses in exposed subjects.

Given the scarcity of evidence supporting the association of chronic multisymptom illness with low-level pesticide exposure in chronically exposed populations such as the Agricultural Health Study population; the lack of clear, persistent CNS effect in animal studies of cholinesterase inhibitors and pesticides; the potential for bias in studies that base conclusions on self-reports of illness and exposure; and the lack of sufficient weight of evidence from studies of Gulf War veterans; the Update committee finds insufficient support for the conclusion that pesticides, PB, insect repellents, or combinations thereof are responsible for multisymptom illness seen in Gulf War veterans.

REFERENCES

Abdel-Rahman, A., A. K. Shetty, and M. B. Abou-Donia. 2002. Disruption of the blood-brain barrier and neuronal cell death in cingulate cortex, dentate gyrus, thalamus, and hypothalamus in a rat model of Gulf-War syndrome. *Neurobiology of Disease* 10(3):306-326.

Aldridge, W. N. 1953. An enzyme hydrolysing diethyl-p-nitrophenyl phosphate (E-600) and its identity with the A-esterase of mammalian sera. *Biochemical Journal* 53:117-124.

Ames, R. G., K. Steenland, B. Jenkins, D. Chrislip, and J. Russo. 1995. Chronic neurologic sequelae to cholinesterase inhibition among agricultural pesticide applicators. *Archives of Environmental Health* 50(6):440-444.

Bardin, P. G., S. F. van Eeden, J. A. Moolman, A. P. Foden, and J. R. Joubert. 1994. Organophosphate and carbamate poisoning. *Archives of Internal Medicine* 154(13):1433-1441.

Benmoyal-Segal L., T. Vander, S. Shifman, B. Bryk, R.P. Ebstein, E.L. Marcus, J. Stessman, A. Darvasi, Y. Herishanu, A. Friedman, and H. Soreq. 2005. Acetylcholinesterase/paraoxonase interactions increase the risk of insecticide-induced Parkinson's disease. *The FASEB Journal* 19(3):452-454.

Beseler, C., L. Stallones, J. A. Hoppin, M. C. Alavanja, A. Blair, T. Keefe, and F. Kamel. 2006. Depression and pesticide exposures in female spouses of licensed pesticide applicators in the Agricultural Health Study cohort. *Journal of Occupational and Environmental Medicine* 48(10):1005-1013.

Beseler, C. L., L. Stallones, J. A. Hoppin, M. C. Alavanja, A. Blair, T. Keefe, and F. Kamel. 2008. Depression and pesticide exposures among private pesticide applicators enrolled in the Agricultural Health Study. *Environmental Health Perspectives* 116(12):1713-1719.

Brophy, V. H., R. L. Jampsa, J. B. Clendenning, L. A. McKinstry, G. P. Jarvik, and C. E. Furlong. 2001. Effects of 5 regulatory-region polymorphisms on paraoxonase-gene (*PON1*) expression. *American Journal of Human Genetics* 68(6):1428-1436.

Burchfiel, J. L., and F. H. Duffy. 1982. Organophosphate neurotoxicity: Chronic effects of sarin on the electroencephalogram of monkey and man. *Neurobehavioral Toxicology and Teratology* 4(6):767-778.

Cherry, N., F. Creed, A. Silman, G. Dunn, D. Baxter, J. Smedley, S. Taylor, and G. J. Macfarlane. 2001. Health and exposures of United Kingdom Gulf War veterans. Part II: The relation of health to exposure. *Occupational and Environmental Medicine* 58(5):299-306.

Costa, L. G., A. Vitalone, T. B. Cole, C. E. Furlong. 2005. Modulation of paraoxonase (PON1) activity. *Biochemical Pharmacology* 69:541-550.

Costello, S., M. Cockburn, J. Bronstein, X. Zhang, and B. Ritz. 2009. Parkinson's disease and residential exposure to maneb and paraquat from agricultural applications in the central valley of California. *American Journal of Epidemiology* 169(8):919-926.

Davies, H. G., R. J. Richter, M. Keifer, C. A. Broomfield, J. Sowalla, and C. Furlong. 1996. The effect of the human serum paraoxonase polymorphism is reversed with diazoxon, soman and sarin. *Nature Genetics* 14:334-336.

De Bleecker, J., K. Van den Neucker, and F. Colardyn. 1993. Intermediate syndrome in organophosphorus poisoning: A prospective study. *Critical Care Medicine* 21(11):1706-1711.

Delgado, E., R. McConnell, J. Miranda, M. Keifer, I. Lundberg, T. Partanen, and C. Wesseling. 2004. Central nervous system effects of acute organophosphate poisoning in a two-year follow-up. *Scandinavian Journal of Work, Environment and Health* 30(5):362-370.

FDA (US Food and Drug Administration). 2009. *Bioterrorism and Drug Preparedness.* http://www.fda.gov/Drugs/EmergencyPreparedness/BioterrorismandDrugPreparedness/ucm130343.htm (accessed October 27, 2009).

Fricker, R. D., E. Reardon, D. M. Spektor, S. K. Cotton, J. Hawes-Dawson, J. E. Pace, and S. D. Hosek. 2000. *Pesticide Use During the Gulf War: A Survey of Gulf War Veterans.* Santa Monica, CA: RAND Corporation.

Friedman, A., D. Kaufer, J. Shemer, I. Hendler, H. Soreq, and I. Tur-Kaspa. 1996. Pyridostigmine brain penetration under stress enhances neuronal excitability and induces early immediate transcriptional response. *Nature Medicine* 2(12):1382-1385.

Fukuda, K., R. Nisenbaum, G. Stewart, W. W. Thompson, L. Robin, R. M. Washko, D. L. Noah, D. H. Barrett, B. Randall, B. L. Herwaldt, A. C. Mawle, and W. C. Reeves. 1998. Chronic multisymptom illness affecting Air Force veterans of the Gulf War. *Journal of the American Medical Association* 280(11):981-988.

Furlong, C. E., R. J. Ritcher, S. L. Seidel, L. Costa, and A. G. Motulsky. 1989. Spectrophotometric assays for the enzymatic hydrolysis of the active metabolites of chlorpyrifos and parathion by plasma paraoxonase/arylesterase. *Analytical Biochemistry* 180(2):242-247.

GAO (General Accountability Office). 2004. *Gulf War Illness: DOD's Conclusions about U.S. Troops' Exposure Cannot Be Adequately Supported.* Washington, DC: GAO, 04-767.

Golomb, B. A. 2008. Acetylcholinesterase inhibitors and Gulf War illnesses. *Proceedings of the National Academy of Sciences* 105(11):4295-4300.

Grauer, E., D. Alkalai, J. Kapon, G. Cohen, and L. Raveh. 2000. Stress does not enable pyridostigmine to inhibit brain cholinesterase after parenteral administration. *Toxicology and Applied Pharmacology* 164(3):301-304.

Gray, G. C., R. J. Reed, K. S. Kaiser, T. C. Smith, and V. M. Gastanaga. 2002. Self-reported symptoms and medical conditions among 11,868 Gulf War-era veterans: The Seabee Health Study. *American Journal of Epidemiology* 155(11):1033-1044.

Haley, R. W., and T. L. Kurt. 1997. Self-reported exposure to neurotoxic chemical combinations in the Gulf War: A cross-sectional epidemiologic study. *Journal of the American Medical Association* 277(3):231-237.

Haley, R. W., S. Billecke, and B. N. La Du. 1999. Association of low PON1 type Q (type A) arylesterase activity with neurologic symptom complexes in Gulf War veterans. *Toxicology and Applied Pharmacology* 157(3):227-233.

Hotopf, M., M. I. Mackness, V. Nikolaou, D. A. Collier, C. Curtis, A, David, P. Durrington, L. Hull, K. Ismail, M. Peakman, C. Unwin, S. Wesseley, and B. Mackness. 2003. Paraoxonase in Persian Gulf War veterans. *Journal of Occupational and Environmental Medicine* 45(7):668-675.

Ishoy, T., P. Suadicani, B. Guldager, M. Appleyard, and F. Gyntelberg. 1999a. Risk factors for gastrointestinal symptoms. The Danish Gulf War Study. *Danish Medical Bulletin* 46(5):420-423.

Ishoy, T., P. Suadicani, B. Guldager, M. Appleyard, H. O. Hein, and F. Gyntelberg. 1999b. State of health after deployment in the Persian Gulf. The Danish Gulf War Study. *Danish Medical Bulletin* 46(5):416-419.

Jensen, F. S., L.T. Skovgaard, J. Viby-Mogensen. 1995. Identification of human plasma cholinesterase variants in 6,688 individuals using biochemical analysis. *Acta Anaesthesiologica Scandinavica* 39:157-162.

Kamel, F., C. Tanner, D. Umbach, J. Hoppin, M. Alavanja, A. Blair, K. Comyns, S. Goldman, M. Korell, J. Langston, G. Ross, and D. Sandler. 2007. Pesticide exposure and self-reported Parkinson's disease in the Agricultural Health Study. *American Journal of Epidemiology* 165(4):364-374.

Kang, H. K., C. M. Mahan, K. Y. Lee, C. A. Magee, and F. M. Murphy. 2000. Illnesses among United States veterans of the Gulf War: A population-based survey of 30,000 veterans. *Journal of Occupational and Environmental Medicine* 42(5):491-501.

Keifer, M. C., and J. Firestone. 2007. Neurotoxicity of pesticides. *Journal of Agromedicine* 12(1):17-25.

Lallement, G., A. Foquin, D. Baubichon, M. F. Burckhart, P. Carpentier, and F. Canini. 1998. Heat stress, even extreme, does not induce penetration of pyridostigmine into the brain of guinea pigs. *Neurotoxicology* 19(6):759-766.

Lallement, G., A. Foquin, F. Dorandeu, D. Baubichon, S. Aubriot, P. Carpentier. 2001. Subchronic administration of various pretreatments of nerve agent poisoning. I. Protection of blood and central cholinesterases, innocuousness towards blood-brain barrier permeability. *Drug and Chemical Toxicology* 24(2):151-164.

Lockridge, O. 1999. Butyrylcholinesterase genetic variants in persons with gulf War illness. www.gulflink.osd.mil/medsearch/GeneticStudies/DoD60.shtml (accessed December 13, 2009).

London, L., V. Nell, M. L. Thompson, and J. E. Myers. 1998. Effects of long-term organophosphate exposures on neurological symptoms, vibration sense and tremor among South African farm workers. *Scandinavian Journal of Work, Environment and Health* 24(1):18-29.

Lotti, M., and A. Morreto. 2005. Organophosphate-induced delayed polyneuropathy. *Toxicology Review* 24(1):37-49.

Mackness, B., P. N. Durrington, and M. I. Mackness. 2000. Low paraoxonase in Persian Gulf War veterans self-reporting Gulf War syndrome. *Biochemical and Biophysical Research Communications* 276(2):729-733.

Mahan, C. M., W. F. Page, T. A. Bullman, and H. K. Kang. 2005. Health effects in Army Gulf War veterans possibly exposed to chemical munitions destruction at Khamisiyah, Iraq: Part I. *Military Medicine* 170(11):935-944.

Medline Plus. 2008. *Pyridostigmine*. http://www.nlm.nih.gov/medlineplus/druginfo/meds/a682229.html (accessed online March 24, 2010).

Nisenbaum, R., D. H. Barrett, M. Reyes, and W. C. Reeves. 2000. Deployment stressors and a chronic multisymptom illness among gulf war veterans. *Journal of Nervous and Mental Disease* 188(5):259-266.

Nishiwaki, Y., K. Maekawa, Y. Ogawa, N. Asukai, M. Minami, K. Omae, and Sarin Health Effects Study Group. 2001. Effects of sarin on the nervous system in rescue team staff members and police officers 3 years after the Tokyo subway sarin attack. *Environmental Health Perspectives* 109(11):1169-1173.

Ohtani, T., A. Iwanami, K. Kasai, H. Yamasue, T. Kato, T. Sasaki, and N. Kato. 2004. Post-traumatic stress disorder symptoms in victims of Tokyo subway attack: A 5-year follow-up study. *Psychiatry Clinical Neuroscience* 58(6):624-629.

Page, W. F., C. M. Mahan, T. A. Bullman, and H. K. Kang. 2005a. Health effects in Army Gulf War veterans possibly exposed to chemical munitions destruction at Khamisiyah, Iraq: Part I. Morbidity associated with potential exposure. *Military Medicine* 170(11):935-944.

Page, W. F., C. M. Mahan, H. K. Kang, and T. A. Bullman. 2005b. Health effects in Army Gulf War veterans possibly exposed to chemical munitions destruction at Khamisiyah, Iraq: Part II. Morbidity associated with notification of potential exposure. *Military Medicine* 170(11):945-951.

Pilkington, A., D. Buchanan, G. A. Jamal, R. Gillham, S. Hansen, M. Kidd, J. F. Hurley, and C. A. Soutar. 2001. An epidemiological study of the relations between exposure to organophosphate pesticides and indices of chronic peripheral neuropathy and neuropsychological abnormalities in sheep farmers and dippers. *Occupational and Environmental Medicine* 58(11):702-710.

RAC (Research Advisory Committee on Gulf War Veterans' Illnesses). 2008. *Gulf War Illness and the Health of Gulf War Veterans: Scientific Findings and Recommendations*. Washington, DC: US Government Printing Office.

Rosenstock, L., M. Keifer, W. E. Daniell, R. McConnell, and K. Claypole. 1991. Chronic central nervous system effects of acute organophosphate pesticide intoxication. *Lancet* 338(8761):223-227.

Sastre, A. and M. R. Cook. 2004. Autonomic Dysfunction in Gulf War veterans. Midwest Research Institute. Fort Detrick, MD: U.S. Army Medical Research and Materiel Command. Award number: DAMD-17-00-C-0018. November.

Savage, E. P., T. J. Keefe, L. M. Mounce, R. K. Heaton, J. A. Lewis, and P. J. Burcar. 1988. Chronic neurological sequelae of acute organophosphate pesticide poisoning. *Archives of Environmental Health* 43(1):38-45.

Spencer, P. S., L. A. McCauley, J. A. Lapidus, M. Lasarev, S. K. Joos, and D. Storzbach. 2001. Self-reported exposures and their association with unexplained illness in a population-based case-control study of Gulf War veterans. *Journal of Occupational and Environmental Medicine* 43(12):1041-1056.

Steenland, K., B. Jenkins, R. G. Ames, M. O'Malley, D. Chrislip, and J. Russo. 1994. Chronic neurological sequelae to organophosphate pesticide poisoning. *American Journal of Public Health* 84(5):731-736.

Stephens, R., A. Spurgeon, I. A. Calvert, J. Beach, L. S. Levy, H. Berry, and J. M. Harrington. 1995. Neuropsychological effects of long-term exposure to organophosphates in sheep dip. *Lancet* 34(8658):1135-1139.

Stephens, R., A. Spurgeon, and H. Berry. 1996. Organophosphates: The relationship between chronic and acute exposure effects. *Neurotoxicology Teratology* 18(4):449-453.

Suadicani, P., T. Ishoy, B. Guldager, M. Appleyard, and F. Gyntelberg. 1999. Determinants of long-term neuropsychological symptoms. *Danish Medical Bulletin* 46(5):423-427.

Telang, F. W., Y.-S. Ding, N. D. Volkow, P. E. Molina, and S. J. Gatley. 1999. Pyridostigmine, a carbamate acetylcholinesterase AchE inhibitor and reactivator, is used prophylactically against chemical warfare agents. *Nuclear Medicine and Biology* 26:249-250.

van Helden, H. P., R. A. Vanwersch, W. C. Kuijpers, H. C. Trap, I. H. Philippens, and H. P. Benschop. 2004. Low levels of sarin affect the EEG in marmoset monkeys: A pilot study. *Journal of Applied Toxicology* 24(6):475-483.

Wesseling, C., M. Keifer, A. Ahlbom, R. McConnell, J. D. Moon, L. Rosenstock, and C. Hogstedt. 2002. Long-term neurobehavioral effects of mild poisonings with organophosphate and n-methyl carbamate pesticides among banana workers. *International Journal of Occupational and Environmental Health* 8(1):27-34.

Wills, A. M., S. Cronin, A. Slowik, D. Kasperaviciute, M. A.Van Es, J. M. Morahan, P. N. Valdmanis, V. Meininger, J. Melki, C. E. Shaw, G. A. Rouleau, E. M. Fisher, P. J. Shaw, K. E. Morrison, R. Pamphlett, L. H. Van den Berg, D. A. Figlewicz, P. M. Andersen, A. Al-Chalabi, O. Hardiman, S. Purcell, J. E. Landers, and R. H. Brown, Jr. 2009. A large-scale international meta-analysis of paraoxonase gene polymorphisms in sporadic ALS. *Neurology* 73(1):16-24.

Wolfe, J., S. P. Proctor, D. J. Erickson, and H. Hu. 2002. Risk factors for multisymptom illness in US Army veterans of the Gulf War. *Journal of Occupational and Environmental Medicine* 44(3):271-281.

Yanagisawa, N., H. Morita, and T. Nakajima. 2006. Sarin experiences in Japan: Acute toxicity and long-term effects. *Journal of Neurological Sciences* 249(1):76-85.

APPENDIX B

COMMITTEE BIOGRAPHICAL SKETCHES

Stephen L. Hauser, M.D. (*Chair*), is Professor and Chair of the Department of Neurology at the University of California, San Francisco. He is board certified in both internal medicine and neurology. He has been President, American Neurological Association and received the 2008 John Dystel Prize for Multiple Sclerosis Research. He is Editor-in-Chief of the journal *Annals of Neurology* and is also an editor of the textbook *Harrison's Principles of Internal Medicine*. His research interests are in the areas of multiple sclerosis, neuroimmunology, autoimmunity, and human genetics. Dr. Hauser is a member of the Institute of Medicine (IOM) and has served on the IOM Membership Committee and on the Committee on Multiple Sclerosis: Current Status and Strategies for the Future. Dr. Hauser received his M.D. from the Harvard Medical School.

Alvaro Alonso, M.D., Ph.D., is Assistant Professor in the Department of Epidemiology and Community Health at the University of Minnesota School of Public Health and Adjunct Assistant Professor in the Department of Preventive Medicine and Public Health, School of Medicine, University of Navarra, Pamplona, Spain. His research interests are in the areas of epidemiology of cardiovascular disease and neurological disorders, specifically multiple sclerosis and neurodegenerative conditions. Dr. Alonso received a Fulbright Fellowship in 2004 to conduct post-doctoral research at Harvard School of Public Health. He obtained his M.D. and Ph.D. in Epidemiology from the University of Navarra, Pamplona, Spain.

Robert H. Brown, Jr., M.D., is Professor and Chair of the Department of Neurology at the University of Massachusetts School of Medicine. Previously, he was Director of the Day Neuromuscular Research Laboratory and Professor of Neurology at the Harvard Medical School. Dr. Brown's research is focused on the molecular basis of selected inherited neuromuscular disorders, particularly gene defects in familial amyotrophic lateral sclerosis, one type of muscular dystrophy, hyperkalemic periodic paralysis, hereditary sensory neuropathy type 1, and adrenoleukodystrophy. He is a member of the Institute of Medicine. Dr. Brown received his M.D. from the Harvard Medical School and his D.Phil. from the University of Oxford.

Douglas A. Drossman, M.D., is Co-Director of the UNC Center for Functional GI and Motility Disorders, and Professor of Medicine and Psychiatry at the UNC School of Medicine, Division of Gastroenterology and Hepatology. He has a long standing interest in the research and evaluation of difficult to diagnose and treat gastrointestinal (GI) disorders. He began a program of research in functional GI disorders at UNC more than 25 years ago, has received large number of NIH grants in this area, and has published more than 500 books, articles, and abstracts relating to epidemiology, psychosocial and quality of life assessment, design of treatment trials, and outcomes of research in GI disorders. Dr. Drossman received his M.D. from Albert Einstein College of Medicine.

W. Dana Flanders, M.D., D.Sc., is Professor of Epidemiology in the Rollins School of Public Health at Emory University. Dr. Flanders teaches courses on epidemiological methodology and study design and conducts research on health risks in many areas, including those related to exposure to environmental Legionella bacteria, development of Legionella sampling strategies, association of hypersensitivity pneumonitis in metal workers with mycobacteria in metal-working fluids, cancer and genetic epidemiology, and health risks associated with indoor exposure to toxigenic fungi and air pollution. He received his M.D. from the University of Vermont, his D.Sc. degree in Epidemiology and Masters Degree in Public Health from Harvard University, and is board certified in Preventive Medicine.

Matthew C. Keifer, M.D., M.P.H., is Co-Director of the Pacific Northwest Agricultural Safety and Health Center and professor in the Occupational Medicine Program at the University of Washington. He practices and teaches occupational and internal medicine at the Harborview Medical Center of the University of Washington, and at the Yakima Valley Farm Workers Clinic. Dr. Keifer is currently the Director of the Fogarty International Scholars program at the University. His research interests focus on the health of agricultural workers, international occupational and environmental health, and the health effects of exposure to occupational pesticides. Dr. Keifer served on the NRC Subcommittee on Methyl Bromide. He is a diplomate of the American Board of Internal Medicine and the American Board of Preventive Medicine-Occupational and Environmental Medicine. He received his M.D. from the University of Illinois and his M.P.H. from the University of Washington.

Francine Laden, D.Sc., is the Mark and Catherine Winkler Associate Professor of Environmental Epidemiology at the Harvard School of Public Health, and an Assistant Professor of Medicine at the Harvard Medical School and the Brigham & Women's Hospital. Dr. Laden's research focuses on environmental risk factors of chronic diseases, including cancer, cardiovascular and respiratory disease. She studies the relationship of exposure to organochlorine chemicals with both breast cancer and non-Hodgkin's lymphoma. She also studies the association of exposure to diesel exhaust and other sources of fine particulate matter with all cause mortality and incidence of and mortality from cardiovascular and respiratory disease and lung cancer. Dr. Laden received her Sc.D. from the Harvard School of Public Health.

Jennifer D. Peck, Ph.D., is Assistant Professor, Department of Biostatistics and Epidemiology, University of Oklahoma Health Sciences Center. Her research focuses on the reproductive health effects of environmental exposures to endocrine active agents. She has also studied exposures to tobacco smoke, nonpersistent compounds such as phthalates, and persistent organic pollutants such as polychlorinated biphenyls and polybrominated biphenyl ethers and their effects on thyroid function and neurodevelopment in human populations. She received her Ph.D. in Epidemiology from the University of North Carolina at Chapel Hill.

Beate R. Ritz, M.D., Ph.D., is Professor, Department of Epidemiology, Department of Environmental Health Sciences and Vice Chair, Department of Epidemiology at the University of California, Los Angeles, School of Public Health. Her primary research interests are the effects of occupational and environmental toxins such as pesticides, ionizing radiation, and air pollution on chronic diseases, including neurodegenerative disorders (Parkinson's disease), cancers, and adverse birth outcomes. Dr. Ritz received her M.D. from the Board of Health in Hamburg, Germany and her Ph.D. from the University of California, Los Angeles.

Rebecca P. Smith, M.D., is Assistant Clinical Professor of Psychiatry at Mount Sinai Hospital and Medical School. She has worked on the development of clinical and research programs for survivors of terrorism, disasters and violence, in the United States and abroad, including India, Sri Lanka, Israel and the Palestinian territories, New Orleans, and the Asian Tsunami). She has done extensive work on monitoring the physical and mental health effects of the World Trade Center disaster. Dr. Smith has also worked in design and analysis of epidemiologic studies and clinical trials of human immunodeficiency virus and the epidemiology of suicide. Dr. Smith attended Brown University Medical School and completed her psychiatric residency and fellowship at New York Presbyterian Hospital.

Ezra S. Susser, M.D., Ph.D., is Professor of Epidemiology, at the Mailman School of Public Health and Professor of Psychiatry at the College of Physicians and Surgeons at Columbia University. His recent research has been primarily on the epidemiology of mental disorders, and on examining the role of early-life experience in health and disease throughout the life course. He heads the Imprints Center for Genetic and Environmental Lifecourse Studies, which fosters collaborative research and intellectual exchange among investigators studying developmental origins in birth cohorts across the globe. As one example, the findings from a series of studies have suggested that exposure to famine in early gestation is associated with increased schizophrenia among offspring. Dr. Susser is Associate Editor of the International Journal of Epidemiology, and Former Chair of the Department of Epidemiology at the Mailman School of Public Health (1999-2008). He received his M.D. and Ph.D. from Columbia University.

Christina M. Wolfson, Ph.D., is Director of the Division of Clinical Epidemiology at the McGill University Health Centre and a Professor in the Department of Epidemiology and Biostatistics and Occupational Health and in the Department of Medicine at McGill University. She is an Associate Member in the Department of Neurology and Neurosurgery, the Department of Mathematics and Statistics, and the Division of Geriatric Medicine at McGill University. Her research lies in the epidemiology of neurodegenerative disorders, including dementia, multiple sclerosis, amyotrophic lateral sclerosis, and Parkinson's disease. She is also Co-Principal Investigator on the Canadian Longitudinal Study on Aging, a nationwide 20-year study of 50,000 participants aged 45 to 85. Dr. Wolfson received her Ph.D. in epidemiology and biostatistics from McGill University.

INDEX

N

O

P

Q

R

W